Bases of Auditory
Brain-Stem Evoked
Responses

Bases of Auditory Brain-Stem Evoked Responses

Edited by

ERNEST J. MOORE, PH.D.

Communicative Disorders Program
National Institute of Neurological and
    Communicative Disorders and Stroke
National Institutes of Health
Bethesda, Maryland

GRUNE & STRATTON
A Subsidiary of Harcourt Brace Jovanovich, Publishers
New York   London
Paris   San Diego   San Francisco   São Paulo
Sydney   Tokyo   Toronto

Library of Congress Cataloging in Publication Data
Main entry under title:

Bases of auditory brain-stem evoked responses.

  Bibliography
  Includes index.
  1. Hearing disorders—Diagnosis.   2. Auditory evoked
response.   I. Moore, Ernest J.   [DNLM: 1. Evoked
potentials, Auditory.   2. Brain stem—Physiology.
WV 270 B299]
RF290.B34   617.8'07547   82-6274
ISBN 0-8089-1465-0   AACR2

Grune & Stratton, Inc.
111 Fifth Avenue
New York, New York 10003

Distributed in the United Kingdom by
Academic Press Inc. (London) Ltd.
24/28 Oval Road, London NW 1

Library of Congress Catalog Number 82-6274
International Standard Book Number 0-8089-1465-0
Printed in the United States of America

To Audrey, Brenda, Ronnie, Marc, Rozalyn, Everett, and Shauna.

Contents

Foreword

In this context, technology transfer, a perfectly apt and cogent expression (but a rather laborious term), has aided the development of computerized tomographic scanners and led to a remarkable revision of methods of neurologic examination. In the same sense, technologic developments in microelectronics now allow us to "see" electrical activity in the peripheral and central nervous system. Even at first glance, it is clear that the process of displaying electrical responses to sound stimulation promises to be of incalculable value to auditory and neurologic clinicians and to clinical investigators in those areas. Since the introduction of this technique, there has been an almost bewildering plethora of information on instrumentation, stimulus modes, electrode placement, recording methods, and interpretation of observations. There has even been talk of attempts to write and adopt standards on some of these topics—talk that for the most part fortunately has been nipped in the bud (it has been recognized that standardization this "early in the game" might serve only to stifle further attempts to explore fully the capabilities of such a new technique).

A volume of this type, comprising the thoughts and appraisals of some of the world's leading experts in the field, should encourage every student, investigator, and practitioner to pause and assess the progress, from the basic to the esoteric, critically examining what we are saying and doing (and perhaps what we should be doing), what we now know, and what new avenues remain to be explored in the area of auditory brain-stem evoked responses.

R. F. Naunton, M.D.
National Institute of Neurological
    and Communicative Disorders and Stroke
Bethesda, Maryland

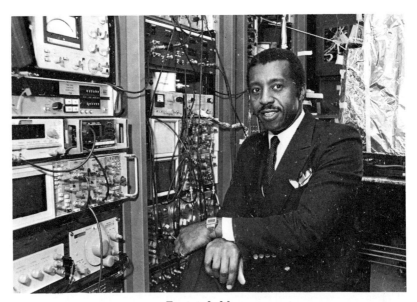

Ernest J. Moore

Preface

Yesterday . . . Today . . . Tomorrow

This volume has been written to serve as a basic introductory text for students and specialists interested in auditory brain-stem evoked responses (BSER). The 15 chapters included represent an undertaking that began in 1971 when I offered my first formal course in auditory evoked potentials to a group of first-year audiology students at Emerson College in Boston. Little did they realize that they were about to experience the unfolding of one of the most exciting areas of audiology since its beginning in the early 1940s. Since there was an apparent lack of enthusiasm for the long list of references (55, to be exact) that I had assigned, which included a number of introductory chapters on fundamental background information, the inevitable question was asked: "Why is not there a textbook available to us that provides, under one cover, the necessary background materials and introductory information needed to understand and appreciate auditory brain-stem evoked responses?" My answer to them at that time was, "The scope of the information on BSER is just too narrow to support such a book."

Since that time, the progress made with the auditory BSER and attendant areas has been impressive. Auditory BSER achievements have been most outstanding, especially when one considers the number of arduous hours spent in experimenting with a group of subvoltage electrical currents (10^{-6}) that can miraculously be evoked from the depths of the human brain.

The fact that many of us who use BSER in the clinic take much for granted—the placement of the electrodes, selection of recording parameters, or watching for the five or six "Jewett bumps"—is perhaps an indication that our research labors have been, and will continue to be, portentious of a success story for those patients who benefit from the several facets of the BSER regimen. It is truly a vital adjunct to the clinician's diagnostic armamentarium.

In the fall of 1970 I approached several auditory research scientists, otologists, and audiologists in the Boston area in a fruitless attempt to convince them that those strange-looking "squiggly lines" that I had recorded as part of my doctoral dissertation had great potential clinical value. Several of these individuals in those early days referred to my work as unimportant; one of them would not even take the time to give me an appointment. One clinician had commented, "There will never be a place in my clinic for evoked potentials because I do not see them as being of any value to my patients." Some of these same individuals today use the BSER to obtain large grants, and some have even attracted major attention from the news media as having introduced to the public this "new and exciting tool."

Fortunately, I was not discouraged by this negativism. In 1971 I proceeded to develop an evoked-response system within the Communication Sciences Laboratory at Emerson College. Shortly thereafter, we proved that the clinician's predictions were wrong by assisting the audiology clinic with a number of difficult-to-test patients. Today, a decade later, there is a significant increase in the number of audiology clinics, otology practices, neurology and pediatric departments, and several basic science laboratories among those who now routinely utilize the BSER technique. This book is an attempt to pull together, in one volume, most of the information that is needed to foster a well-planned use of the BSER in the clinic.

It is my hope that the contents of this book will assist students and residents in otology, neurology, and pediatrics in their quest for background information and fundamental knowledge about the various facets of the BSER. Certain segments of this volume will serve as a review for the already practicing clinician, while basic scientists may find that some of the discussions will influence them into probing deeper into some of the unanswered questions still facing the BSER story.

This book is divided into four sections: Part I provides the necessary background information. Part II discusses fundamentals of auditory brainstem evoked responses. The clinical use of auditory brain-stem evoked responses is reviewed in Part III, and Part IV reports on other evoked responses and utilization.

Chapter 1 provides a historical perspective, beginning with the discovery of animal electricity and ending with a wealth of contemporary articles. The purpose of this chapter was to provide the reader with meticulous reviews of relevant publications that have assisted in the unfolding of the BSER story, combined with some of my personal experiences. This historical review is not exhaustive since I am certain that some references have been overlooked. Several were purposely not cited since these results were a superfluous repetition of previous work.

Chapter 2, written by John D. Durrant, is both lucid and interesting. Dr. Durrant applies his excellent background in basic acoustics, auditory evoked responses, neurophysiology, and audiology to the subject of physical acoustics. The reader thus has little need to consult other basic books on the physics of sound and attendant areas in order to understand and appreciate the role that acoustical factors play in the overall schema of BSER techniques.

Chapter 3 provides a functional approach to the anatomy of the auditory system. D. Kent Morest is well suited to this task; his long-standing contributions to the neuroanatomy of the auditory system are well known. He brings to the book an excellent knowledge of gross, macro- and microstructure of the mamallian auditory system. What Dr. Morest offers for the reader is information about the necessary "hard-wiring" structures, pathways, and collateral areas. With these properties in hand, the student can trace the anatomic pathway from its most peripheral origin, through the brain stem, and up to more central structures and not get bogged down with unnecessary neuroanatomic terms and methodology that often tend to confuse the anatomically uninitiated.

Function is an integral part of structure. Chiyeko Tsuchitani methodically approaches each of the peripheral and central auditory nervous system structures and assigns the appropriate physiologic functioning. Dr. Tsuchitani's chapter (Chapter 4) is particularly laudatory when one sees that she relates the BSER gross waves to the neurophysiology of single-unit or slow wave activity in nuclei, axons, dendrites, and collateral endings. It is both fitting and proper that Dr. Tsuchitani does this in an excellent manner since she brings to the assignment a strong background in physiology and several years of experimentation within the brain stem of the cat in her own laboratory.

In practice, the student of audiology, otology, neurology, and pediatrics is bound to confront the pathologic auditory system. Michael Paparella and Timothy Jung provide the reader with the necessary pathologic conditions that occur in the auditory system. Drs. Paparella and Jung are practicing otolaryngologists and they both conduct their own laboratory-based research. Their excellent knowledge of temporal bone pathology led them to organize a systematic approach to peripheral and central auditory nervous system pathology. Chapter 5 (the last chapter in Part I) is a vital adjunct to the normal anatomy outlined in Chapter 3 and the neurophysiology section of Chapter 4.

Chapter 6 offers a pragmatic description of several auditory evoked potentials. The approach taken by Terence Picton and Peter Fitzgerald reflects their strong background in recording all of the auditory evoked responses. The choice of explicating the potentials into endogenous and exogenous categories is instructive, given the fact that the major focus of this book is on the "first" or "fast" exogenous responses. In this chapter, an appropriate tone is set and a workable outline that explains the potentials based on the widely accepted categorization using latency measurements is provided.

Chapter 7, by Jennifer Buchwald, relates what is currently known about the origin or generator(s) of the BSER. This chapter allows one to gain a better understanding of possible contributions of various waves to the clinical test situation. Jenifer does a first-rate job with her assignment. She borrows heavily from her own laboratory experiences, but does not ignore the balanced contributions made by others in her field. The BSER waves are discussed based on anatomic divisions. This chapter is definitely state-of-the-art; reading it in conjunction with the anatomy chapter by Dr. Morest and the physiology chapter by Dr. Tsuchitani is well worth the investment.

Because of the rapid advances in electronic technology, any book or chapter on instrumentation runs the risk of being outmoded before the printing press stops rolling. In Chapter 8, Alfred Coats avoided this dilemma by preparing a treatise that provides the basic information without reference or prejudice toward any commercially available systems. The basic principles provided by Dr. Coats, therefore, will be around in subsequent years. Dr. Coats also made excellent use of illustrative materials allowing the student to visualize the basic concepts posited and simultaneously gaining an appreciation for the basic factors underlying BSER instrumentation systems.

The interaction of stimulus parameters has occupied a great deal of attention by the earlier BSER investigators. Since the bases for selecting and specifying the experimental stimuli depend heavily on the use of the resultant data, it follows that a thorough knowledge of the effects on the BSER to the physical stimulus is of paramount importance. In Chapter 9, I have attempted to provide an organized schema for understanding the three-dimensional nature of the acoustic stimulus. Considering that frequency, intensity, and the several variables of time interact to influence the morphology, latency, and amplitude of the various BSER waves, a full treatment of these effects was thought to be in order. Many of the illustrations and text are presented for the first time. Where others have investigated similar phenomena, I have attempted to include their fundamental observations. This chapter concludes the fundamental information and lays the groundwork for Part III, in which the clinical use of the BSER is treated.

Chapter 10 is written by two respected professionals in the neurologic clinic. Janet and Jim Stockard's clinical caseload of both children and adults provides an enormous and unprecedented amount of clinical case reports. Several well selected illustrations complement their clinical findings. It can also be seen that Drs. Janet Stockard and Jim Stockard wasted no time in warning the reader of numerous pitfalls that must be avoided, or at least taken into account, if interpretations of the resultant data are to be meaningful. They can be proud of their complementary observations to several other sections of this volume, such as Chapters 7, 8, 9, 11, and 12.

Chapter 11, by Jos Eggermont, on the audiologic aspects of BSER, is both intuitive and insightful. Interestingly, his treatment of both ECochG and BSER leaves the reader with no doubt that there still remains an appropriate place in the clinic for both techniques. Dr. Eggermont's discussion also points up his substantial background in the basic sciences; his meticulous attention to details of laboratory research is quite evident.

Chapter 12 draws upon the experience of a long-time BSER professional, Harvey (Chaim) Sohmer, who has been with the field since its contemporary beginnings. Not only has Dr. Sohmer published first-class prospective studies, but he also has provided the reader with substantial laboratory-based research. It can also readily be seen that Dr. Sohmer has had a wide range of experiences with numerous clinical patients, including children and adults. Furthermore, he has been able to corroborate several of his clinical findings with autopsy findings.

Part IV is comprised of three chapters on other evoked potentials and animal work. They are presented so as to complement the background information, the fundamental materials, and the clinical use of the BSER.

The middle-, late-, and long-latency auditory evoked potentials were in use as a clinical tool long before BSER became widely accepted. In view of this fact, and in view of a renewed interest in more cortical functioning, I asked two researchers, John Polich and Arnold Starr, to write this chapter. Drs. Polich and Starr spend the majority of their research time in recording not only the short-latency BSER, but also the longer latency middle-, late-, and event-related evoked responses. Dr. Starr's neurologic applications of various evoked potentials have certainly not gone unnoticed. The addition of Dr. John Polich, whose interests are in neuropsychologic functioning of patients, made a natural team to provide this volume with an essay on the longer-latency responses.

Continuing the search for the contribution that other evoked potentials might provide, I asked Roger Cracco and Gastone Celesia to introduce our readers to the importance of somatosensory (Dr. Cracco) and visual (Dr. Celesia) evoked potentials to the diagnostic armamentarium. While the audiologist and otologist are less likely to employ somatosensory and visual evoked responses, a working knowledge of the contribution of other sensory modality responses will nevertheless be beneficial. Certainly, the neurologist and pediatrician may have more of a need for the information provided in this chapter. Drs. Cracco and Celesia have done a commendable job; from their chapter, it is again apparent that these clinician-researchers are experts in their respective areas.

The concluding Chapter 15 is tantamount to all of the others. Most, if perhaps not all, BSER work can be traced to fundamental observations made with animal preparations. Mike Merzenich, John Gardi, and Mike Vivion have all labored with the intricacies of recording various auditory evoked potentials from animals. These three researchers know their subject well and have substantial experience with basic gross and single-unit neurophysiologic recordings in animals. Their work has served as the basis for findings in a number of chapters such as 4, 7, 9, 11, and 12. Fundamental contributions from animal work shall continue to be of interest to students of this field in subsequent years.

In summary, to have been among the first audiologists deeply involved in the growth of this area, I take pride in having been given an opportunity by the publisher of this volume to organize this venture. Several individuals were instrumental in assisting me to reach this goal: Ernest J. Moore, Sr., Irene Edwards, Rosie Jones, Sarah Moore, Lorenza Jones, Betheul Brown, George Jones, Allen Counter, Leo Buchanan, Donna Bonner, Howard Bartner (cover illustration), Marva Babin, Joe Hind, Walter Grengg, John Reneau, and Bobby Logan.

Yesterday: I never thought that these efforts would come to fruition. *Today:* I am quite proud of the contributions my colleagues have made. *Tomorrow:* I hope that those inspired by our contributions will continue the exciting story of the auditory brain-stem evoked response.

Contributors

JENNIFER S. BUCHWALD, PH.D.
Department of Physiology
Brain Research Institute and Mental Retardation Research Center
School of Medicine
University of California Medical Center
Los Angeles, California

GASTONE G. CELESIA, M.D.
Department of Neurology
University of Wisconsin for the Health Sciences
William S. Middleton Veterans Memorial Hospital
Madison, Wisconsin

ALFRED C. COATS, M.D.
Departments of Otorhinolaryngology and
Communicative Sciences and Neurology
Neurosensory Center of Houston
Baylor College of Medicine
Houston, Texas

ROGER Q. CRACCO, M.D.
Department of Neurology
State University of New York
Downstate Medical Center
Brooklyn, New York

JOHN D. DURRANT, PH.D.
Department of Otorhinology
Temple University School of Medicine
Philadelphia, Pennsylvania

JOS J. EGGERMONT, PH.D.
Department of Medical Physics and Biophysics
Catholic University of Nijmegen
Nijmegen, The Netherlands

PETER G. FITZGERALD
Department of Medicine
Ottawa General Hospital
Ottawa, Canada

JOHN N. GARDI, PH.D.
Department of Otolaryngology
Coleman Memorial Laboratory
University of California School of Medicine
San Francisco, California

DON L. JEWETT, M.D., D.PHIL.
Departments of Orthopedics and Physiology
University of California School of Medicine
San Francisco, California

TIMOTHY T. K. JUNG, M.D., PH.D.
Department of Otolaryngology
University of Minnesota Medical School
Minneapolis, Minnesota

MICHAEL M. MERZENICH, PH.D.
Department of Otolaryngology
Coleman Memorial Laboratory
University of California School of Medicine
San Francisco, California

ERNEST J. MOORE, PH.D.
Communicative Disorders Program
National Institute of Neurological and Communicative Disorders and Stroke
National Institutes of Health
Bethesda, Maryland

D. KENT MOREST, M.D.
Department of Anatomy and Communication Sciences
University of Connecticut Health Sciences Center
Farmington, Connecticut

MICHAEL M. PAPARELLA, M.D.
Department of Otolaryngology
University of Minnesota Medical School
Minneapolis, Minnesota

TERENCE W. PICTON, M.D., PH.D.
Department of Medicine
Ottawa General Hospital
Ottawa, Canada

JOHN M. POLICH, PH.D.
Neuropsychology Laboratory
The Salk Institute
La Jolla, California

HARVEY (HAIM) SOHMER, PH.D.
Department of Physiology
Hebrew University
Hadassah Medical School
Jerusalem, Israel

ARNOLD STARR, M.D.
Department of Neurology
California College of Medicine
University of California
Irvine, California

JAMES J. STOCKARD, M.D., PH.D.
Electrocochleography and Evoked Potential Laboratory
San Diego Medical Center
University of California
San Diego, California

JANET E. STOCKARD, B.A.
Electrocochleography and Evoked Potential Laboratory
San Diego Medical Center
University of California
San Diego, California

CHIYEKO TSUCHITANI, PH.D.
Sensory Sciences Center
Graduate School of Biomedical Sciences
University of Texas Health Sciences Center
Houston, Texas

MICHAEL C. VIVION, PH.D.
Nicolet Biomedical Instruments
Nicolet Instrument Division
Madison, Wisconsin

Introduction

Don L. Jewett

Readers whose eyes have reached this page probably fall into one of two categories: (1) those who know little about auditory evoked potentials and (2) those with considerable knowledge in this area. Strangely, both readers may, from different vantage points, share an interest in answers to questions addressed in this book such as, "Why a book about *evoked* potentials?" "Why a book about *auditory* evoked potentials?" and "Why a book about auditory *brain-stem* evoked potentials?" In his preface, Dr. Ernest Moore has carefully described the nature of the contribution of each of the chapters to this new field. I will therefore attempt to answer each of these questions from a broader perspective.

Why is there interest in *evoked* potentials? Certainly the brain, as an object of study, has its own fascinating quality of being an almost unfathomably complex organ of behavior, memory, and learning as well as creativity and consciousness. Study of the spontaneous activity of the brain has a long history and a well established place in clinical medicine, and so does brain electrical activity, which is brought about by an experimenter or clinician (and hence "evoked"). The advent of the averaging computer permitted detection of responses from the scalp that would otherwise have required surgical skull penetration, with its attendant problems of anesthesia, infection, and technique. While generally limited to sensory systems, evoked responses detected by averaging stimulated considerable interest among those interested in brain function because responses could be elicited by specific stimuli. Measurement of the activity of only a fraction of the brain's neurons was thus possible, these neurons being distinguished by functional groupings related to a specific sensory input rather than by spatial (anatomic) separation. It should be noted that the averaging process, which can recover a signal buried in random noise, requires numerous repetitions of the stimulus, so that only those signals that are time-locked to the stimulus can be recovered. This limitation may or may not be important, depending on the use intended. Certainly, it must also be admitted that averaged evoked responses have been studied because they are new and therefore offer the investigator a greater chance of making an important discovery than do investigations of better known and well understood phenomena.

Why *auditory* evoked responses? For each of the major sensory inputs (and therefore evoked responses), there are different groups of investigator proponents. In some ways, more is known about the auditory system evoked response than about the visual evoked response and somatosensory evoked response in both technical detail and clinical applications for a number of circumstantial reasons: (1) the auditory system contains neurons that are highly responsive to transient, brief, repetitive inputs and responds with highly time-locked responses; and (2) these neurons exist in sequential short-axon pathways that give rise to a sequence of responses that, in the brain stem, last less than a millisecond. The axons of the somatosensory system, in contrast, are very long, with correspondingly long potentials. The generator potentials of the auditory system are brief and small, and this is in contrast to the long-lasting generator potentials of the visual system.

Why the auditory *brain-stem* evoked response? At this point in the development of evoked response knowledge, the auditory brain-stem response provides, on balance, a better trade-off between a variety of factors that determine usefulness (discussed below) compared with the middle or late responses as presently recorded. For the purposes of this discussion, the division of the auditory evoked response into logarithmic decades (as originally summarized by Picton, Hillyard, Krausz, and Galambos, 1974) is useful: the first logarithmic decade (in milliseconds) after the stimulus (i.e., 10^0 to 10^1 msec, or from 1 to 10 msec after the stimulus) is the domain of the auditory brain-stem response (based on evidence that this is the region of the brain containing the electrical generators of the response). The second logarithmic decade (10^1 to 10^2, i.e., 10 to 100 msec) is the time interval for thalamic and cortical activation and the associated middle responses. The third logarithmic decade (10^2 to 10^3, i.e., 100 to 1,000 msec) encompasses the late response; the location of the generators of this response is unknown, but is presumed to be neocortical, probably in multiple, widely separated locations. In any sensory system there is a progressive increase in the number of neurons as one ascends from the sensory receptor through the brain stem to the cortex. This arrangement tends to provide larger potentials (if sufficient synchrony is preserved through multiple synapses and divergence occurs) as activation ascends the neuraxis; such is the case in the auditory system—the late waves are larger than the middle waves, which are larger than the early waves. As one traverses more and more synapses, however, there is greater temporal variability, which translates to variable latencies of the response from stimulus to stimulus, i.e., "jitter." When such variability is averaged together, the peaks and valleys of the responses may sum together to give little or no response at times, or variable waveforms and latencies. Parenthetically, the late responses may be characteristic of parts of the nervous system whose very function is to provide variability, rather than reliability. On a biologic basis, the brain-stem responses (occurring after passing from one to six or seven synapses) are the most accurately time-locked to the stimulus and therefore the most reliable components of the auditory evoked response. However, since the auditory brain-stem evoked responses are much smaller than later waves, more repetitions are required, and greater technical care is needed in their detection.

As one ascends a sensory system, stimulus-synchronized neurons occur in more widely spaced anatomic locations. In these circumstances, it is difficult to ascribe an abnormal waveform to a change in activity of a specific anatomic location. Because the location of the generators of the auditory brain-stem response are better known than are those of the middle and late responses and are located in a restricted region, it is more fruitful to make comparisons of changes in wave shape with localized diseases or with experimental manipulations that affect specific groups of cells. (Indeed, my current view is that in the brain-stem response, the first wave represents the first-order neurons, the second wave the second-order neurons, and so forth, wherever such neurons may be, since simultaneous activity in differing anatomic locations must algebraically sum, and the time course of the brain stem is consistent with it being generated by short axons separated by a synaptic delay of about 0.5 msec.)

Finally, since the brain-stem response originates in a region of vital functions, the motivation to understand pathology in the region of the brain stem is very high. These responses are little affected by sleep, wakefulness, tension, awareness of stimuli, etc., and this provides an advantage when dealing with infants or others who have difficulty in communicating or cooperating; by the same token, this insensitivity to marked differences in CNS "activation" does limit the usefulness of the brain-stem response in studying these interesting brain functions (whereas the late waves are sometimes affected by such conditions).

In summary, the auditory system can be repetitively and rapidly stimulated for averaging purposes, and its physiologic and anatomic pathways have sufficient reliability and freedom from jitter to allow recording of the brain-stem response, as well as more variable middle and late responses. The auditory brain-stem responses are characterized by high reliability (narrow limits of normality), as contrasted with the middle and late responses. The

xxiv   Introduction

auditory brain-stem responses, like all auditory evoked responses, are significantly affected by changes in stimulus input and disease processes of the primary sensory organ. The changes with postnatal maturation are quite regular, offering a means of following maturation of response in an individual. The similarity of responses across species as diverse as the human, rat, bat, and porpoise has also been of considerable impetus in the development of this field because cross-correlation of results in different species (including humans) are easy, thus permitting a large variety of experimental manipulations.

Should the history of science be "x-rated," i.e., restricted to only the eyes of the "mature?" Here is a question raised by Stephen Brush (1974), a historian of science who suggested (tongue in cheek) that perhaps a realistic history of scientific discovery should be kept secret from the young scientist because he or she might be too "immature" to tolerate an accurate description of the ebb and flow of this human activity. I strongly favor as much honesty in the history of science as is possible within the limits set by the ego of the writer and, in some cases, the laws of libel. Watson (1968) has, I think, set a good example in his book *The Double Helix*, and I would like to follow his example here, as best I can, in setting forth the evolution of the science of the auditory brain-stem response as I remember it. Thus, this is *not* a history presented as a story of logical thought, brilliant deductions, and direct progression toward a desired goal, which could only serve as an organized fiction to spur young scientists to endure patriotic glories of self-sacrifice for the good of a God called "Science." Instead, really, it is a story of bumbling and mistakes, false starts, and delays.

In 1963, I was a bright-eyed postdoctoral student fresh off the boat with my Oxford Ph.D. (D.Phil.) when I moved to New Haven to work at Yale in the laboratories of Dr. Robert Galambos. I had worked on the neural control of the heart rate and had come to Yale to start my study of the CNS, which I felt to be much more interesting and challenging than the simpler reflexology I had been studying. Dr. Galambos seemed to me to combine both research compulsiveness (attention to detail) with a broader picture of research strategies needed to unravel the secrets of brain function. He had published beautiful studies on single units in the auditory system, and he was then trying to develop ways of studying glial cells that, he hoped (because they were a largely unstudied cell type), might be the basis of interesting mental functions such as remembering, forgetting, associations, etc., and that might modulate, direct, or control brain functions in ways we could only guess at. Over the years, I have come to realize that *reductio ad absurdum* approaches postpone problems, but do not solve them. Thus, to explain the mysteries of how a union of egg and sperm can develop into a human being by assuming (as was once done) that the sperm contains a miniature person who will grow within the egg seems to solve the initial problem, but leaves the conundrum that the testes of the miniature person must contain sperm in which there are miniature persons with testes, with sperm, and so on ad infinitum. The "solution" is really little more than a way of avoiding the problem. Similarly, imagining the earth is supported by Atlas solves the immediate problem, but a little thought raises the disquietude, "What does Atlas stand on?" And again the giant turtle gives temporary respite, but no permanent solution. (The most ingenious solution I have heard of was the reply of the true believer, when pressed to describe what the turtle stands on, who said: "Don't try to fool me with your arguments—I know that it is turtles all the way down!") So, my present view is that putting the problems of memory into glial cells was attractive, but no real solution, since they were harder to study than neurons.

Dr. Galambos's lab was quite busy with postdoctoral students, graduate students, and undergraduates, all flowing through at different stages of learning. I immersed myself in techniques of round window recording, stereotaxic implantations, and such, still wondering what project to take up as mine. After several false starts, Dr. Galambos and I agreed that I would work on figuring out why auditory evoked responses had been detected in nonauditory brain areas in some preliminary experiments by Wolf and Chimiento, using computer averaging of evoked responses in awake, chronically implanted, freely moving animals. It was Dr. Galambos's hope that these potentials might be created by some unsuspected process involving glial cells and thus be a new mechanism by which information was flowing through the brain. So I began a series of experiments, starting with anesthetized animals, using stereotaxic electrodes to find and map out these waves. Initially, I started on what I now guess were early middle components, but there always seemed to be a wave at the far left of the display screen, so I worked hard at increasing the sweep rate, digging into the equipment manual to find alternative ways of circumventing the limitations of the averager. Only later was I to realize that as I pushed for faster sweep rates, the accuracy of the A to D converter was decreasing, so that at the maximum rate I could detect no signal at all in the average; but I did find a compromise sweep rate that would give results in anesthetized animals, where the EEG variability was significantly reduced compared with awake, moving animals. Dr. Galambos pushed for experiments in awake animals, but I stuck to anesthetized preparations despite his urgings.

By pushing the averager to its limits, I was able to get small, early potentials throughout the brain, whether I probed in the cortex or deeper into the thalamus and then into the midbrain. What were they? After some initial puzzlement, I had gotten a recording from the cortex in which the waves were exactly time-synchronous with the N_1 response at the round window, so it was pretty clear that the generator of this response was the eighth nerve and that the potentials were nothing but the result of distant current flow in a volume conductor. And then I made a major error—those of you who are sensitive to nuances will have caught it in the preceding sentence: the words "nothing but" bespeak an attitude that determined my behavior. I had classified these potentials in my mind as "artifacts" because they really had nothing to do with glial cells or cortical functioning at all. Of course, "artifacts" should be either ignored or eliminated, like weeds. Only later was I to realize that a rose in a wheat field is a "weed," i.e., the concept of weed is relative and operational—the weed of the wheat field can become the pride of the rose garden. But this was not apparent to me as I finished my work in a rush during my last few weeks at Yale and packed away the data of the brain-stem response helter-skelter with other inconsequential baggage to move to my first faculty appointment in the Physiology Department of the University of California, San Francisco. Before leaving Yale, I gave an informal seminar to four or five individuals in the laboratory, proving the "artifactual" nature of the potentials. As I drove off west, I did not realize that the results would lie unattended for five years while I immersed myself in the joys of teaching and the despair of trying to make a new line of experiments work. I was trying to use rapid, localized cooling of the corpus callosum as a means of reversibly blocking interhemispheric transfer of information, hoping to thereby temporally trap the memory engram in one cortex or the other so that its mechanism might be elucidated. Through a mixture of bad luck, negative serendipity, misdirection, and misjudgment, my efforts produced a few papers, but inadequate progress, and it became clear that I should switch research directions. And while the Yale auditory brain-stem response experiments would from time to time fleetingly pass through my consciousness, I regularly and tenaciously stuck to my view that they were "artifacts" in which only a few electrophysiologists would have but a slight, momentary interest. I recall driving back from Davis, California, one night after I had delivered a talk on the auditory brain-stem response to a small group. Van Peeke (a former postdoctoral fellow) and Mike Romano (a graduate student at the time) both were urging me to further study of the brain-stem response, and I pontifically gave my judgment that it did not seem likely to be a fruitful line of research, that not much could be done once it was clear that it was an "artifact." But I needed some publications, so I wrote up the Yale cat experiments while Dr. Romano started to work on his dissertation on the development of the postnatal brain-stem response in kittens and rat pups.

I am really not exactly sure how we got started on the auditory evoked response in humans. We had borrowed an averager for Dr. Romano to do his thesis, and all I recall is that one day Dr. John Williston (who was a postdoctoral fellow in my lab) and Dr. Romano told me that they had been trying to get some recordings on each other in the animal box, without any luck. Why were they doing that, I asked? John Williston argued that there would be much more interest in the auditory brain-stem response animal data if it could also be shown to occur in humans. I thought about it a bit, then readily agreed, and so began with them to try to get the response which we were sure must be there, though we could not show it.

Our only "shielded room" was a monkey box of about one cubic meter, and since 60-cycle interference can be a problem with these recordings, we squeezed our bodies into contorted wads in the box, electrodes on scalp, earphones on ears, spending long, boring hours with stiff limbs as we tried to record the response. I do not recall any visitors to the lab at this time and this was fortunate since it would have been difficult to explain why we were hunched into this box trying to record an artifact while our legs were cramped, our feet asleep, and trying very hard to relax our neck muscles (Bickford had shown that tight neck muscles could contaminate middle auditory responses). Discouragement mounted along with the hours of unproductive work. I began to sense that this line of research might also need to be abandoned, and then one day I realized something while in the shower.

I digress to say that I have found that some of my most creative thinking has occurred in unexpected places (often associated with water): by waterfalls, gazing at the ocean, or watching water currents in a stream. So the shower was, and still is, a place where my mind runs in a slightly different channel.

So as I was taking this shower, my mind turned to the technical details of the averager we had borrowed, which on paper should have been fine for the job (an all-analog capacitative-storage averager), and as I mulled over how the machine worked, it suddenly occurred to me to try a very counterintuitive approach—to turn *down* the sensitivity of the averager and to turn *up* the sensitivity of the read-out. I went to the laboratory that day, repositioned the knobs, and "presto!," there were the waves we were seeking!

So then we were really quite buoyed up, got replications on three subjects, and sent off a paper to *Science* magazine because brain-stem responses off the scalps of humans seemed a scientific breakthrough. The editorial policy of *Science* magazine is that the authors provide a list of possible reviewers for articles submitted. We thought about whom to nominate for the review and finally decided that we would list those who worked prominently on the auditory evoked response—up to that time a highly variable and elusive electrical phenomenon whose clinical use was frustrated by its unreliability. Certainly they would understand and appreciate the importance of our work! It was all very beautiful, if you think naivete is beautiful. For it was not long before we received a rejection letter from *Science* thanking us for letting them review the paper, indicating how many good papers they had to turn down, and so forth.

I was incensed and wrote a blistering letter back to the editor complaining that *his* reviewers were markedly in error for many reasons, and I listed them. A long wait then ensued, followed by a reply from the editor—a reply that he must have enjoyed writing—that said, "I do not agree with you that my reviewers were in error since your paper was rejected under the advice of *your* reviewers. I sent the paper out to *my* reviewers and they considered it of scientific merit and we will publish it in due course." And they did (Jewett, Romano, and Williston, 1970).

It was only a couple of years ago that George Moushegian told me how he was one of *Science* magazine's reviewers on that second review. He read that paper and said to himself, "This is absurd, one cannot record at such a distance from brain stem to scalp," so he set the paper aside to write the critique in a few days. Then he got to thinking about it and figured that if the paper was right, it could be important, so he decided to see if he could get the response in his laboratory. He went into the lab and set up to replicate the experiment, but he set the parameters of the stimulating equipment wrong, and instead of generating clicks the system generated a prolonged, low-frequency tone burst. And that is how, George told me, he first stumbled on the frequency following response (FFR)! Meanwhile, back in my laboratory, Burt Rutkin, an engineer-advisor, helped us label the phenomena as "far-field," and John Williston (Jewett and Williston, 1971) did the very careful studies that became the paper published in *Brain* without a single correction or modification. But we had not submitted those results to *Brain* originally; we had sent them to *Electroencephalography and Clinical Neurophysiology*, sure that they would publish the paper on the auditory brain-stem response in humans since they had published the original cat paper on the same response (Jewett, 1970). Is not naivete beautiful? "No," they replied. There "was not anything new in the paper worth publishing." Well, I thought I knew how to deal with this. I wrote a blistering letter back to the editor, saying what a mistake it was to reject the paper, but this editor, relying on his advisors, sent me a rather formal reply rejecting the paper again and commenting that, "Time will tell whether this is an important contribution." I only wish that I had saved that letter. I threw it away along with the several NIH grants we had submitted that had all been rejected for reasons such as, "It has all been done before."

So John Williston went to teach at San Francisco State University (a university that unfortunately could not utilize his research skills), and I moved on to Orthopedic Surgery to use my clinical background in new directions. Dr. Romano finished his Ph.D. thesis on the development of the brain-stem response and went on to what he wanted to do—go to veterinary school. Meanwhile, Dr. Galambos had moved to the University of California, San Diego, and, seeing a preprint copy of the human auditory brain-stem response, realized it could be the clinical tool he had been looking for in studying hearing deficits in infants. In addition, Arnold Starr had taken a position at the University of California, Irvine, and recalling a talk of mine on the brain-stem response that he had heard some years before, began to develop the technique for clinical applications in neurology. These two have done a great deal to further the clinical usefulness of the brain-stem response and to popularize the method.

At an earlier period I visited Hallowell Davis in St. Louis and arranged to tell him of the human findings, at that point only published in *Science*. He did not arrange for a seminar, but gave me an "audience" in his office with only himself and Dr. Osterhammel as listeners. Dr. Davis was polite, but at that point was not to be deterred from his work on the late waves, while Dr. Osterhammel returned to Denmark to report that the brain-stem response was likely to be better for clinical purposes. That is how Dr. Terkildson and his group got into brain-stem responses. The main point here is that human contacts have been important throughout the early spread of the technique. Granting agencies that worry about the costs of underwriting scientific meetings should be aware of how crucial such face-to-face meetings are to the development of a scientific field.

What would have happened if I had not taken that shower? It is clear that others would have had the privilege of writing the early papers on the human response. Ernest Moore had, working alone, found the responses that ultimately were an important part of his Ph.D. thesis (1977). In the introduction to this text, Dr. Moore gives further description of his early findings and how they were negatively received. What goes unrecorded was what must have been his deep disappointment in seeing our papers on the human response reach publication before his—since his papers also were rejected by several journals. Dr. Sohmer and his coworkers would also have "discovered" the brain-stem responses, though his published wave shapes have always been somewhat different from those obtained in my laboratory, a result (I think) of technical differences. Dr. Sohmer, from his perspective, always emphasized the importance of the contribution of the potentials at the ear lobe to the recorded auditory brain-stem response. It took us several years before we were no longer blinded by the "far-field" analogy that we had nurtured and realized that he was right. At this point the rather narrow story line expands exponentially: it is too large an undertaking to follow the work of multiple laboratories, various commercial companies, and international communications, but this book gives some indications of that expansion. Certainly I am proud to have been a part of the early efforts in which animal experimentation has led rather directly to human clinical applications.

Perhaps I should end by trying to put the auditory brain-stem response into an appropriate context. The context is that of a reader, holding an open book, reading these words, seated in a room in a building; in a city located in a land of variegated mountains, fertile plains, seashores, deserts, and urban sprawls; in one of a number of intercommunicating, cooperating, and competing countries; twirling on a small, blue orb that is partly covered by white clouds that circles a hot, burning-out, third-rate star; off in the corner of a huge star cluster that is but one of numerous galaxies; separated by inconceivable, un-understandable distances are groups of such galaxies, moving at fantastic speeds away from each other, playing out their roles in the cosmic bubble that itself may expand forever, or burst, or reach an apogee, only to reverse and start a return, slowly at first, then progressively faster, of a movement back together, a rushing of all toward the ultimate black hole singularity that will mix and unite the matter and energy of the universe in an indescribable "soup" for timeless "eons," until the moment of a sudden triggering that in a millionth of a millionth of a millionth of a second will announce the asymmetric big bang that will start the process anew.

"That's it?" the reader may ask. "He puts the brain-stem response in the context of the universe and ends in a black hole?" No, what I am saying is that making sense out of chaos requires the imagination you have just evidenced by following the preceding "cosmic zoom." Scientific endeavor involves generating, experiencing, and enjoying these flights of imagination, cooperating with men and women separated in both space and time to build these models in our minds. By reading this book you are joining the small percentage of humanity that is exploring this part of our intellectual universe.

I BACKGROUND

Ernest J. Moore

1 History

It is always instructive to glimpse backward when considering contemporary issues such as electrocochleography (ECochG) and auditory brain-stem evoked responses (BSER). In order to put the past into proper perspective, several lines of historical evidence must be examined. One line of historical importance germane to this book is the discovery of bioelectrical potentials in animals, first described by Galvani, circa 1791. In 1848, du Bois-Reymond published his seminal paper on the discovery of negative action potentials in nerves. This was followed in 1875 by the first published evoked potential recordings by Caton. Following this, we see the first recording of brain electrical potentials from the human scalp, by Berger in 1929, which came to be known as the electroencephalogram, or EEG.

THE WEVER-BRAY EFFECT

In 1930, a different kind of bioelectrical potential became known to the scientific community—electrical potentials from the cochlea. This monumental discovery was made by Wever and Bray (1930) and came to be known as the *Wever-Bray effect*, or cochlear microphonic (CM). This discovery is particularly significant since the investigators erroneously concluded that the phenomenon they observed was generated by the auditory nerve. This

I wish to thank Dr. M. A. Styx for library research and technical assistance during the preparation of this chapter.

discovery may in fact have been the first observation of what is now known as the *frequency following responses*, or FFR. The FFR will be addressed in a later section and in Chapter 6.

ELECTRICAL ACTIVITY IN ANIMALS

While Wever and Bray were making inroads into the neurophysiology of animal electricity, other investigators were recording rhythmic slow potentials from various animal preparations, such as the caterpillar (Adrian, 1930), the water beetle (Adrian, 1931), and the goldfish (Adrian, 1932; Adrian and Buytendijk, 1931). These investigations pioneered the gradual change and acceptance of the concept that a form of electrical activity other than the classical "spike" potential existed in nervous system structures (Lindsley, 1969). Other notable contributions were being made as well about the neurophysiology of neural and muscle properties (Bartley and Newman, 1930a, 1930b; Bartley, 1933; Perkins, 1933; Travis and Herren, 1930; Travis and Dorsey, 1931).

Following the lead of Wever and Bray, the Harvard group (Davis and Saul, 1931; Saul and Davis, 1932; Derbyshire and Davis, 1935) investigated numerous auditory sites. What Wever and Bray called the cochlear microphonic, Davis and Saul called the *cochlear spread* (Davis, 1976b). Fundamental to these discoveries were other important events, such as the use or improvement of the string galvanometer, the electronic amplifier, and the cathode-ray oscilloscope (Braun tube, Karl Ferdinand Braun, 1850-1918). These all contributed enormously to the recording of electrical events of nerves and muscles.

While fundamental observations were continuing in animal preparations (Fischer, 1932; Kornmuller, 1932; Gerard, Marshall, and Saul, 1933; Derbyshire and Davis, 1935; Stevens, Davis, and Lurie, 1935), others sought to confirm the observation of EEG waves in humans, as made by Berger (Adrian and Matthews, 1934; Adrian and Yamagiwa, 1935; Jasper and Carmichael, 1935). Several researchers concentrated their efforts on laying the experimental groundwork for recording more direct indicants of auditory functioning: the cochlear microphonic (CM), and auditory nerve action potentials (AP) in humans (Fromm, Nylén, and Zotterman, 1934).

COCHLEAR POTENTIALS IN HUMANS

Fromm and colleagues were perhaps the first investigators to employ the ECochG technique. By inserting a wire electrode through tympanic membrane perforations, these investigators reported successful CM recordings from the niche of the round window and portions of the promontory. The response diminished in amplitude when recorded from the external auditory meatus and mastoid process. It is of interest that this discovery, made again during the 1970s, served as a lively debate by those who advocated the use of ECochG over BSER. Fromm, et al. also demonstrated that potentials recorded in humans were smaller in amplitude than those recorded from animals. It is sobering to realize that this observation too was "re-discovered" in the 1970s.

In 1939, a second group of investigators (Andreev, Arapova, and Gersuni, 1939) recorded CM from humans. They are believed to be the first group of investigators to publish a graphic record of CM recordings, although Ruben and co-workers (Ruben, Knickerbocker, and Sekula, et al., 1959) gave this credit to Perlman and Case (1941). Andreev, et al. observed that CM amplitude was quite variable, that lower frequencies (around 200 Hz) yielded larger responses, and that CM was not obtainable from patients exhibiting auditory thresholds in excess of 50 decibels (dB) (no physical reference given). The presence of scars or thickening in the region of the promontory and round window hindered CM detection. The resultant plot of the intensity of sound vs the magnitude of CM yielded an S-shaped curve. These findings led the investigators to conclude that the intensity of the stimuli can continue to be increased, while auditory sensation, or loudness, may continue to increase, although the magnitude of CM has already reached a saturation level.

SURGICAL RECORDING TECHNIQUES

The first Americans to record CM in humans from the promontory were Perlman and Case (1941). These researchers conducted extensive investigations on rabbits and monkeys prior to employing the technique on human subjects with perforated tympanic membranes. Later, unsuccessful attempts were made on a group of normal hearing human subjects with an electrode placed against the tympanic membrane. The active electrode consisted of a "hair-thin," enamel-insulated copper wire about 15 cm in length. Insulation was removed from both ends, and a cotton pellet dipped in Ringer's solution was attached to one bared end (see Cullen, Ellis, and Berlin, et al., 1972, using a similar technique some 30 years later). This was placed near the round window membrane. The experimental case reports of the nine patients studied led to the general conclusions that: (1) CM can be obtained in humans when nearly normal auditory thresholds exist; (2) the potentials are quite small, on the order of a few microvolts, but can be heard over a loudspeaker or via headphones with sufficient amplification; (3) CM reaches a maximum amplitude at certain intensity levels; (4) the limited dynamic range and magnitude of CM may be comparable to a limited range of auditory sensation resulting from electrical stimulation; (5) CM is not a physiologic reaction of the organ of Corti or synonymous with auditory sensation; and (6) CM recordings in humans may aid in the diagnosis of "functional or hysterical deafness" (Perlman and Case, 1941).

Some 6 years elapsed before another reported human CM recording attempt was documented (Lempert, Wever, and Lawrence, 1947). Lempert and co-workers were interested in developing the procedure for both general diagnostic purposes and for surgical guidance during middle-ear explorations. They stated that even if CM is successfully elicited, it has two basic limitations. First, the responses were neither a direct nor an absolute representation of cochlear mechanism activity, but more of relative significance, since the recorded potentials would be affected by the conductive mechanisms of the middle ear. Secondly, CM reflected end-organ activity and not auditory nerve activity or more central processes. Thus, CM is a representation of inner-ear activity, reflecting properties of the ear up to and including the hair cells.

Lempert, et al. (1947) carried out tests on 11 ears during the course of operations for otosclerosis, tinnitus, or Ménière's disease. They positioned the electrode in the round window niche, making contact with the round window membrane. Clearly positive responses were elicited from four ears and "faint responses from two others." The remaining ears yielded negative results. Three years later, Lempert and his colleagues (Lempert, Meltzer, and Wever, et al., 1950) published a final report, in which they concluded that since there were so many inherent technical difficulties posed by the procedures employed, use of CM recordings for practical clinical utility was of limited value. During the same period, two other publications appeared in the European literature which also reported the successful recording of CM in humans (Krejci, 1949; Krejci and Bornschein, 1950).

The paucity of literature on this subject following the pessimistic report of Lempert, et al. (1950) perhaps suggests a general discouragement in attempts to record human CM. It was nearly a decade later that a series of germane papers were generated by a group at Johns Hopkins University (Ruben, Knickerbocker, and Sekula, et al., 1959; Ruben, Sekula, and Bordley, et al., 1960; Ruben, Bordley, and Liberman, 1961; Liberman, Ruben, and Bordley, 1962; Ruben and Walker, 1963; Bordley, Ruben, and Liberman, 1964). Most of these investigations are summarized by Ruben (1967).

The work reported by the Hopkins group was carried out under conditions of middle-ear surgery. Recordings were taken in most instances from or near the round window and associated structures. Ruben, et al. (1960) were the first to report and publish pictures of the round window recordings of VIIIth cranial nerve APs in humans. They found that, in general, two types of responses could be obtained from the round window niche: CM, which they attributed to the electrical activity of hair cells; and AP, which was attributed to the neural activity of the auditory nerve.

Ruben and co-workers (1967) also tested patients having conductive, sensorineural, and "central" deafness. In general, they observed that patients with conductive pathologies showed both CM and AP, but that their input-output functions were shifted to the right on the intensity axis. Patients with cochlear lesions showed neither CM nor AP, while patients with neural abnormalities exhibited only CM.

Independent investigations, by Brinkman and Tolk (1961, 1962), Gavilan and Sanjuan (1964), and Ronis (1966), were also conducted. Gavilan and Sanjuan (1964) overcame numerous technical difficulties, such as induction potentials from the earphone and electrode placement directly on the tympanic membrane. Their results yielded microphonic potentials from a number of normal subjects and ears exhibiting otosclerosis.

Ronis (1966) was the first investigator to report the use of an electronic averager for recording CM and AP in humans. In general, electronic summing allows small, time-locked, periodic signals to emerge out of a background of noise; the latter, being random in nature, tends to "average" out (see Chapter 8). Thus, a *summed* CP or AP is obtained, and a division by the sum of responses yields an *average response*.

Ronis (1966) recorded from a group of patients undergoing stapedectomy. The active electrode consisted of a thin silver wire, while a hypodermic needle subcutaneously placed behind the pinna served as an indifferent electrode. Pure tones and clicks were used; they were delivered by a loudspeaker driver unit attached to a mount on an operating microscope. The sound was finally led to the ear by an aluminum tube attached to a speculum that was inserted in the external auditory meatus. Ronis found that: (1) CM amplitude increased after stapedectomy, (2) post-stapedectomy CM amplitude was larger for low-frequency stimuli than for high-frequency stimuli, (3) response identification was easier after stapedectomy, and (4) amplitude as well as latency of the click AP were sensitive to improved middle-ear conduction. Similarly, CM recordings during surgery also were reported by Flach and Seidel (1968) and Finck, Ronis, and Rosenberg (1969).

Within a similar framework, extensive investigations of *electrical stimulation* of the cochlea and eighth cranial nerve were reported (Simmons, Epley, and Lummis, et al., 1965; Simmons, 1966). In examining the published results, it would appear that these investigators were apparently unsuccessful at *recording* potentials from the cochlea and eighth nerve.

NON-SURGICAL RECORDING TECHNIQUES

In 1966 and 1967, several groups of investigators adopted the technique of Lempert, et al. (1950), i.e., inserting a needle electrode through the tympanic membrane and recording CM and AP from the vicinity of the round window niche (Suzuki, Yoshie, and Ohashi, 1966; Portman, Aran and LeBert, 1967; Sohmer and Feinmesser, 1967; Spreng and Keidel, 1967; Yoshie and Ohashi, 1967; Yoshie, Ohashi, and Suzuki, 1967).

Within this frame of reference, the intratympanic electrode technique or non-surgical approach dominates the results of the available literature. Particularly noteworthy were a series of papers by Yoshie and his collaborators (Yoshie, 1968; Yoshie and Ohashi, 1969; Yoshie and Okudaira, 1969; Yoshie and Yamura, 1969).

The early non-surgical techniques can best be described in the following manner (see Fig. 8-15B): An electrode, usually fabricated from a hypodermic needle, is inserted either into or near the annulus of the tympanic membrane, or into the posterior/inferior external ear canal wall within close proximity to the tympanic membrane. The shaft of the electrode is then glued into the notch between the tragus and antitragus. An indifferent electrode is usually attached to the ipsilateral or contralateral earlobe, or a needle electrode is subcutaneously inserted behind the auricle. Prior to insertion of the ear-canal electrode, the skin of the external auditory meatus is anesthetized. Yoshie, at times, used a somewhat different electrode arrangement for the active lead. His procedure permitted insertion of the needle through the tympanic membrane, where it was placed directly on the promontory or near the round window niche (see Fig. 8-15A).

In 1967 Portman, et al. reported CM results recorded from humans with an electrode at the round window niche. They presented clicks generated by electrical square waves of 0.1 msec duration at a repetition rate of 6/sec and at acoustic levels as high as 140 peak-equivalent dB sound pressure level (db SPL). It was only necessary to present from 20-100 clicks as CM responses obtained were readily visible, ranging from 4-40 μv.

Spreng and Keidel (1967) obtained AP with latencies ranging from 1.5-4.0 msec. The cochlear microphonic was recorded to a 1000 Hz tone. These researchers, however, failed to discuss amplitude, or to publish calibration markers along with their data; consequently, response magnitude could not be evaluated.

Yoshie and his colleagues obtained both CM and AP using intratympanic and extratympanic techniques, and obtained summating potentials (SP) using the intratympanic approach (see Suzuki, Yoshie, and Ohashi, 1966). The CM records showed faithful following of the input signal from 500-1500 Hz in 100 Hz steps, but were limited (at 1500 Hz) by the frequency restrictions of the electronic averager. The classic AP response consisted of three negative peaks, N_1, N_2, and, at times, N_3; these neural responses were usually preceded by CM. Yoshie and co-workers obtained extensive results from normal hearing subjects, and from subjects with either conductive or sensorineural hearing losses. In fact, they were successful in differentiating between various pathologic conditions on the basis of response characteristics , i.e., changes in morphologic features, amplitude, and latency, and on the basis of input-output curves.

Sohmer and Feinmesser (1967) tried a variety of electrodes and recording sites, including: (1) a ball-tipped electrode at the round window, (2) a similar electrode at the tympanic membrane, (3) a needle electrode inserted in the earlobe, (4) a surface electrode (clip-on type) on the earlobe, and (5) a surface electrode on the bony bridge of the nose. However, AP recordings from surface electrodes were so successful that they abandoned the technique of placing an electrode in the external auditory meatus.

Sohmer and Feinmesser made a significant statement, which may have gone unnoticed by most researchers. They stated: ". . . the recorded responses were usually made up of *four* negative peaks. The first two . . . [are] the N_1 and N_2 components of the cochlear action potential. The succeeding negative peaks . . . may be due to repetitive firing of auditory nerve fibers . . . or may be due to the discharge of *neurons in brain-stem auditory nuclei* . . ." (author added italics for emphasis). These fundamental observations led the authors to conclude that they were the first to record auditory nerve APs from extracochlear sources (tympanic membrane, ear canal, and earlobe) in humans. Not withstanding, however, the reader is referred to Figure 4 in a report by Kiang (1961). Geisler and Kiang (1960) recorded several analog "bumps" (as in "Jewett bumps") that may well be BSERs. It is apparent that their active electrode position (behind the ear) was not the most advantageous for optimizing the detection of the BSER waves and that their analysis time was perhaps too long. We also see extensive investigations of BSER in animals (Bullock, Grinnell, and Ikezono, et al., 1968).

The first investigators to report consistent success with the nonsurgical technique in the U.S. were Coats and Dickey (1970, 1972). Their method was quite similar to Yoshie et al. The electrical stimuli consisted of 0.01 msec square waves, which were led to a set of speakers mounted 34 cm from the ear. As Yoshie did, Coats and Dickey tape-recorded their data at 60 inches/sec (ips) and reproduced it at 7½ ips. Thus, the effective analog-to-digital conversion rate during the averaging process was increased by a factor of 8 ($60 \div 7.5$). These data were compared with equivalent recordings from cats. Control procedures were employed to establish the validity of CM and AP responses, such as (1) acoustical monitoring of the clicks, (2) employment of masking noise, (3) increasing click intensity, and (4) reversing click polarity.

CM and AP (N_1 and N_2) ranged from 1-4 μv. Latency of N_1 ranged from 1.8-3.6 msec as click intensity decreased. The waveform, latency, and input-output functions closely paralleled those derived from animal experiments. Masking noise reduced the amplitude of the neural responses, but had no effect on CM. As in animals, reversal of click polarity reversed the polarity of CM, a non-neural response, but failed to reverse the polarity of N_1 and N_2, a neural response.

SURFACE ELECTRODE TECHNIQUES

Excluding the reports of Sohmer and Feinmesser (1967, 1970), there appear to be three other investigations that reported successful recording of AP responses with surface electrodes during this era. Two were unpublished doctoral dissertations (Hood, 1971; Moore, 1971); the third is the now-monumental publication by Jewett, Ramano, and Williston (1970). They presented the first full description of the scalp responses, postulated to be generated by brain-stem nuclei (Jewett, et al., 1970). Jewett also provided us with the widely used numbering system (I, II, III, etc.) for the BSERs (Jewett and Williston, 1971).

Jewett, et al. (1970) attached electrodes to the vertex and lateral posterior neck. To ascertain which electrode was the more active lead, recordings were also taken from the vertex-wrist and neck-wrist. It was found that the vertex lead was detecting most of the brain-stem activity. Several of the control recordings noted above were taken into consideration. The responses obtained showed a series of waves between 2 and 7 msec. N_1 occurred at approximately 2.0 msec; N_2 at 3.0 msec. Much larger deflections were noted about 0.5-1.0 msec later. The later waves (from about 3.5-7.0 msec) were interpreted by Jewett and his colleagues as generated by the brain stem. Waves preceding 3.5 msec were thought to arise from the auditory nerve.

Combining the human work with animal work on the cat and the rat, Jewett and his colleagues (Jewett, 1969, 1970; Jewett, et al., 1970; Jewett and Williston, 1971; Jewett and Romano, 1972) posited fundamental findings that have stood the test of time—that waves that resemble those of humans can be recorded from both the cat and the rat; that the waves detected at the scalp are volume-conducted events from diverse areas of the brain stem, and can therefore be designated as "far-field" potentials; that an electrode positioned at or near the vertex that is referenced to the ipsilateral mastoid or earlobe will reveal the best results; and that the potentials undergo changes in both latency and amplitude as nervous system maturational changes occur.

Moore (1971) recorded from a total of 38 human subjects in five experiments. While the primary focus was directed toward investigating CM and AP from humans using surface electrodes, the potential value of the brain-stem waves did not go unnoticed. A number of stimulus variables were manipulated, such as click intensity, repetition rate, number of data samples averaged, and frequency of tone pips. Two methodologic experiments were conducted both to establish the validity of the responses and to develop an artifact-free earphone system. It would appear that Moore (1971) was the first investigator to record CM from surface electrodes. The bulk of his work unfortunately was never published (see the introduction by D. Jewett). Nevertheless, it was not "buried" as had been suggested (Davis, 1976). That is, several attempts were made to publish these data, but they were rejected by several journals as mere epiphenomena. We can therefore surmise that most investigators are perhaps not aware of its existence, since several have published similar studies since that time without citing the initial work.

From 1971 to 1981, we have observed four parallel lines of short latency evoked potential development: ECochG, BSER, endocochlear potential (EP), and FFR. There were those, however, who supported the continued development and use of ECochG techniques using intratympanic electrodes (Aran, 1971, 1973; Aran and DeLaunay, 1971; Aran and Negrevergne, 1973; Aran, Pelerin, and Lenoir, et al., 1971; Aran and Portman, 1972; Aran, Portman, and Portman, et al., 1972; Brackman and Selters, 1976; Eggermont, 1977a, 1977b, 1977c, 1979a, 1979b; Eggermont and Odenthal, 1974a, 1974b, 1974c, 1974d; Eggermont, Odenthal, and Schmidt, et al., 1974; Naunton and Zerlin, 1976a, 1976b, 1977; Portman and Aran, 1971a, 1971b; Portman and Aran, 1972; Portman, Portman, and Negrevergne, 1974; Simmons, 1974, 1975; Simmons and Glattke, 1975; Yanz, 1976; Yoshie, 1971, 1973; Yoshie and Ohashi, 1971). Others concentrated on ECochG procedures, using extratympanic electrodes variously placed in the outer ear or near the tympanic membrane (Coats, 1974; Cullen, Ellis, and Berlin et al., 1972; Cullen, Berlin, and Gondra, et al., 1976; Elberling, 1973, 1974, 1976a, 1976b, 1976c; Elberling and Salomon, 1973; Khechinashvili and Kevanishvili, 1974; Khechinashvili, Kevanishvili, and Kajaia, 1973; Khechinashvili, Kevanishvili, and Khachjdze, et al., 1974; Montandon, Megill, and Kahn, et al., 1975; Montandon, Shepard, and Marr, et al., 1975; Salomon and Elberling, 1971). Also, several investigators continued to record from the surface of the earlobe using clip-on type electrodes (Thornton, 1974, 1975a, 1975b, 1975c, 1976; Thornton and Coleman, 1975).

DISCOVERY OF THE FFR

A logical sequel to these developments was an interest in low-frequency hearing, below about 2000 Hz. This revived an interest in "volleying" potentials from the inner ear and/or brain stem, and are known in the evoked-potential vernacular as *frequency-following responses* (FFR), or *frequency-following potentials* (FFP).

The FFR was first demonstrated by Tsuchitani and Boudreau (1964) and Boudreau (1965a, 1965b) followed by Marsh and Worden (1968) and Marsh, Worden, and Smith (1970). (In some recent published work on humans, these researchers are not given credit for being the first to investigate these potentials. The findings of Tsuchitani and Boudreau may, however, have been preceded by Wever and Bray in 1930.) Suffice it to say, attempts have been made to introduce the FFR to the clinical setting (Kruidenier, 1979). Studies have been conducted on their origin, effects of various stimulus parameters, and the influence of type and level of hearing (Daly, Roeser, and Moushegian, 1976; Gardi and Merzenich, 1979; Gardi, Merzenich, and McKean, 1979; Gardi, Salamy, and Mendelson, 1979; Gerken, Moushegian, and Stillman, 1975; Glaser, Suter, and Dashieff, et al., 1976; Hall, 1979; Marsh, Brown, and Smith, 1975; Marsh, Smith, and

Worden, 1972; Moushegian, Rupert, and Stillman, 1973, 1978; Smith, Marsh, and Brown, 1975; Sohmer and Pratt, 1976; Sohmer, Pratt, and Kinarti, 1978; Stillman, Crow, and Moushegian, 1978; Stillman, Moushegian, and Rupert, 1976). K. Terkildsen (personal communication, 1974) pointed out the possibility of FFR in several of Moore's records (Moore, 1971). Moore had interpreted the several periodic oscillations as CM, not noticing the delayed onset latency of about 6 msec (Sohmer and Pratt, 1976).

There are two problems associated with the FFR; its *origin*, whether it is generated from neural structures (inferior colliculus or other brain-stem structures) or sensory structures (cochlear); and the *region* of the basilar membrane which gives rise to the neural pathway. That is, it has been demonstrated that FFR in normal hearing subjects is made up of a short-latency CM and a longer-latency neural FFR. In fact, the post-auricular muscle (PAM) response also may contribute to the long latency (≥ 10 msec) FFR (Sohmer, Pratt, and Kinarti, 1978). Sohmer and his colleagues attribute CM to cochlear basal activity, and FFR to apical turn activity. While Gardi, Merzenich, and McKean (1979) and Gardi, Salamy, and Mendelson (1979) implicated multiple generator sites (cochlea, cochlear nucleus, superior olivary complex, and lateral lemniscus) and not the inferior colliculus (IC) as the sources of FFR, they nevertheless suggest that scalp-recorded FFRs can be useful in assessing low-frequency hearing sensitivity. However, Yamada and his colleagues (Yamada, Kodera, and Hink, et al., 1978, 1979; Yamada, Marsh, and Potsic, 1980; Yamada, Yamane, and Kodera, 1977) suggest an IC origin.

BSER IN AUDIOLOGY, OTOLOGY, NEUROLOGY, AND PEDIATRICS

Since 1970, the BSER technique has emerged as a vital adjunct to the clinical armamentarium of the audiologist, otologist, neurologist, neurosurgeon and pediatrician, who jointly determine hearing sensitivity, lesion site, and central nervous system (CNS) integrity, pathology, and maturation. In practice, however, there is a great deal of interaction among all of these disciplines, since no single diagnostic protocol is exclusive to any one discipline. Furthermore, investigators have continued their interest in gathering additional information on machine recognition of the potentials (Elberling, 1979a, 1979b; Weber and Fletcher, 1980).

BSER applications in audiologic-otologic disorders and site-of-lesion testing have shown that the responses are well-suited for the detection of hearing abnormalities (Shaia and Albright, 1980). They became popular in clinical audiology and otology because of reproducibility, ease of administration, low inter- and intra-subject variability, and accuracy in estimating hearing sensitivity (Clemis and McGee, 1979; David, 1976a; Davis and Hirsh, 1976; Emmett and Shea, 1980; Mokotoff, Schulman-Galambos, and Galambos, 1977; Morgon, Charachon, and Gerin, 1971; Sohmer and Feinmesser, 1970, 1973, 1974; Sohmer, Pratt, and Feinmesser, 1974, among others).

Still another recent application has been the use of BSER in neurological diseases (Starr, Sohmer, and Celesia, 1978). Given that a patient exhibits a normal functioning cochlea and auditory nerve, the BSER has been of great assistance in diagnosing various brain-stem lesions, the determination of CNS integrity, and the assessment of patients with various CNS abnormalities. That is, brain-stem lesions cause a selective absence or alteration of one or more of the response components; patients with brain stem damage (due to various types of tumors, demyelinating diseases, diminished brain-stem circulation, and even brain death) show either an absence of certain components, or prolonged latency and reduced amplitude of response components. Many of the pathological conditions have been corroborated with findings at autopsy (Berry, Briant, and Winchester, 1976; Chu, Squires, and Starr, 1978; Shagass, 1972; Sohmer, Feinmesser, and Bauberger-Tell, 1972; Starr, 1976; Starr and Achor, 1975; Starr and Hamilton, 1975, 1976; and Chapters 10, 11 and 12).

An interest in the hearing of children led investigators to discover that norms applied to adults were not appropriate for various developmental stages in children. This led to a series of systematic studies in premature infants, full-term infants, and preadolescent children (Ellingson, Danahy, and Nelson, et al., 1974; Engel, 1971; Galambos, 1978; Galambos and Hecox, 1977, 1978; Hecox, 1975; Hecox and Galambos, 1974; Hecox, Squires, and Galambos, 1976; Jewett and Ramano, 1972; Leiberman, Sohmer, and Szabo, 1973a, 1973b; Monod and Garma, 1971; Salamy and McKean, 1976; Salamy, McKean, and Buda, 1975; Salamy, McKean, and Pettett, et al., 1978; Starr, Amlie, and Martin, et al., 1977). A related application is an attempt to discover electrophysiologic correlates underlying demyelinating diseases such as multiple sclerosis (Chiappa, Harrison, and Brooks, et al., 1980). The majority of these investigators subscribe to the well-known relationship that as the peripheral and central nervous systems mature, (e.g., as additional myelinization takes place, and perhaps as axon diameter increases), latency of BSERs tend to decrease until an adult norm is achieved. In addition, the magnitude of the potentials are observed to increase with age.

The 1970s saw the introduction and recommended use of BSER testing in certain clinics (Goldstein, 1979). However, there is still an interest in determining the origin of certain of the BSER waves (Allen and Starr, 1978; Achor and Starr, 1980a, 1980b; Buchwald and Huang, 1975; Cohen and Sohmer, 1977; Galambos, 1979; Goff, Allison, and Lyons, et al., 1977; Hashimoto, Ishiyama, and Tozuka, 1979; Hashimoto, Ishiyama, and Yoshimoto, et al., 1981; Hashimoto, Ishiyama, and Mizutani, 1980; Plantz, Williston, and Jewett, 1974; and this volume), for determining the effects of sedation in animals and children (Bobbin, May, and Lemoine, 1979; Crowley, Davis, and Beagley, 1975), and determining the effects of various stimulus and other recording parameters (Amadeo and Shagass, 1973; Anthony, Durrett, and Pulec, et al., 1979; Blegvad, 1975; Boston and Ainslie, 1980; Brama and Sohmer, 1977; Hyde, Stephens, and Thornton, 1976; Mouney, Cullen, and Gondra, 1976; Mouney, Berlin, and Cullen, et al., 1978; Terkildsen, Osterhammel, and Huis in't Veld, 1973, 1974a, 1974b, 1975a, 1975b, 1978). The logical concomitant to these studies has been several descriptive and review articles and chapters that assimilate and synthesize the voluminous results of the accumulated literature (Adams and Roeser, 1979; Bochenek, Fialkowska, and Bochenek, et al., 1974; Berlin, 1978; Berlin and Dobie, 1979; Berlin and Gardi, 1981; Davis, 1976a; Fria, 1980; Gardi and Mendel, 1978; Gerull, Giesen, and Mrowinski, et al., 1974, 1979; Hood, 1975; Jerger, Hayes, and Jordan, 1980; Mendel, 1977, 1978; Moore, 1978; Picton, Hillyard, and Krausz, 1974; Picton, 1978; Skinner and Glattke, 1977; Simmons and Glattke, 1975; Terkildsen, 1978; Weber, 1979).

DISCUSSION

The "information explosion" in the area of auditory brain-stem evoked responses has been, to say the least, a most remarkable event. In previous years, one could certainly keep up with the published articles by simply browsing through a few well-selected journals. Today, a MEDLINE search using the most sophisticated data entry and interactive retrieval systems still miss a few germane articles attendant to the subject of this volume, and, therefore, one should be reminded of possible gaps in this account. Any account of an area of historical significance will slight certain topics. The approach here was to point out some of the most important highlights, leaving to the reader the task of drawing his or her own conclusions about those events most important to the discovery and widespread use of the auditory BSER.

John D. Durrant

2 Fundamentals of Sound Generation

This book is devoted to the general subject of auditory brain-stem evoked responses. Implicit in the term "evoked response" is the presence of a stimulus. Presentation of an appropriate stimulus elicits a response by the organism, assuming that the organism is capable of responding. The nature of the stimulus can, and generally does, have substantial influence on the nature of the response. It is therefore fitting, in a book addressing BSER, that some discussion be given to acoustics.

It is unfortunate that chapters of texts entitled "Acoustics," "Physics of Sound," etc., often provide the reader a real approach-avoidance situation, with avoidance often winning out. The enthusiastic reader, for instance, would like to get to the heart of the matter and forget these preliminaries. Other readers bear a preconceived notion that they have an inability to handle physical concepts. The current reader is strongly encouraged to put aside such preconceptions and to give this chapter a chance. First, the physical principles treated here will largely be approached on an intuitive basis; only a limited physical background and no substantial mathematics background is assumed. With these physical principles in hand, the reader will ultimately find various aspects of the nature and behavior of auditory evoked responses to be less mysterious, especially the auditory BSER to which the

The author wishes to express his appreciation to Dr. Sandra Gabriel, Temple University, for her comments and criticisms and to acknowledge her contribution to research upon which portions of this chapter are based.

15

majority of this book is dedicated. Finally, the reader will gain a realistic impression of the limitations imposed by the sound stimuli themselves in obtaining desired results with evoked-response audiometry.

VIBRATORY MOTION

Sound involves the motion of the minute particles making up the medium through which it is transmitted (i.e., air). The motion in question is not linear, but cyclic or vibratory. A concrete example of vibratory motion is found in the movement of the grandfather clock pendulum. There is no net displacement gained by the swing of the pendulum. Nevertheless, work can be accomplished by such motion; the oscillation of the pendulum provides a driving force (in addition to that of the mainspring) to keep the clock working. In all forms of motion, the elements of *mass, elasticity,* and *friction* determine how much *motion* will be realized for a given applied force, and how much *energy* will be required to maintain the motion. However, in vibratory motion, these factors— mass, elasticity, and friction—interact in a special manner.

Natural Response

The most fundamental vibratory machine is the simple spring-mass system or simple harmonic oscillator (Fig. 2-1A). If the mass is left untouched, nothing will happen; a force must be applied to start this machine, accomplished by pushing or pulling the mass to either side of the point of equilibrium (E), and then releasing it (Fig. 2-1B). If the mass is momentarily brought to one point and abruptly released, only the *magnitude* of this displacement will have any specific influence on what transpires; the further the mass is displaced, the greater the subsequent motion (assuming that the

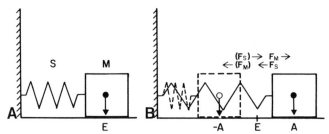

Figure 2-1. Simple harmonic oscillator. A. At rest. B. At two instances in time during oscillation, specifically at +/− peak amplitudes (A) of displacement of the mass (M). Key: equilibrium position (E), spring (S), opposition to change in motion due to inertia (F_M), restoring force (F_S). (Adapted with permission from Durrant, J. D. and Lovrinic, J. H., *Bases of hearing science.* Baltimore, Maryland: Williams and Wilkins, 1977.)

elastic limits of the spring are not exceeded). When force is applied to reposition the previously "resting" mass, for instance, pulling it to the right (point A in Fig. 2-1B), a restoring force is developed in the spring. The release of the mass now permits the energy stored in the spring, known as *potential energy*, to do work; the restoring force tends to pull the mass back toward the resting position. However, masses too have their nuance—*inertia*. Via inertia, the mass opposes changes in motion, so at the first instance the mass is released it just sits there. Slowly but surely, though, it begins to move and gather momentum. Indeed, it picks up enough momentum to speed past point E. The instant it passes this point, all the *potential energy* (originally stored in the spring) has been converted into *kinetic energy* of the moving mass. Having passed point E the spring begins to be compressed; this causes a restoring force to develop. As time goes on, the energy is gradually reconverted to

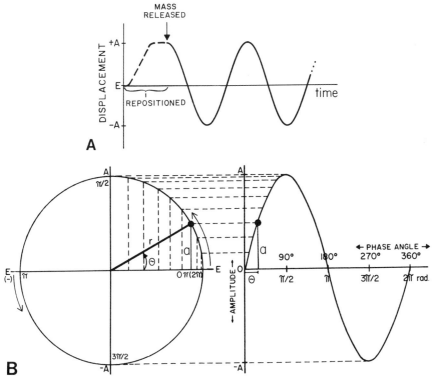

Figure 2-2. A. Time course of displacement of the mass of the simple harmonic oscillator as it is repositioned from E to A (see Fig. 2-1) and subsequently released. B. Generation of the sinusoid from the motion of a point or dot moving around a circle. The phase (θ) and amplitude (a) of displacement at one instant are highlighted. (Adapted with permission from Durrant, J. D. and Lovrinic, J. H., *Bases of hearing science.* Baltimore, Maryland: Williams and Wilkins, 1977.)

potential energy, the mass slows down, and for an instant the mass comes to a halt. In the next moment, the entire process is initiated in reverse, as the mass begins to move in the opposite direction. This describes cyclic motion, which continues as the mass oscillates back and forth. A graph of the time-course of these events is shown in Figure 2-2A; the wave will be recognized as a sinusoid.

There are several parameters by which this form of motion can be characterized and, indeed, quantified. The first is its *amplitude*, which is represented by the distance from A to $-$A in Figures 2-1 and 2-2, that is A $-$ ($-$A) = A + A = 2A. This is actually the peak-to-peak amplitude of displacement. Note that the distance between A and E and E and $-$A are equal. Therefore, amplitude could be just as accurately represented by either A $-$ E or E $-$ ($-$A), that is, the peak amplitude. The time required for the completion of one cycle of motion is also of interest; it is known as the *period* (T = 1/f). Directly dependent upon period is *frequency*, the number of cycles completed/unit of time (f = 1/T) (Hz = cycles/sec). Period (T) and frequency (f) are inversely related; as frequency increases the period decreases (and vice versa). For example (shown in Table 2-1), a 1000-Hz sinusoid has a period of 1/1000 sec, which equals 0.001 sec, or 1 msec. Conversely, in one msec, only one cycle of a 1000-Hz sine wave is completed.

Another parameter is *phase* (angle), which can better be appreciated from Figure 2-2B. Referring for a moment to Figure 2-1, and imagining the mass were vibrating, its movement could be tracked by watching the dot on the side of the mass. The movement of the dot could be conceived as a point traveling around a circle, as the mass travels from E to A, A back to $-$E, and so on, as it completes each cycle (Fig. 2-2B). At every instant, a different angle is subtended by the radius connecting the center of the circle to the

Table 2-1
Relationship between Frequency of a Sound
and Its Corresponding Period and Wavelength*

Frequency (Hz)	Period (sec)	Period (msec)	Wavelength† (meters)
100	0.01	10.0	3.43
250	0.004	4.0	1.37
500	0.002	2.0	0.69
1000	0.001	1.0	0.34
2000	0.0005	0.5	0.17
4000	0.00025	0.25	0.09
8000	0.000125	0.125	0.04

*Note that as frequency increases, period and wavelength decrease.
†Speed of sound = 343 m/sec at 20°C.

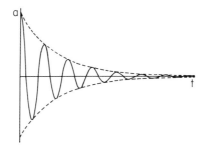

Figure 2-3. Graph of a damped sinusoid (a, amplitude; t, time).

point and the E axis. Each point along the sine wave, therefore, has its own phase, ranging from 0° to 360° (Fig. 2-2B).

The most intriguing aspect of simple harmonic motion is its natural frequency—that is, even though no specific frequency of vibration is imparted to the system during the initiation of the motion, the system vibrates at one specific, inherent frequency. This frequency is uniquely determined by the stiffness and mass in the system. However, there is another factor which must be considered—friction. Whereas energy can be stored in either the motion of the mass or in the compressed spring, friction siphons off energy and dissipates it, in the form of heat. This energy, of course, is not destroyed, but it is lost for purposes of doing useful work. Consequently, after starting up the simple harmonic oscillator, the oscillations will ultimately die out (Fig. 2-3). The rate at which this occurs depends upon the amount of friction involved. The effect of friction is called *damping*. (Think of the influence of shocks on automobile suspension systems; were these dampers not present, automobiles would shimmy constantly, given the numerous potholes and other imperfections of highways.) Again, the time-course of events is not influenced by any specific aspect of how the motion was initiated. The frequency of vibration and the rate at which it decays are all part of the natural response of the system.

Forced Vibration

The solution to the problem posed by friction is to continually supply energy to replace that which is lost in the form of heat. This is called *forced vibration*. Now, there is no rule that the driving force has to be of the same frequency as the natural frequency. However, when they differ, it becomes increasingly difficult to transfer energy from the driving source to the system being driven (often referred to as the *load*). This is because motion is not "in phase" in components of mass and stiffness (Fig. 2-4A). Recall that mass (due to inertia) opposes changes in motion or acceleration which, in turn, leads velocity. By the same token, displacement is opposed by stiffness

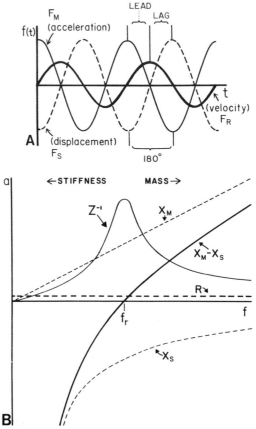

Figure 2-4. A. Phase differences between acceleration, velocity, and displacement, associated with different forms of opposition to motion due to inertia (mass component, F_M), friction (resistive component, F_R), and stiffness (elastic component, F_S). B. Relationship between mass (X_m) and elastic reactance (X_s) in the forced response of a simple harmonic oscillator. The transfer of power to the system is inversely related to its impedance (Z); hence, Z^{-1} reflects the response of the system, which is maximal at the resonant frequency (f_r) (namely, where $X_m - X_s = 0$). At frequencies below the resonant frequency, the response of the system is dominated by stiffness; above, by mass. (Adapted with permission from Durrant, J. D. and Lovrinic, J. H., *Bases of hearing science*. Baltimore, Maryland: Williams and Wilkins, 1977.)

(due to the restoring source) and velocity leads displacement. These forms of opposition are mass and elastic reactance, respectively. The term *reactance* is used to distinguish this form of opposition to motion from that which is due to friction—*resistance*. Unlike resistance, reactance depends upon the driving frequency. Figure 2-4B shows how the magnitude of each type of reactance changes with frequency in the simple spring-mass system.

Parallel to the case of the natural response, there is one frequency at which the response of the simple spring-mass system to an externally applied force is optional (Fig. 2-4B). This is the *resonant frequency*. It is at this frequency that mass and elastic reactances cancel one another; all that is left to oppose the driving force is friction. The more the friction (viz. a highly damped system), the less selective the system will be for frequencies at or near the resonant frequency. The combined opposition afforded by the reactances and the resistance in the system is called *impedance*.

While most practical vibratory systems are more complicated than the simple spring-mass system, they too can be characterized by their impedances. In any event, the transfer of vibratory energy from one system to another will depend upon their impedances. Optimal transfer will occur only when the impedance of the source agrees with that of the load. Of course, impedance, like reactance, depends on frequency. This raises the possibility that the impedances may be matched reasonably well at some frequencies, but not at others. In general, when impedances do not match, devices (called transformers) can be used to "bridge the gap." This is the role of the middle ear, for instance. Unfortunately, the middle-ear transformer operates efficiently only over a limited range of frequencies; therefore, the limits of hearing (along the frequency scale) are imposed by impedance mismatches, viz. at frequencies starting below about 500 Hz and above about 5,000 Hz.

SOUND

It is beyond the scope of this work to comprehensively explore acoustics; rather, it will suffice to use the physical principles just introduced, embellish them with a few aspects particularly relevant to sound, and then continue with some matters of specific interest regarding the elicitation of auditory potentials.

Nature of Sound

The vibratory motion which underlies sound is a bit more complicated than that characterized by the moving mass in the simple harmonic oscillator. Here, the vibratory motion involves innumerable particles of the medium through which sound is transmitted or propagated (i.e., air). If these particles

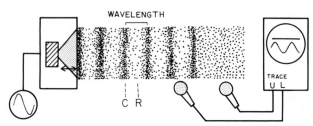

Figure 2-5. Sound waves initiated by vibration of a speaker diaphragm; the speaker is being driven by a sine-wave generator. A cross-section of the medium is represented as though it were magnified many times to reveal the particles comprising it and their positions at one instant in time. The sound wave has reached the microphone nearest the speaker (upper (U) chanel of the oscilloscope) and records the minute pressure variations created by the propagated disturbance. The sound has not yet reached the furthest microphone (lower (L) channel); nothing can be seen on the oscilloscope. (The oscilloscope provides a running plot of the pressure changes detected by the microphones.) Peaks of condensation (C) and rarefaction (R) are indicated. (Adapted with permission from Durrant, J. D. and Lovrinc, J. H., *Bases of hearing science*. Baltimore, Maryland: Williams and Wilkins, 1977.)

could be made visible, they might appear as shown in Figure 2-5. A "slice" of medium is represented, and the positions of the various particles of the medium have been frozen for an instant. The propagation of sound is not so much a matter of how an individual particle is moving but how the particles are distributed at any one instant. As the speaker cone (the source in this case) vibrates, it alternately compresses the particles together on one side of the cone, and in the next half-cycle creates a partial void which the particles rush to fill. These alternating periods of condensation (compression) and rarefaction, as they are known, result in alternating increases and decreases, respectively, in pressure. However, these pressure variations are minute for sounds of practical interest. Due to the inevitable inertia of the particles and the elasticity of the medium, this disturbance in the ambient pressure is relatively local with respect to the speaker during the first few instances after the cone starts to vibrate. Nevertheless, the disturbance is quickly transferred to the adjacent particles and is, thus, propagated (Fig. 2-5). The medium itself does not move as a whole; only the disturbance moves. The propagation of the disturbance is not instantaneous. This can be appreciated from the familiar analogy of hearing thunder some time after seeing the lightning with which it is associated. Light travels many times faster than sound, hence the delay.

Since it takes a certain amount of time for sound to travel from one point to another, and since it also takes a certain amount of time to complete one cycle of vibration of the speaker cone, it is not surprising that a certain distance is covered with the completion of one cycle of any given sound. This distance is called the *wavelength* (Fig. 2-5). Also, since higher-frequency sounds have shorter periods, they also have shorter wavelengths. Because the speed of sound is constant regardless of frequency, increasing frequency means that less distance is covered during the completion of one cycle. Therefore, frequency and wavelength are reciprocally related, as follows:

$$\text{wavelength} = \frac{\text{speed of sound}}{\text{frequency}}$$

Some specific examples of the relation between wavelength and frequency are presented in Table 2-1.

The speed of sound intimately depends upon the properties of the medium—its mass and elasticity, or, more specifically, *density* (mass/unit volume) and *bulk modulus* (a sort of spring or stiffness constant/unit area). These properties, of course, also underlie impedance. Indeed, various media are characterized by their impedances. Thus, both the speed of sound and the characteristic impedance of the medium reflect the properties of the medium (although they themselves are not directly related). Much of the behavior of sound waves and what happens to sound energy in a particular environment is determined by the speed of sound, its relative wavelength, and/or the impedances involved. When sound attempts to pass from one medium to another, for example, most of the sound will either be transmitted or reflected at the boundary between the media, depending upon how the characteristic impedance of one medium compares with the other. It is well known that very little sound energy is transmitted from air to water (or vice versa). Under ideal conditions only about 0.1 percent is transmitted; 99.9 percent is reflected. The presence of fluid in the middle ear (serous otitis media) generally causes hearing loss. There is also a third possibility; sound can be totally or partially absorbed. Absorption is "acoustical friction," that is, the occurrence of absorption causes sound energy to be dissipated as heat. So-called "acoustic" tile is very good at causing this to happen, as are heavy drapes, rugs, and porous materials.

Sound Wave Phenomenon

The main point of the previous paragraphs is that the transmission of sound can be hindered. Any barrier which is either highly absorptive and/or which has a much-different characteristic impedance than that of the adjacent medium can disturb the progression of the sound wave. However, the details of how this occurs depends upon wavelength. If the barrier (in acoustics, it is called a *baffle*) is of relatively small dimensions compared to the wavelength, it will have little effect; the sound will simply scatter around it. This is called *diffraction*. By the same token, if the barrier is relatively large but has a hole in it which is small compared to the wavelength, the sound will be scattered in all directions on the other side of the barrier by virtue of the diffraction caused by the hole. Of course, in this case, the total sound energy will be less on the other side of the barrier, depending upon whether any sound energy was transmitted directly through it. Diffraction is thus what permits the detection of sounds from behind objects. The absence of diffraction, i.e., for very high-frequency sounds in general, is what makes sounds highly directional or "spotty."

For simplicity, the nature of the interaction between incident and reflected sound waves has been avoided up to this point. In reality, the presence of reflected waves can appreciably alter the nature of the "field" in which sound is present. The sound fields commonly experienced are characterized by the presence of reflected waves. Since time is required for the waves to travel to the reflecting surface and back to a certain point of observation, a time delay is inevitable between the incident and reflected waves. When this delay is long, an echo is perceived. Under more routine conditions, the delays are themselves unnoticed, but their effects, called reverberations, are still appreciated. Indeed, the absence of reverberation is generally felt to be unpleasing; everything sounds "dead."

Besides reverberation, there may be situations in which the incident and reflected waves interfere with one another in a constructive manner, and produce a form of resonance. This is the principle by which organ pipes work, and by which a tonal sound can be produced by blowing over the mouth of a bottle. Much like the formation of standing waves on a string (e.g., the strings of a violin), such waves can be set up in acoustical volumes. The establishment of a standing wave depends upon the wavelength of the vibration or sound in question and the length of the string, pipe, etc. Figure 2-6 shows one possible situation of interest here (and discussed in more detail below); this is the occurrence of standing waves in a pipe with one end closed. The fundamental mode for this type of pipe is the frequency whose wavelength is four times that of the pipe; thus, the wave "standing" in the pipe is one-quarter of a wavelength, that is, one-quarter cycle. Higher frequencies will excite the pipe, but only when they are *odd* multiples of the fundamental. It is only at these frequencies (e.g., $3f_o$, $5f_o$, etc., where f_o is the fundamental) that a mode can occur at the open end of the pipe and an antinode at the other. The important points here, however, are that (1) the pipe is quite selective in its response, and (2) such a pipe can act as a sort of transformer. This is a natural consequence of the fact that at the fundamental mode, small sound pressures at the mouth of the pipe are expressed as relatively large sound pressures at the closed end. This is exactly what happens in the ear canal, which is of course "closed" by the tympanic membrane.

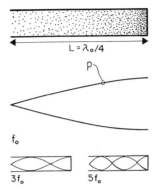

Figure 2-6. Formation of standing waves in a pipe with one end closed. Top: Cross-section of pipe and distribution of air particles at the fundamental mode (f_o, lowest frequency at which standing waves can be established), specifically at the instant of peak condensation at the closed end. This occurs at a frequency (f_o) with a corresponding wavelength (λ_o) four times the length (L) of the pipe; in other words, the standing wave is ¼ wavelength ($\lambda_o/4$) long. Middle: Envelope of pressure amplitude variations (P) along the length of the pipe. Bottom: Standing waves at higher frequencies occur only at odd multiples of the fundamental mode, e.g., $3f_o$ and $5f_o$.

APPLIED ACOUSTICS

Having developed some basic acoustical principles, some consideration can be given to basic sounds and their production. The measurement and quantification of sound is of great interest here. This concerns not only the determination of the magnitude of the sound stimulus but also its frequency content, that is, spectrum analysis, which greatly facilitates understanding of the basic types of sound.

Analysis of Sound

Spectrum analysis is fundamentally a matter of representing a particular signal, expressed in terms of amplitude vs frequency. That is, any given sound or vibration is comprised of one (as in the case of simple harmonic motion) or more frequencies, each with its own amplitude. The graph in Figure 2-2A is the result of the time analysis of the vibration of the simple spring-mass system; the time-course of the motion of the mass is graphed in terms of amplitude time. A sound whose time-analysis is similarly characterized by the sinusoid is called a *pure tone* (a 200 Hz tone), as illustrated in the upper panel of Figure 2-7A. Its amplitude spectrum is shown in the corresponding panel of Figure 2-7B. (Incidentally, the phase spectrum also exists—phase vs frequency—but for our purposes, only the amplitude spectrum will be con-

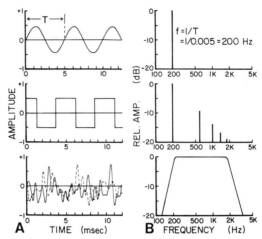

Figure 2-7. Time (A) and spectrum (B) analyses of a 200 Hz sine wave (top), 200 Hz square-wave (middle) and 200-2000 Hz band of noise (bottom). Two time epochs of the noise are shown to demonstrate the lack of repeatability which characterizes noise.

sidered.) As expected, the spectrum analysis of the pure tone reveals that all the energy in the sound is ideally concentrated at one frequency; in other words, the spectrum appears as a straight line, in this case at 200 Hz.

In nature, sounds tend to be much more complex but still may appear to have been synthesized by adding many individual tones together. For example, the square wave (center panel of Fig. 2-7A), which when reproduced by a speaker or earphone has a "buzzing" sound, has such a spectrum, as shown in Figure 2-7B (center). Complex tones, as a class, are characterized by this kind of spectrum; their spectral contents are discrete and are represented by vertical lines on the graph. The spectra of periodic sounds/vibrations (namely pure and complex tones) are called *line spectra*.

In contrast to the spectra of periodic sounds are the spectra of noises, an example of which is shown in the bottom panel of Figure 2-7. In this case, the frequency "contents" are not discrete but vary continuously, at least over a certain range of frequencies or bandwidth. For convenience, a unit bandwidth of 1 Hz is usually assumed, and, through the use of computers, noises also can be synthesized by adding many of these units together. It may be tempting to view noise as an infinitely complex tone with a fundamental of 1 Hz. However, herein lies another important aspect of noise—there is no fundamental. Examining the time analysis from one moment to the next (Fig. 2-7A, bottom), no repeatable pattern is evident. In other words, there is no basic period within which the signal repeats itself, as in the case of pure and complex tones. From one frequency component to the next, amplitude and phase vary at random. The noise spectrum illustrated in Figure 2-7 would actually result only after averaging numerous samples of the noise, so that the long-time average, or overall amplitude, at each frequency would emerge. Just as there is a pure tone, there is also pure noise—Gaussian noise. Its spectrum is generally described as being continuous with equal amplitude at all frequencies; ideally, its bandwidth is infinite. The graph of its spectrum analysis appears simply as a flat horizontal line, but, again, this implies "in the long run." At any given instant, the spectrum of a noise will be just as erratic as its waveform.

Thus far, amplitude has been treated in rather simple terms, namely peak and peak-to-peak values. In evoked-response work, this method of measurement is often applied to the responses (or electrical potentials) themselves, as well as the sound stimulus. However, for many purposes a value, which is more reflective of the equivalent steady magnitude, is preferable. This is analogous to determining the direct-current equivalent of the alternating-current voltage used to power household appliances (i.e., as if measuring the voltage of a car battery). One such measure is the root-mean-square (RMS) magnitude. For example, sound level meters record RMS sound pressures. For pure tones, the RMS amplitude (A_{RMS}) is related to peak (P) amplitude (A_p) by a constant ($A_{RMS} = 0.707\ A_p$); however, for more complex signals the computation is more demanding. Fortunately, RMS detector circuits are well known in electronics, so the measurement of the RMS sound pressure of noise is no more difficult than the measurement of tones.

Actually, sound pressure is rarely specified directly; enter the all-too-familiar, but often mystifying, decibel (dB). The basic unit of the decibel, the *bel*, is defined as the logarithm of the intensity of the sound, divided by a reference intensity (a power-like quantity, i.e., watts/m²). The decibel, one-tenth of a *bel* (1 bel = 10 dB), is considered a more practical unit, so the log ratio of the intensities is multiplied by 10. Furthermore, sound pressure is more practical to measure than intensity, so the equation for sound pressure level (SPL) in decibels must be adjusted to reflect the relationship between sound pressure and intensity. The resulting equation follows:

$$SPL = 20 \log P/P_O$$

where P is the pressure measured, and P_O is the reference, e.g., 2×10^{-5} newtons/m², or 20 μPa (micropascals). (Note: the logarithm is the common log, or log to the base 10.)

The reference sound pressure need not be a commonly agreed upon value, such as 20 μPa. It can be any value, for example, the average sound pressure at which a sample of young adult listeners can just detect sound. This will be recognized as the basis of the audiogram; values so referenced are named hearing levels (HL). Alternatively, it may be desirable to reference sound pressures to an individual's threshold of hearing, in which case one obtains sensation levels (SL). In any event, it must be realized that the physical dimensions are not directly reflected, since the physical units of sound pressure are cancelled in the dB equation. For this reason, the decibel is said to be a "dimensionless" number. Therefore, unless it is sufficient to show only the relative magnitude of a sound (i.e., as in Fig. 2-7B), or a relative change (i.e. 20 dB reduction or attenuation), the quantity in dB should always be accompanied by a reference (e.g., 40 dB SPL re: 20 μPa).

Sound Stimulus Generation

The Tone Burst

This subsection might well be titled "Shaping Sound Spectra." The production of sound stimuli for hearing testing, etc., typically involves taking a signal from a sine wave or function generator and gating it "on" and "off" at a certain rate and with specific rise and decay times. These manipulations are viewed as occurring in the time domain; yet, they can profoundly affect the spectrum of the stimulus, as illustrated by Figure 2-8, which shows the spectra of 2 and 20 msec tone bursts. The spectra of sounds which are sinusoidal are expected to be line spectra (as much as can be approximated by machine analysis). This is clearly not the case here. Turning a sinusoid "on" for such brief intervals causes energy to be scattered to other frequencies, although the main lobe of the spectrum is still centered around the frequency of the sinusoid. The more brief the duration of this sine wave burst, the more impulsive its nature, the more scattering of energy, and, consequently, the broader the main lobe of the spectrum. This is evidenced by comparing the 20 and 2 msec condition in Figure 2-8. The onset and offset of the tone burst (its

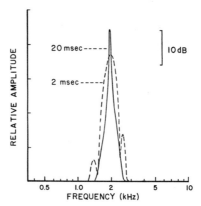

Figure 2-8. Spectra of 2000 Hz tone bursts transduced by an earphone; durations are as indicated (with, nominally, 1 msec rise-decay durations and cosine envelopes).

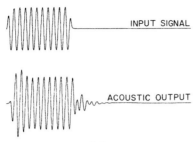

INPUT SIGNAL

ACOUSTIC OUTPUT

Figure 2-9. Comparison of the acoustic output of an ear-phone to the electrical input signal driving it. The rise-decay duration of the input signal is 0.1 msec, thus providing an essentially rectangular envelope.

shape, or *envelope*), are also influential. Some envelopes cause more scatter than others. Generally speaking, the more gradual the time-course of the rise/decay, the less spectral "splatter." Also, less scattering will occur when the sine wave is turned "on" at phases of 0° or 180°, where the instantaneous amplitude is zero.

Now, it is one thing to generate a sinusoidal pulse or tone burst with certain characteristics, and another to accurately reproduce it acoustically. Consider, for instance, the production of a tone burst with a rectangular envelope, as illustrated in Figure 2-9. "Ringing" is evident at the onset and offset of the tone burst. In other words, the forced response of the transducer (in this case an earphone) is accompanied by some natural response which, in turn, is elicited by the abruptness of the onset and offset of the input signal. In some cases, the natural response becomes the dominant factor. Consider the ability of a common earphone to follow the signals shown in Figure 2-10. For a frequency well within the operating limits of this transducer, two different envelopes are distinguishable and well preserved in the sound created or acoustic output (Fig. 2-10A,D). At other frequencies, e.g., near the upper limits of the frequency response of the transducer (8 kHz), this distinction can no longer be made, and the acoustic "response" appreciably outlives the duration of the input signal (Fig. 2-10 B,E). Shortening the duration of the input signal makes the involvement of the natural response even more evident (Fig. 2-10 C,F). The envelope of the offset of the sound (acoustic output) appears to be following an exponential time-course, which may be thought of as the "natural" decay function (compare with Fig. 2-3).

The Click

It is now apparent that abruptly switching a sinusoid "on" and "off" for very brief intervals (i.e., approaching or less than the period of the sinusoid) inevitably creates an impulsive sound. The ideal impulse, however, rises to its peak amplitude infinitely fast; its duration is infinitely short. In general, as

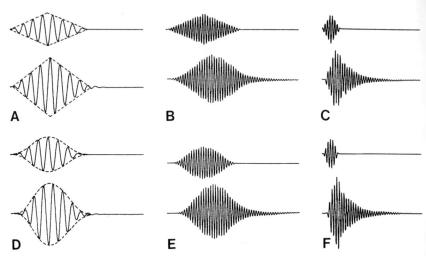

Figure 2-10.   Reproduction of brief tone bursts by an earphone. The upper, smaller amplitude traces in each case are the input signals; the lower traces represent the acoustic output of the earphone. Rise-decay functions: A-C. rectilinear; D-F. cosine. Other parameters: A, D. 2 kHz, 1 msec rise-decay; B, E. 8 kHz, 1 msec rise-decay; C, F. 8 kHz, 0.5 msec rise-decay. In A and D, the envelopes of the stimuli have been outlined for clarity.

duration approaches zero, bandwidth approaches infinity. The impulse can be of interest in a way similar to Gaussian noise, as both provide the means to stimulate over a wide range of frequencies. The brevity of the impulse makes it of special value in evoked-response work (described in later chapters).

Whereas tones, tone bursts, and noises are created from alternating current, the particular impulsive sounds of interest here are created by rapidly switching direct current (DC) on and off, as illustrated in Figure 2-11A (input signals). When a DC pulse drives an earphone or loudspeaker, a broad-spectrum sound is produced, although its spectrum is not identical to that of the DC pulse (Fig. 2-11B). This is first evidenced in the waveform (time analysis) of the acoustic output of the earphone/speaker, as shown in Figure 2-11. The resulting sound is known as the *acoustic click*. The spectrum of the click, obtained utilizing a conventional earphone (Telephonics TDH-39), is shown in Figure 2-11B.

The spectra of the input and output signals are likely to differ for several general reasons. First, the earphone/speaker is not capable of responding equally well at all frequencies. Mechanical and electrical limitations make it rather inefficient outside of a certain bandwidth (roughly 100-10,000 Hz for earphones typically used in clinical audiometry). Secondly, the transducer's response is often "colored" by resonances, depending on how well it is damped (note the major peak in the click spectrum between 2-3 kHz in Fig.

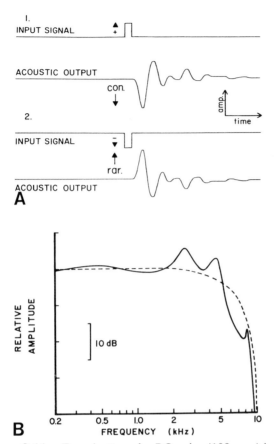

Figure 2-11. Transduction of a DC pulse (100 μsec) by an earphone (Telephonics TDH-39): A(1). Condensation (con); A(2). Rarefaction (rar). (Note that the relationship of the polarity, or phase of the click, to the polarity of the pulse is dependent upon several factors and cannot therefore be expected to be the same for all systems.) B. Spectrum of the acoustic click versus the input DC pulse, up to 10 kHz. (Energy is also present at higher frequencies, namely between "dips," at every 10 kHz (the reciprocal of 100 μsec).

2-11B). The resulting output represents the combined forced and natural response of the transducer. The resulting spectrum thus is the product of the spectrum of the input signal and the frequency response of the transduction system. Also, what you "get" is not always what you "see." In analyzing sounds, there will likely be some infidelity in the sound monitoring/measuring system, which may be introduced by the microphone, electronics, and/or acoustic coupler. The frequency response characteristics of the monitoring system itself therefore must be known if spectral and/or discrete sound pressure measurements are to be completely trusted. For example, in Figure 2-11B, the output of the earphone is underestimated at frequencies above 5 kHz, whereupon the sensitivity of the (measuring) microphone progressively decreases (namely, from 1 dB at 6 kHz to 5 dB by 10 kHz). Consequently, the high-frequency roll-off in the click spectrum is slightly exaggerated.

Referring again to Figure 2-11A, it is obvious that the acoustic click can be excited by pulses of positive (Fig. 2-11A(1) or negative (Fig. 2-11A(2)) polarity. The starting phase of the click is accordingly altered; it will be initiated with condensation or rarefaction (Fig. 2-11 A(1) and A(2), respectively). Note that the relationship of the pulse polarity to the phase of the click depends on the specific system employed, and may not appear as shown in the figure. The clicks produced by the two pulse polarities are indistinguishable in terms of their amplitude spectra, as long as the sound system employed responds equally as well to both polarities. Accordingly, the two "polarities" of clicks sound alike. Yet their starting phases are of concern in auditory-evoked response work. This interest lies in the fact that, just as the inward and outward movements of the diaphragm of an earphone create rarefaction and condensation, the tympanic membrane is pushed inward during condensation and pulled outward during rarefaction. The ossicular chain and, ultimately, the cochlear partition, follow suit. Discharges of the auditory neurons, however, tend to be more effectively triggered during the rarefaction phase, so the two polarities of clicks do not initiate the auditory system's response in exactly the same manner. (Further discussion and practical applications of these facts are presented in Chapters 8 and 10.)

One final practical matter regarding click generation deserves attention—the influence of the input pulse duration. The spectrum of the DC pulse is systematically affected by its duration (specifics are discussed in Chapter 9). In practice, the spectrum *per se* is not the only consideration. There must be sufficient acoustic output which is also influenced by duration (Fig. 2-12B). Due to the limited frequency response of the typical earphone/loudspeaker, not all changes in duration will have equally significant effects. Note the relatively small changes in the waveform of the clicks shown in Figure 2-12A with increasing duration (at least above 20 μsec), although the amplitude changes appreciably. The longer the duration, the more energy in the acoustic output, resulting in a higher overall (specifically, impulse) SPL (shown in Fig. 2-12B). However, SPL growth tends to be asymptotic. This can be understood by looking at clicks produced by what, in practical terms, are unusually long pulses (Fig. 2-12C). By 500 μsec (0.5 msec), a sort of double-click begins to emerge, wherein clicks are effectively being separately produced by the onset and offset of the input pulse. This is clearly evident by 2.0 msec duration; it happens because the earphone (in this case) cannot transduce direct current. There is a consequent "relaxation" of the diaphragm after

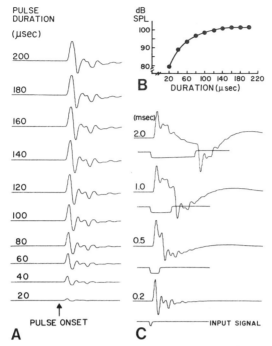

Figure 2-12. Effects of input pulse duration on click amplitude and waveform. A. Click waveforms for durations as indicated (microsecond, μsec, equals 10^{-6} sec). B. Sound pressure levels (impulse RMS; see text) of clicks in A. C. Clicks for relatively long durations, beginning with 0.2 msec (2/1000 sec or 200 μsec). (Note that waveforms shown for the input signals are not perfectly reproduced, due to the limited temporal resolution of the digital monitoring system employed to record them.)

the onset during the steady-state phase of the pulse; to this transducer, the offset looks simply like another pulse of opposite polarity. It is interesting to note that 100 μsec has become all but standardized in auditory-evoked response work. At least for the earphone used to obtain the data in Figure 2-12, this pulse duration is within a range over which SPL is sharply duration-dependent (Fig. 2-12B). Unless there is some provision for the precise control and monitoring of the pulse duration, a more prudent choice might be 180 μsec, in which case the duration could vary considerably without significantly changing the SPL, although some click spectrum changes would occur. However, for an earphone like the TDH-39, those changes would not be a very significant factor for durations under 200 μsec.

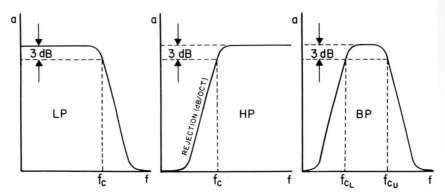

Figure 2-13. Comparison of low-pass (LP), high-pass (HP), and band-pass (BP) filter functions; frequency cut-off (fc), determined at the 3 dB-down point(s). (Reprinted with permission from Durrant, J. D. and Lovrinic, J. H., *Bases of hearing science*, Baltimore, Maryland: Williams and Wilkins, 1977.)

Filtering

Aside from the spectral effects of switching (that is, manipulating the driving signal in the time domain), spectra also may be shaped through the use of filters (see also Chapter 8). Filters cause energy to be passed either above a certain frequency (*high-pass*), below a certain frequency (*low-pass*), or between two frequencies (*band-pass*), as illustrated by Figure 2-13. (There is a type of filter known alternatively as a notch, stop-band, or band-reject filter that pass all but a certain band of frequencies). Although there are acoustic filters, filtering is generally performed on the electrical signal used to drive the earphone or speaker employed due to the versatility and economy of electronic filtering. An example of filtering is the production of the narrow-band noises typically utilized for audiometric masking. Filtering can also be used to "clean up" sounds. For instance, when tone bursts are generated via computers, only a finite number of points along the sine function can be calculated. The waveform of the stimulus is merely approximated in a stepwise fashion (in contrast to the continuous function represented by the true sinusoid). As a consequent artifact of the stimulus waveform digitization, there is some high-frequency noise added to the tone burst. A low-pass filter can solve this problem. It may be tempting to propose, "Why not use band-pass filtering to narrow the spectra of brief tone bursts?" However, its use in this situation is excessive; when an impulsive stimulus is fed to a narrow band-pass filter, the output will ostensibly represent the ringing of the filter. Indeed, the waveform of a DC pulse, say of 100 μsec duration, which has been band-pass filtered (one-third octave bandwidth), resembles that of a brief tone burst (Fig. 2-14). In essence, the filter "rings" at a frequency in the middle of the passband.

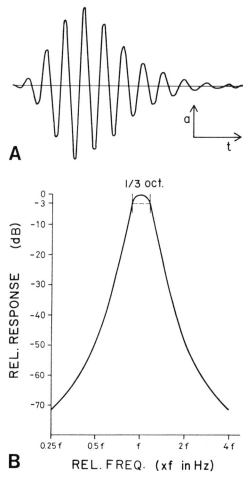

Figure 2-14. A. Filtered click obtained by passing a direct-current pulse through a ⅓ octave band-pass filter. B. Response characteristics of the filter and, in essence, the spectrum of the filtered click. (Based on figures from Zerlin, S. and Naunton, R. F., Physical and auditory specifications of third-octave clicks, *Audiology*, 1975, *14*:135-143.)

Instrumentation

Space does not permit a thorough treatment of the instrumentation available to generate the various stimuli typically used in auditory evoked-response recording. There are many facets to this subject, from the type of transducer utilized to computer control of the stimulus. Nevertheless, some general concepts will be helpful in understanding the basic components of the typical sound systems employed in this area.

In the broadest terms, there are two ways of generating sound stimuli: (1) utilizing discrete electronic components, and (2) using a computer. Note that the distinction is based upon the electronic devices utilized to create the stimulus waveform; in either case, an earphone, a speaker, or even a bone vibrator will be used to transduce this signal into the sound energy. Another part of this final common pathway will be an attenuator, (preferably one calibrated in dB steps) to control the level of the stimulus, and an audio power amplifier and/or impedance-matching transformer. A power amplifier may be necessary only for high levels of sound stimulation, depending upon the magnitude of the signal available from the source of the driving (input) signal. A basic, widely applicable system is block-diagrammed in Figure 2-15. (Similar instrumentation is presented and further discussed in Chapter 8.) This system can be completely instrumented from discrete electronic devices or discrete components in conjunction with an audiometer equipped with an auxilliary input (often labelled "tape," etc.).

The simplest stimulus used in auditory evoked-response work (at least in terms of instrumentation) is the click. The DC pulse used to drive the transducer to produce the click may be obtained from a pulse generator, a device which produces pulses of different durations, pulse rates, or frequency, and delays with respect to a synchronizing pulse. A function generator may also be used; this instrument often produces sine, triangle, and square waves as

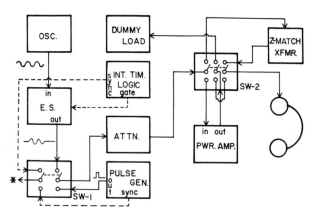

Figure 2-15. Block diagram of system for generation of tone bursts and clicks utilizing discrete electronic components. Flow of audio signals is shown by solid lines; timing signals are shown by broken lines. Key: sine oscillator (Osc); electronic switch (ES); pulse generator (Pulse Gen); step attenuator (Attn); interval timing logic (Int Tim Logic); audio power amplifier (Pwr Amp); impedance matching transformer (Z-match Xfmr); manual switches (SW-1, SW-2); synchronizing or trigger pulses (sync); * to computer.

well. These devices are more versatile than pulse generators, but they typically do not provide as much control of the timing parameters involved. As mentioned earlier, feeding a pulse to a narrow-band filter produces a stimulus somewhat like a brief tone burst. Tone bursts can also be created using a sine wave or function generator in conjunction with an electronic switch and interval timer (Fig. 2-15). The former turns the sine wave "on" and "off" with certain rise-decay functions and thus controls rise-fall time. A certain amount of timing logic is necessary to control the duration of the tone burst and the interstimulus interval (the interval between successive stimuli).

In the previous examples, discrete electronic components were employed. A digital computer can also be used to create pulses for clicks or to synthesize tone bursts. The word "synthesize" is important here, because a true sinusoid is a continuous function in time, and so its electrical analog must be continuous as well. Indeed, devices producing such signals (i.e. sine oscillators) are called analog devices. The electronic signal used to generate the sound varies continuously and in proportion to the stimulus waveform. As discussed earlier, true sinusoids can only be approximated through the use of digital electronics. But through suitable filtering (part of which is inherent in the limits of the transducer itself), rather "clean" stimuli can be digitally created. The computer can then control all of the timing, the level of the stimulus (in conjunction with a programmable attenuator), and the entire stimulus and response-measurement sequence; the system is highly versatile. Any desired waveform can be computed and rendered in analog form through a digital-to-analog converter. Whichever approach is taken in the generation of the sound stimulus—analog or digital—depends on intent, technical competency, familiarity with computers, facilities available, technical support available, and, of course, budget.

SPECIAL CONSIDERATIONS

Various acoustical factors must be considered with regard to the specific situations in which sound stimuli are to be generated. The acoustics of the ear and the frequency response characteristics of the auditory system have considerable bearing on just what the effective stimulus will be.

Sound Travel

In auditory evoked-response work, much emphasis is given to the time at which certain electrical events occur (discussed in Chapters 9-13). Some consideration must thus be given to time delays. These delays may be introduced by the method of sound stimulation, given the understanding that time is required for the propagation of sound waves. The further removed the subject from the transducer, the greater the delay, as expressed in the following equation:

$$\text{time delay} = \frac{\text{distance}}{\text{speed of sound}}$$

For example, if the speaker is located 1 meter away (and assuming the speed of sound to be 343 meters/sec), it will take 2.9 msec (1/343 = 0.0029 sec) for the sound to arrive at the subject's ear. This is not the entire delay between the time at which the speaker is first actuated and that at which the tympanic membrane is first set into vibration. This is due to the location of the eardrum at the end of the ear canal, about 0.025 meter (2.5 cm or 1 in) from its opening at the concha. Therefore, an additional delay of approximately 0.07 msec (0.025/343 = 0.00007 sec) is required for sound to propagate down the ear canal. This also indicates that, even with the use of earphones, some sound-travel delay is inevitable. For most purposes, this delay is negligible, although in some areas of evoked-response measurement (i.e., in ECochG or in the measurement of the auditory BSER), time differences on the order of 0.1 msec (100 μsec) can be resolved and may be meaningful.

Transduction Systems

Each transducer has its own idiosyncracies. First, an electromechanical system (such as an earphone, loudspeaker, or bone vibrator), by virtue of its frequency response, impedance, and distortion characteristics, will produce a sound with a unique spectrum for any given driving signal. For steady tones, the differences between the spectra of the sounds produced by two different transducers may be minimal and insignificant. Even if significant, corrections often can be made, as is done in the calibration of audiometers. Where broad spectrum sounds are being produced (such as a click), the idiosyncracies of the transducer may become much more significant, and corrections can be much less easily applied. No two clicks from two transducers, even of the same make and model, are identical. Differences also may be introduced by how a transducer is used. For example, an earphone fitted with a cushion and directly positioned on the ear produces a slightly different spectrum at the tympanic membrane than that which is produced by the same earphone held, say, 0.1 meter (about 4 in) away. There will be relatively more sound pressure at low frequencies with the earphone held firmly against the ear, but there will be a relative loss of sound pressure at high frequencies. The former is due to the fact that the earphone can work more efficiently when loaded by the small volume of air between the earphone and the eardrum than when it works into an open room. The relative reduction in the high frequencies with the earphone placed over the ear, on the other hand, is due to the loss of the head- and auricle-baffle effects. The directionality of sound can also be a significant factor in sound field stimulation; it also is most evident for high-frequency sounds, as less diffraction occurs as the sound is radiated from the speaker.

Influence of the Acoustics of the Ear

Even if the sound transduction system were capable of true high-fidelity performance (that is, completely faithful reproduction of the input signal), the spectrum of the sound actually reaching the inner ear would not necessarily be identical to that produced by the transducer. The ear has its own particularly dramatic acoustic properties with respect to sound field presentation of stimuli (i.e., utilizing a loudspeaker). The ear and its anatomical location make it somewhat analogous (acoustically) to a microphone mounted in a solid spherical baffle, e.g., a wooden ball. At relatively low frequencies, the baffle has no significant effect due to diffraction; the sound waves simply scatter around the ball. However, at frequencies whose wavelengths are less than the diameter of the ball, sound will be reflected back into the sound field and, thus, can contribute to the sound pressure detected by the microphone. For "head-sized" spherical baffles this begins to happen above 1-2 kHz.

The spherical baffle actually is an over-simplification of the real ear situation. First, there is the presence of another baffle, albeit small—the auricle. This baffle can significantly influence the spectrum only above 5 kHz. Secondly, the eardrum (analogous to the microphone diaphragm), is located below the surface of the skull (baffle) at the end of a tube—the ear canal. (As noted earlier, this is analogous to a pipe with one end closed; such structures can resonate due the formation of standing waves.) The fundamental mode of the ear canal occurs at approximately 3.4 kHz. The enhancement of the sound pressure at the eardrum, afforded by the combination of the head/auricle baffle and the ear-canal resonance effects, can be appreciated from the top graph (B) in Figure 2-16. A substantial boost in sound pressure occurs from about 2-7 kHz. (The actual gain realized depends upon the orientation of the head; these data are for the situation in which the loudspeaker is directly in front of the head or $0°$ azimuth.) Sound energy must finally be conveyed to the inner ear via the middle ear. Despite the impressive efficiency, frequency response, and low distortion of the middle ear mechanism, it is imperfect. It too has a resonant frequency of around 1 kHz. The combination of these factors is reflected in the minimum audibility curve (MAC) (plotted upside-down in Fig. 2-16A, to make it analogous to a frequency response curve.) The net result is that sound delivered to the inner ear is inherently band-pass filtered.

Other factors ultimately determine the effective spectrum of the auditory stimulus as it is manifested in the response of the auditory system to sound and ultimately reflected in the MAC. The acoustic or middle-ear muscle reflex can alter the sound spectrum, since it somewhat selectively attenuates sound transmission via the middle ear at frequencies below about 1 kHz. For very

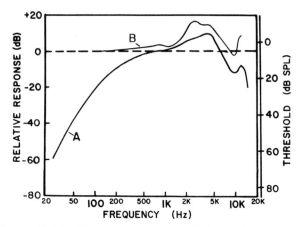

Figure 2-16. Frequency response of the auditory system (curve **A**), approximated by inverting the minimum audibility curve. (From Robinson, D. W. & Dadson, R. S., A redetermination of the equal loudness relations for pure tones. *British Journal of Applied Physiology*, 1956, 7:166-181. Contribution of the combined head-baffle and ear-canal-resonance effects indicated by curve B (Adapted from Shaw, E. A. G. The external ear. In Keidel, W. D. & Neff, W. D. (Eds.). *Handbook of sensory physiology. Vol. V/1. Auditory System: anatomy, physiology (ear).* Berlin: Springer-Verlag, pp. 455-490, 1974.) (Adapted with permission from Durant, J. D. Anatomic and physiologic correlates of the effects of noise on hearing. In Lipscomb, D. M. (Ed.), *Noise and Audiology.* Baltimore, Maryland: University Park Press, pp. 109-141, 1978.)

impulsive stimuli, such as clicks, the reflex may have no effect at all. The frequency response characteristics of the total auditory system also change according to the overall level of the stimulus, as evidenced by the equal loudness contours. Namely, as the level of the sound is increased, the frequency response characteristics of the auditory system are "flatter." At high-level sounds, all frequencies are perceived as being more nearly equal in loudness than would have been expected from the outer/middle ear response characteristics and the MAC.

As noted, the use of earphones appreciably alters the situation, mainly by way of the elimination of the head/auricle-baffle effect. Nevertheless, the ear-canal and middle-ear resonances are still in effect. The acoustic effects of the structure of the ear and how the transducer is coupled to it can substantially influence the spectrum of the stimulus. These factors also substantially contribute to the spectral differences observed in the past example of the earphone held against (versus away from) the ear; the differences are perceptible. Holding the earphone away produces a click that is slightly more "sharp" in quality; conversely, holding the earphones against the ear makes it sound more dull, or "flat." (This phenomenon should be borne in mind by anyone involved in testing newborns, small infants, or in those situations in which a standard earphone headset cannot be worn by the subject and the earphone must be hand-held or otherwise supported.)

Response of the Auditory System to Brief Stimuli

In auditory evoked-response work, it is sometimes of interest to stimulate the auditory system at specific frequencies while using a fairly impulsive stimulus. Since such brief stimuli have continuous and not line spectra, however, it is difficult "to have your cake and eat it, too." Although very brief tone bursts elicit a sense of pitch, they do not sound tonal. Thus the question arises, "How well does the auditory system 'tune in' on these stimuli?" One

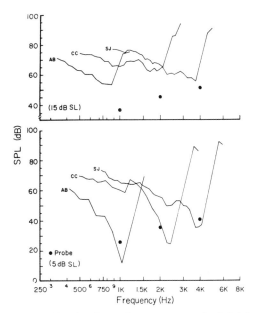

Figure 2-17. Psychophysical tuning curves for brief-duration probe stimuli (tone bursts of 1.2 msec effective duration; cosine envelope) for two sensation levels and three probe frequencies (data from three different subjects: AB, CC, and SJ). A sweep-frequency automatic threshold-tracking paradigm was employed. Masked thresholds were taken as the descending reversal points in the tracings and graphed via point-to-point extrapolation; the masker was continuous. (Reprinted with permission from Durrant, J. D., Gabriel, S., & Walter, M. Psychophysical tuning functions for brief stimuli: Preliminary report. *American Journal of Otolaryngology*, 1981, 2:108-113.

way to examine this issue is to determine psychophysical tuning curves for these stimuli.

To obtain the psychophysical tuning curve the test or probe stimulus is presented at a fixed level above threshold. Tones of different frequencies are used as maskers; the sound pressure level at which the probe is just masked is determined as a function of frequency. The graph of these masked thresholds, examples of which appear in Figure 2-17, reveals that the masker is most effective at one characteristic frequency (CF). The CF usually occurs at or very near the probe frequency, and the effectiveness of the masker decreases dramatically at frequencies above and below the CF. The psychophysical tuning curve closely resembles tuning curves for individual auditory neurons, especially primary neurons. The shape of the graph therefore largely reflects the frequency selectivity of the peripheral auditory system, beginning at the level of the basilar membrane (in other words, the hydromechanical events of the cochlea) and the response of the hair cells to its motion.

The psychophysical tuning curves shown in Figure 2-17 were obtained utilizing probe stimuli of 1.2 msec duration (effectively; nominally, 2 msec total duration, with 1 msec rise-decay durations and cosine envelope). The maskers were continuous. The data plotted in the lower part of Figure 2-17 were obtained with the probe stimuli presented at 5 dB SL. These graphs do not reflect the sharper tuning that would be observed utilizing probe stimuli of longer duration. However, the brief tone bursts must be presented at levels substantially above the threshold of effectively continuous tones (namely, greater than 200 msec) in order to be detected. This is due to the threshold power integration phenomenon: The auditory system can summate the power in the stimulus over durations up to about 200 msec. Up to this limit, the longer the stimulus, the less intensity required to reach threshold. Conversely, the shorter the stimulus, the greater the intensity of the stimulus required to reach threshold. As shown in Figure 2-18, in which tuning functions are compared for probes of 1.2 and 7.2 msec effective duration, there seems to be a level-dependent degradation in tuning sharpness. This is further demonstrated by the tuning functions shown in top panel of Figure 2-17 (1.2 msec probes presented at 15 dB SL). Yet, when compared at equal sound pressure levels (as in Fig. 2-18), very similar functions are obtained, regardless of duration. These data demonstrate that it is indeed possible to obtain reasonably discrete stimulation (vis-à-vis frequency) using very brief tones. However, the "tip" of the psychophysical tuning function for these stimuli is not well preserved for levels of stimulation much above those representative of normal hearing thresholds.

These observations suggest that some frequency spread in the stimulus is tolerable, even when attempting to stimulate the hearing organ in a manner analogous to utilizing steady pure tones (at least at very low levels of stimulation). Just how much spread can be tolerated? Intuitively, the limit might be expected to be set by the *critical bandwidth*, which is a manifestation of the

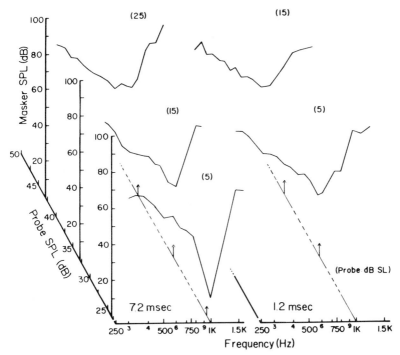

Figure 2-18. Psychophysical tuning curves for two brief-duration probe stimuli (effective durations as indicated: cosine envelopes). Parameter in parentheses is sensation level expressed in decibels. All data obtained from one subject. Method as described in Fig. 2-17. (Reprinted with permission from Durrant, J. D., Gabriel, S., & Walter, M. Psychophysical tuning functions for brief stimuli: Preliminary report. *American Journal of Otolaryngology*, 1981, 2:108-113.

auditory system's ability to resolve different frequencies of sound or simultaneously occurring spectral components. Of interest in this regard are data from an investigation carried out in our laboratory to directly study the influence of the bandwidth of the probe stimulus on the characteristics of the psychophysical tuning function (Fig. 2-19). The auditory system can be seen here to respond almost as selectively to a 150 Hz band of noise centered around 2 kHz as it can to a tone of 2 kHz [bandwidth (BW) = 1 in Fig. 2-19]. For bandwidths equal to or greater than the critical band for 2 kHz (namely, about 300 Hz), however, the tuning function begins to deteriorate. These observations indicate that considerable compromises can be accepted in terms of the spectrum of the tone burst stimuli employed, i.e., in the interest of using a fairly impulsive stimulus to better synchronize the response of auditory neurons— as long as the spectral splatter does not exceed one critical band-width (in the interest of stimulating effectively one "place" along the hearing organ.)

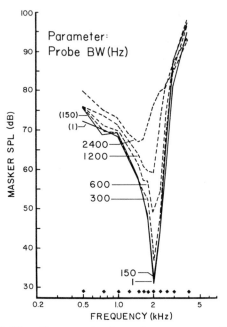

Figure 2-19. Mean psychophysical tuning curves (N = 6) for probe stimuli of different bandwidths (BW), as indicated, chosen to be below (solid), and approximately at or above (broken lines), the average critical bandwidth (approximately 300 Hz). The probe stimuli were 200 msec duration (10 msec rise-decay) and were presented in the presence of continuous maskers. The masked thresholds were measured utilizing a fixed-frequency tracking procedure; the test frequencies are marked along the abscissa. (Based on data from Gabriel, S. Dependence of Psychophysical Tuning Curves on Probe Bandwidth: Relation to Critical Bandwidth. Unpublished Ph.D. dissertation, Temple University, Philadelphia, Pennsylvania, 1981.)

This method of analysis can be taken one step further. Since the spectrum of the acoustic click is quite removed from that of the ideal impulse, and given the combined resonances of the typical earphone (assuming this mode of transduction), ear canal, and middle ear, it might be anticipated that the spectrum of the click reaching the cochlea will not be very broad and may in fact have a prominent spectral peak which the auditory system can "tune" on. Indeed, utilizing the click for a probe stimulus, some degree of tuning can be demonstrated, as shown by the psychophysical tuning curves in Figure 2-20. But relatively sharp tuning is again seen only at low levels of the probe stimulus which, in turn, are near the normal hearing threshold of this stimulus. Note that the actual CF of "click tuning functions" is probably quite indi-

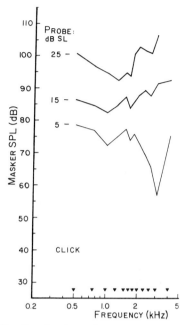

Figure 2-20. Psychophysical tuning curves obtained from one subject utilizing the acoustic click as the probe stimulus (100 μsec DC pulse driving a Telephonics TDH-49 earphone at a rate of 3 pulse/sec; spectrum shown in Fig. 2-8). Procedure as described in Fig. 2-19. (Reprinted with permission from Durrant, J. D., Gabriel, S., & Walter, M. Psychophysical tuning functions for brief stimuli: Preliminary report. *American Journal of Otolaryngology*, 1981, 2:108-113.)

vidual, depending on the actual ear-canal resonance, characteristics of the earphone, and the chosen masking frequencies. At higher levels, tuning greatly deteriorates and the "tip" is lost.

Standardization of Stimuli

It is essential to have some sense of the magnitude of the stimulus when recording and measuring auditory evoked responses, just as in psychoacoustic research and clinical audiometry. For most practical purposes, this is a matter of determining the SPL of the stimulus. For types of work wherein tonal stimuli of relatively long duration are to be used, the RMS SPL of a steady tone of the same frequency can be determined and utilized. When earphones are employed, the advisability of using a 6-cc cavity to represent the typical ear vs (at the opposite extreme) making real-ear measurements must be considered. In other words, all the debates of years of audition literature concerning standardization practices in psychoacoustics and audiometry apply here as well. The simplest approach, of course, is to settle for the measurements in a cavity, a so-called artificial ear. This practice is still widely accepted, particularly in clinical audiology, and these measurements can be made simply by using an audiometric calibration unit.

For situations demanding more impulsive stimuli (i.e., brain-stem evoked-response audiometry), a substantially different approach is required; few guidelines and no standards have been developed. The sound level meters, typically a part of audiometric calibration units, are not made to accurately measure impulsive sounds. If measurements of, say, the SPL of a click is attempted with such instruments, little if any deflection will be seen, unless the clicks are presented at relatively high rates of repetition. What is then observed on the meter will probably be proportional to the magnitude of the stimulus; it will not be very representative of its true amplitude. This is because the meter movement is too sluggish to follow the instantaneous magnitude. It will "smooth over" the click, register something proportional to the average SPL of the click- or pulse-train created by the repeated presentation of the clicks (in conjunction with the RMS detection circuitry in the instrument).

One solution to the measurement problem posed by clicks and the like is to use an oscilloscope connected to the recorder or oscilloscope output of the sound level meter, and match the click to a continuous tone in terms of peak-to-peak amplitude. The comparison tone might be chosen to have a frequency whose period is approximately the same as that of the first "cycle" of the click (see Fig. 2-11A), i.e., about 3 kHz, or a frequency equal to the resonant frequency of the earphone/speaker, i.e., around 2 kHz (see Fig. 2-11B). The RMS SPL of this comparison tone is then measured. This measurement has come to be known as the peak equivalent SPL (peSPL). From the peSPL, one can derive the actual peak or peak-to-peak sound pressures, by working back through the decibel and RMS-vs-peak magnitude equations (presented earlier). There are, however, sound level meters and some spectrum analyzers which are useful in their ability to measure the RMS SPL of impulses. There generally is a "hold" function available which permits the measurement of isolated clicks; the sound is captured and stored by a sample-hold circuit. Nevertheless, limitations are involved; the metering circuits assume certain characteristics of the impulse. The instrument used also will have one or more weighting networks, i.e., the A-weighting network, which is so popular for carrying out noise surveys. In short, there are likely one or more "fudge factors" which affect the SPL measured; not all will be appropriate for the intended application.

A particularly important aspect of the calibration process when utilizing click stimuli or tone bursts with fixed starting phases (so-called *phase co-*

herent) is to determine whether the stimulus is, nominally, condensation or rarefaction in phase. This cannot be determined by a sound level meter alone; again, an oscilloscope is required. Next, it must be determined which direction of deflection of the tracing on the oscilloscope corresponds to condensation (as in Fig. 2-11A). The technical literature accompanying the sound level meter (or whatever instrument is being employed) may provide this information. If this is not known, however, it must be determined. One way is to lightly tap on the microphone with a cotton wisp and watch the initial direction of deflection. (A storage oscilloscope or someone who can watch the scope helps.) This initial deflection is the direction for condensation, since the diaphragm of the microphone is being inwardly displaced, analogous to the buildup of air particles against it. In other words, a relative increase in pressure is being simulated. Note the delicacy of this procedure; the reader should consider seeking technical assistance in determining the phase of their stimulus. Also, the polarity/phase of the electrical signal driving the transducer should be carefully determined, along with the polarity of the connection of the transducer to the electronic instrumentation. If this is done, the determination of the phase of the stimulus should be required only once in the lifetime of any given evoked-response system (see also Chapter 8).

The determination of the physical characteristics of the stimulus clearly is important, but what is generally of greater importance in the application of evoked response techniques is the level of the stimulus relative to normal levels of stimulus detection. Here, too, no firm standards have developed. For work with stimuli which can reasonably be treated as steady tones (i.e., 200 msec or more, to permit full threshold power integration) (see Chapter 9), the standards which have been developed for clinical audiology are reasonable. Hearing levels can thus be derived from SPL measurements. Again, the greater problems arise concerning the more impulsive stimuli. The SPLs of these stimuli, regardless of how they are determined, are less directly interpretable, since higher SPLs are inherently required for these sounds to be detected. The detection of these stimuli is also keenly dependent upon the rate at which they are presented and, to some extent, the number of stimuli presented in any given time frame.

Perhaps the simplest way to reference the level of the stimulus is to use the subject's own behavioral threshold (i.e., for a continuous string of clicks presented at the rate used for recording the evoked electrical potential of interest). The use of sensation level is, however, limited to cooperative subjects; it is of limited value if the general status of hearing is not known. Besides, once thresholds have been determined for a group of subjects which have been found to have normal hearing sensitivity (via conventional audiometry), the basis for specifying the stimulus magnitude in terms of hearing level is extant. In other words, the level can be referenced to the average threshold of this group of normal listeners. It is beyond the scope of this writing to discuss the psychophysical methods employed to determine these thresholds; suffice it to say that variations of the method of limits are generally felt to be the most practical and reasonably reliable (e.g., the staircase or up-down method). The interested reader is encouraged to refer to a psycho-physics or sensory psychology text if unfamiliar with psychophysical method-ology (e.g., G. A. Gescheider's *Psychophysics: Method and Theory*).

Some workers are compelled to designate hearing levels derived in this manner by the letters "nHL" (meaning "normal" hearing level), presumably to avoid any implication of standardization by the American National Stan-dards Organization or the International Standards Organization. This is un-necessary and confusing; HL implies average/normal hearing sensitivity as the standard of comparison. A fundamentally more important consideration is that HL, like SPL and all measures expressed in dB, is relatively mean-ingless without the proper reference, e.g., SPL re: 20 μPa, HL re: ISO 1964, etc. An explicit specification of the reference is requisite. Since no standards currently exist for clicks, etc., the reference can be adequately specified only by providing complete descriptions of the subjects, stimulus parameters, and psychophysical methods employed in each standardization process. This specification might read as follows: The reference level for our click stimulus was standardized utilizing a group of young adult listeners (N = 10, mean age = 20 years), with normal hearing (within 10 dB of 0 dB HL re: ANSI 1969, 250 to 8000 Hz). Thresholds for the clicks (100 μsec, presented at 10/sec) were determined utilizing the staircase method (reference or details here). At this juncture, just like click spectra, one person's HL may be some-what different from another's. This possibility fortunately has not led to the chaos that might be expected, since the same audiometric standards are widely accepted and form the basis for criterion by which subjects in the stan-dardization sample are selected.

DISCUSSION

From an understanding of basic physical principles and simple harmonic motion, it is possible to arrive at an understanding, at least intuitively, of various other physical or acoustical concepts which underlie sound stimuli production. This prompts the realization that the specific characteristics of the sound stimulus are products of various factors, besides those of the input signal used to generate the sound. There are two general classes of factors in-volved. The first is physical. Any given stimulus is a product of both the natural and forced response of the sound production system. The latter is governed by the impedances acting at each stage of the system, wherein op-timal performance occurs only when there is a reasonable match between the impedances of each stage (e.g., between an audio power amplifier and a speaker). Impedance, in turn, depends on the components of mass, elasticity, and friction (or their electrical counterparts), which also determine the characteristics of the natural response of the system. These physical properties determine the frequency response characteristics of the system and, subsequently, the spectrum of the stimulus. For instance, a rectangular, DC, pulse (input signal) is transduced into a brief oscillatory sound and described as a "click." Yet, these things do not completely determine the final form of the stimulus as it is received and processed by the auditory system.

There is another class of factors attributable to the structure and functioning of the auditory system. (In some situations there may be even more than the ear involved, as in the case of the head-baffle effect.) The ear canal fosters standing waves, and the middle-ear mechanism is a less-than-perfect impedance-matching transformer. In short, the stimulus is prefiltered by the peripheral auditory system. The initial stage of information processing of the stimulus also occurs in the periphery and thus places constraints on how finely the system can resolve stimulus detail. Through the use of appropriate psychophysical methods, it is possible to analyze the characteristics of the auditory system's response to the various stimuli of interest, and its ability to resolve differences between them. In the final analysis, some degree of compromise will likely be required in any given stimulus situation, due to practical limitations in the generation of a specific stimulus and limits in the auditory system's ability to respond to the stimulus in the desired manner.

Lastly, the standardization of stimuli for the measurement of auditory brain-stem evoked responses, with respect to both production and calibration, is still awaited. Until standards are available, each individual must decide which stimulus parameters, methods of production, and calibration procedures are to be used. Even if standards are developed and widely adopted, some specific applications may mandate other methodology. These decisions should be facilitated by a basic understanding of the concepts set forth in this chapter.

D. Kent Morest

3 Functional Anatomy of the Auditory System

The purpose of this chapter is to acquaint the reader with the functional anatomy of the peripheral and central auditory system. Primary emphasis is on the afferent auditory system beginning at the cochlea, or end organ, and ending at the primary auditory cortex. This discussion centers on the neural "wiring" diagram, with a brief review of outer and middle ear anatomy. Details of cytoarchitecture and techniques used to study anatomy are not included. Within this framework an attempt is made to provide a working knowledge of the gross auditory structures, pathways, and collateral systems, as well as some physiologic applications (see Chapter 4). This approach should lead to an understanding of the physiologic and neural substrates that have been either demonstrated or implicated as generators or sources (see Chapter 7) of electrocochleographic (ECochG) and brain-stem evoked responses (BSER). For a more complete review of the gross anatomy of the outer and middle ear, consult more extensive treatments, such as those of Bloom and Fawcett (1975) and Polyak (1946).

OUTER AND MIDDLE EAR

The receptors of the inner ear in the petrous portion of the temporal bone relate to two different systems (Fig. 3-1). The vestibular labyrinth serves

The preparation of this chapter was supported in part by Grant R01 NS 14347, awarded by the National Institute of Neurological and Communicative Disorders and Stroke, NIH.

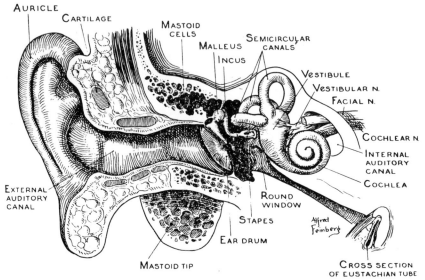

AURICLE
CARTILAGE
MASTOID CELLS
MALLEUS
SEMICIRCULAR CANALS
INCUS
VESTIBULE
VESTIBULAR N.
FACIAL N.
COCHLEAR N.
INTERNAL AUDITORY CANAL
COCHLEA
EXTERNAL AUDITORY CANAL
ROUND WINDOW
STAPES
EAR DRUM
MASTOID TIP
CROSS SECTION OF EUSTACHIAN TUBE
Alfred Feinberg

Figure 3-1. Representation of the human ear. The cochlea has been rotated slightly from its normal position. (Reprinted with permission from Davis, H. (Ed). *Hearing and deafness: A guide for laymen*. New York: Murray Hill Books, 1947.)

as a transducer and proprioceptor for angular and linear acceleration of the head. The cochlea is a distance receptor for sound waves. Airborne sound waves impinge upon the tympanic membrane, which delimits the external canal, or external auditory meatus, from the middle ear. The sound waves set the tympanic membrane in motion. The resulting vibrations are normally conveyed to the cochlea by way of the middle ear bones, or ossicles, which consist of the malleus, incus, and stapes. The head of the malleus inserts on the tympanic membrane, and joints connect the malleus to the incus and the incus to the stapes. The stapes, which has a plunger shape, inserts into one of the openings of the cochlea, the oval window. The cochlea consists of an epithelial duct filled with fluid and suspended within a fluid-filled cavity, the perilymphatic space.

The middle ear ossicles are very important for matching sound waves conveyed through air to the inner ear receptors, which are immersed in a fluid medium. There is great attenuation of sound when energy is transferred from one medium to another, in this case from air to fluid. One could think of the middle ear ossicles as a system of levers, jointed levers, with a very high mechanical advantage that match the impedance (a measure of resistance) of the air medium to that of the cochlear fluids. More simply, one could think of the middle ear ossicles as a kind of amplification system helping to counteract the loss of energy that naturally occurs when sound waves pass from air to fluid. A great deal is known about the transfer function and resonant properties of the middle ear (Guinan and Peake, 1967; see also Chapters 4 and 10 of this book).

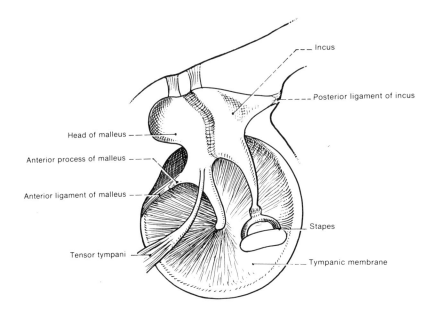

Incus

Posterior ligament of incus

Head of malleus

Anterior process of malleus

Anterior ligament of malleus

Stapes

Tensor tympani

Tympanic membrane

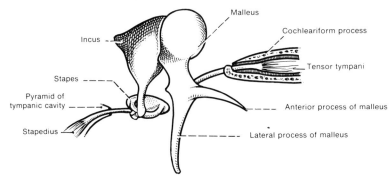

Malleus

Cochleariform process

Incus

Tensor tympani

Stapes

Pyramid of
tympanic cavity

Anterior process of malleus

Stapedius

Lateral process of malleus

Figure 3-2. Drawing of the middle ear muscles and ossicles. Top: medial aspect; bottom: lateral aspect after removing the tympanic membrane. (Reprinted with permission from Bossy, J. *Atlas of neuroanatomy and special sense organs*. Philadelphia: W. B. Saunders, Co., 1970, p. 267.)

There are two muscles in the middle ear that are related to the ossicles: the stapedius and the tensor tympani (Fig. 3-2). The tensor tympani inserts on the malleus, and its action is to tense the tympanic membrane so as to dampen sound vibrations. It is innervated by the motor component of the trigeminal nerve. The stapedius, which inserts on the stapes, is innervated by the motor facial nerve. These are the phylogenetic derivatives of the first and second gill arches. The action of the stapedius muscle is to pull the stapes away from the oval window and thus dampen the vibrations transmitted to the inner ear. The middle ear muscles subserve regulatory reflexes. In the case of high-intensity sounds, for example, they would tend to protect the ear or function as a kind of control mechanism for the CNS to modulate the amplitude of its own input. The dimensions of the vibrations transmitted are minute—fractions of nanometers. If one used an electron microscope to view the stapes vibrating, one might not even see it move. The excursions of the stapes have to be measured using very sophisticated techniques, such as laser interferometry (Törndorf and Khanna, 1968). Molecular dimensions are involved.

INNER EAR

The cochlear duct is an epithelial tube, filled with fluid (the endolymph), in continuity with the vestibular labyrinth (Fig. 3-3). The endolymph is characterized by an elevated potassium ion concentration, compared to blood or cerebrospinal fluid. The tube is suspended within another fluid-filled space, the perilymphatic space. The perilymphatic space in the cochlea is continuous with that of the vestibular labyrinth and contains perilymph, having a composition similar to that of cerebrospinal fluid, with which it can exchange materials in the region of the endolymphatic duct and sac, next to the brain. Thus, there is an intimate relationship between the perilymphatic space of the inner ear and the brain, providing a route for infections to spread.

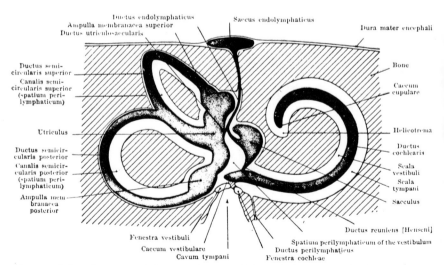

Figure 3-3. Diagram of the membranous labyrinth illustrating the perilymphatic (white) and endolymphatic (black) spaces. The *Fenestra vestibuli* is also called the oval window; the *Fenestra cochleae*, the round window. (Reprinted from Spalteholz, W. *Hand-atlas of human anatomy.* Vol. 3. (5th ed.) Philadelphia: J. B. Lippincott.)

The cochlea responds to sound by causing the footplate of the stapes to vibrate at the oval window, and changes in pressure are transferred to the perilymphatic space. The perilymphatic space is a tube closed at one end by the footplate of the stapes in the oval window and at the other end by the round window. The round window separates the middle ear cavity, containing air, from the perilymphatic space, containing fluid (Fig. 3-3). At the base of the cochlea the oval window opens into the vestibule, from where the scala vestibuli spirals apically for 2½ turns to the heliocotremia and then comes back to the base as the scala tympani, which ends at the membrane of the round window.

The cochlea, although a coiled structure, is essentially a fluid-filled cylinder, with one end closed by the stapes (Fig. 3-4A). Inserting a membrane into the middle of this model cylinder produces a device roughly analogous to the cochlea. The membrane could, for example, represent the cochlear duct. Pressure on the stapes would displace the membrane, but it would stay displaced until the stapes were released. Thus this is not very good for responding to vibrations. A more effective response to vibrations results by making a hole in this membrane, so that pressure can equalize (Fig. 3-4B). Now if the stapes is pressed, the membrane will be initially displaced, but the pressure can be equalized through the hole and the membrane will soon return to its original position. If the stapes vibrated very rapidly, the membrane would flap, because it has a loose end. By extending the cylinder into a long tube containing the membrane, one can make a model of the cochlear duct (Fig. 3-4C). One can even coil it so that it will fit into a relatively small space, but basically it will behave in the same way. The hole is called the helicotrema. The space above the duct represents the scala vestibuli, and the space below, the scala tympani. In the center the cochlear duct forms the cochlear or partition.

Direct observations have been made of the cochlear partition with a variety of techniques, including laser interferometry (Tönndorf and Khanna, 1968), the Mössbauer technique (Johnston and Boyle, 1967; Rhode, 1971), and stroboscopic light (von Békésy, 1953) to show the areas of displacement under a variety of stimulus conditions. When sounds or vibration are applied to the partition, it vibrates in a characteristic manner, much as a sheet might if held at one end and repeatedly jerked at the other end. The resulting constellation of movements could be described as a traveling wave (Fig. 3-5). In other words, the envelope of all the vibrations has a maximum displacement at some particular point along the cochlear duct. The higher the frequency, the nearer the point of maximum displacement is to the base of the cochlea and the stapes. At lower frequencies, the point of maximum displacement travels toward the apex. This phenomenon is a function of the physical properties of the cochlear partition and basilar membrane. One of the most significant structures in the cochlear duct is the basilar membrane, a connective tissue layer with complex elastic and viscous properties. This membrane is stiffer and narrower at the base of the cochlear duct, a feature that may con-

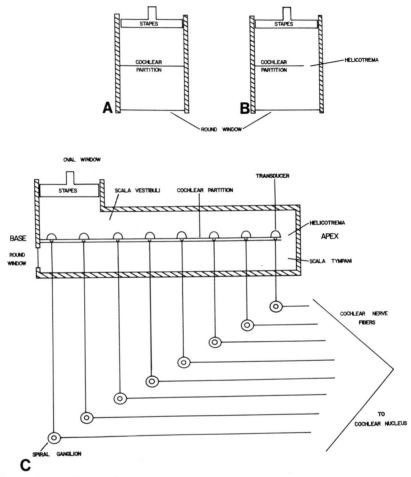

Figure 3-4. Models of the cochlea. A. A fluid-filled cylinder enclosed by a piston on top and a membrane at the bottom. An elastic partition is capable of registering piston displacement. B. Making a hole (helicotrema) in the partition will cause it to flap in response to a displacement of the piston, thus rendering it sensitive to vibrations. C. In a model of the cochlea, the cylinder is extended on one side, while the elastic partition is replaced by the cochlear partition, including the basilar membrane and the organ of Corti. Perturbations are localized on the cochlear partition as a function of stimulus frequency. Localized perturbations of the cochlear partition activate local transducers, which are innervated by a localized portion of the spiral ganglion. The cochlear nerve projects an accurate topographic map of the cochlear receptor surface to the cochlear nucleus in the CNS.

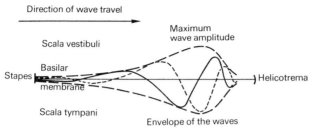

Figure 3-5. A diagram of traveling waves on the basilar membrane in response to a pure tone stimulus. Two individual waves (solid and dashed curves) are shown at two different instants in time. The envelope of all of the possible individual waves corresponds to the maximum wave amplitude occurring at each point along the basilar membrane. (Reprinted with permission from Klinke, R. Physiology of hearing. In Schmidt, R. F. (Ed.). *Fundamentals of Sensory Physiology*. Heidelberg: Springer-Verlag, 1978, p. 180.)

tribute to frequency analysis. Thus the cochlea can function as a frequency analyzer by localizing the place of maximum displacement. To translate this information into electrical signals one needs receptor cells on the basilar membrane (Fig. 3-4). Cochlear nerve fibers that innervate the hair cells can carry information about frequency to the CNS as a function of the place of maximum displacement (place principle). However, fiber discharge rate will also vary with frequency up to 3 kHz (so-called phase-locking or temporal principle).

Figure 3-6 is a cross-sectional drawing of the internal structure of the cochlear duct. On the basilar membrane is an epithelial lining, consisting of receptor hair cells and several varieties of supporting cells (phalangeal, pillar, Hensen's, Claudius', and Böettcher's cells), which together make up the organ of Corti. The supporting cells hold the receptor cells in position and help to maintain the ionic composition of the endolymph, with its characteristic high potassium ion concentration. The hair cells are responsible for the transduction of mechanical energy into electrical potentials. The so-called hairs, or stereocilia, are essentially microvilli that extend from the apices of the hair cell. There are many hairs set in rows on the surface of each cell. There are two types of hair cells: the outer hair cells, which are arranged in three or more rows, and the inner hair cells, which are confined to one row. The stereocilia of the hair cells protrude from the surface of the organ of Corti toward a ribbon-shaped structure above, the tectorial membrane. The tectorial membrane, or cuticle, is an acellular structure. It is a rather stiff structure, attached at one end to the spinal limbus (Fig. 3-6, top). When the basilar membrane vibrates, hairs of the cells bend against the tectorial membrane or are perturbed by fluid displacement. This is thought to produce the transduc-

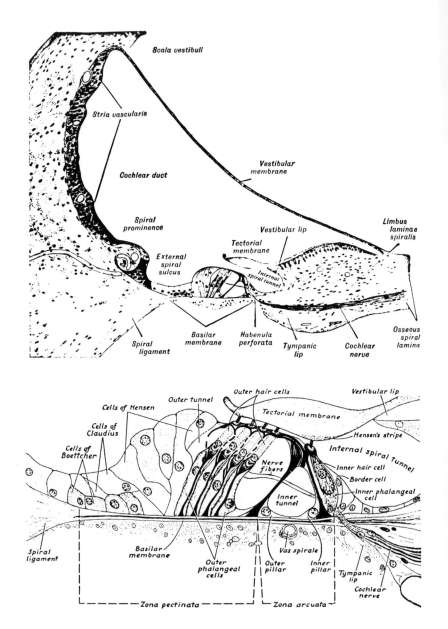

Figure 3-6. Top. Radial transection through the cochlear duct of the basal turn of a human cochlea. The separation of the free end of the tectorial membrane from the organ of Corti is artifactual. Bottom. Radial transection of the organ of Corti from the basal turn of a human cochlea. (Reprinted with permission from Bloom, W., & Fawcett, D. W. *A textbook of histology* (8th ed.). Philadelphia: W. B. Saunders, 1962.)

tion that leads to the generation of receptor potentials in hair cells. It is not known exactly how this happens, but perhaps the bending of the hairs distorts the surface membrane so as to change its ionic permeability. In any case, the electrical potentials generated in the hair cells ultimately result in the release of a chemical transmitter that produces action potentials in the nerve fibers innervating the hair cells.

There are at least two types of nerve fibers that innervate the hair cells. One type innervates the outer hair cells, crossing the organ of Corti through a tunnel that separates the inner from the outer hair cells. When they reach the outer hair cells, the fibers then turn and run lengthwise toward the base and send off small branches that synapse on the bases of the hair cells. These branches are called spiral fibers because they run lengthwise in the cochlea, which, of course, is a spiral structure. One outer spiral fiber can innervate many outer hair cells. The inner hair cells, on the other hand, have a different kind of innervation. A separate set of ganglion cells sends radial fibers to the inner hair cells. A number of these fibers converge on a single hair cell. Inner and outer hair cells differ morphologically as much as rod and cone cells in the retina differ—they presumably also have different functions. It is known that the greater the intensity of stimulation, the larger the number of hair cells excited and the greater the number of cochlear nerve fibers firing, and the higher the rate of firing for individual fibers. Thus, information about stimulus frequency and amplitude is conveyed to the CNS by cochlear nerve discharge patterns.

Two types of nerve endings contact the bases of the hair cells: (1) the afferent nerve fibers of the spiral ganglion cells and (2) the endings from efferent fibers which have their cell bodies in the superior olivary complex of the CNS and feed back upon the hair cells. These neurons form the olivocochlear tracts. The efferent fiber is inhibitory to the hair cell and may provide a method by which the CNS controls the sensitivity of the receptor. Several olivocochlear neurons synapse on the radial afferent fibers, innervating inner hair cells. Some of these efferent olivocochlear axons run lengthwise in the cochlea, forming the inner spiral and tunnel spiral bundles.

COCHLEAR NERVE AND NUCLEUS

Information is brought to the brain by cochlear nerve fibers (Figs. 3-4, 3-7, and 3-8). The bipolar cell bodies of these fibers are located in the spiral ganglion of the middle of the cochlear axons (Figs. 3-4C, 3-6). When the cochlear nerve root enters the cochlear nucleus (CN) in the medulla, it forms ascending and descending branches, or roots (Fig. 3-8). Many of the axons branch into ascending and descending collaterals, which synapse in different parts of the CN. There are three cochlear nuclei: dorsal, posteroventral, and anteroventral, each with several subdivisions.

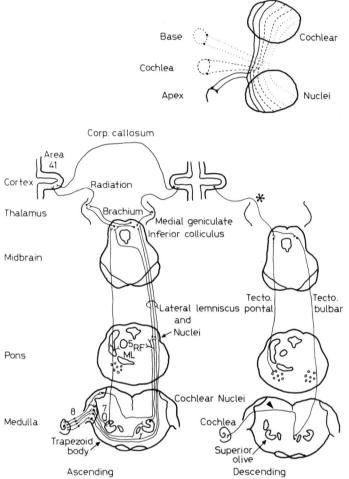

Figure 3-7. Top. Scheme of the tonotopic organization of the dorsal and ventral cochlear nuclei. Cochlear nerve fibers establish an orderly correspondence of successively more apical regions of the cochlea with progressively more ventrolateral sectors in each part of the cochlear nucleus. Bottom. The main ascending and descending pathways of the central auditory system. Key: corticotectal tract (*); crossed olivocochlear tract (*arrowhead*); medial lemniscus (*ML*); reticular formation (*RF*); motor trigeminal nucleus (*5*); motor facial nucleus (*7*); spiral ganglion (*8*). (Reprinted with permission from Morest, D. K. Structural organization of the auditory pathways. In Tower (Ed.), *The Nervous System*. New York: Raven Press, 1975, p. 20.)

There is an orderly arrangement of the cochlear nerve fibers in the cochlear nucleus (Fig. 3-7, top). What is the significance of this order? The location of the nerve fibers in the sequence depends upon where they arise within the cochlea. The neurons that innervate the apical turn of the cochlea project to one side of the CN, neurons that innervate the basal turn of the cochlea

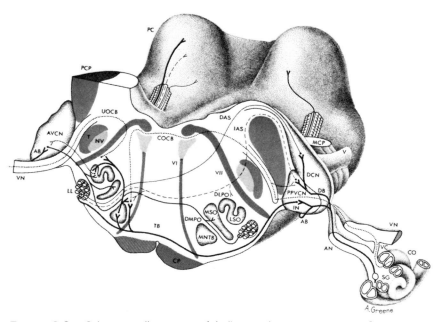

Figure 3-8. Schematic illustration of bulbar auditory connections. In a wiring diagram such as this, the cochlear nerve is represented by a single channel, although the existence of two populations of spiral ganglion cells innervating inner and outer hair cells separately adds another consideration in interpreting central processes. Key: ascending branch of cochlear nerve (*AB*); cochlear (auditory) nerve (*AN*); anteroventral cochlear nucleus (*AVCN*); cochlea (*CO*); crossed olivocochlear bundle (*COCB*); cerebral peduncle (*CP*); dorsal acoustic stria (*DAS*); descending branch (*DB*) of cochlear nerve; dorsal cochlear nucleus (*DCN*); dorsal periolivary region (*DLPO*); dorsomedial periolivary nucleus (*DMPO*); intermediate acoustic stria (*IAS*); posteroventral AVCN (interstitial nucleus) (*IN*); lateral lemniscus (*LL*); lateral superior olive (*LSO*); middle cerebellar peduncle (*MCP*); medial trapezoid nucleus (*MNTB*); medial superior olive (*MSO*); inferior colliculus (*PC*); posterior cerebellar peduncle (*PCP*); posteroventral cochlear nucleus (*PPVCN*); spiral ganglion (*SG*); trapezoid body (*TB*); descending trigeminal tract and nucleus (*T, NV*); uncrossed olivocochlear bundle (*UOCB*); vestibulocochlear (*VC*) anastomosis (Oort); vestibular nerve (*VN*); abducens nerve root and nucleus (*VI*); facial nerve root (*VII*). (Reprinted with permission from Morest, D. K. Structural organization of the auditory pathways. In Tower (Ed.), *The Nervous System*. New York: Raven Press, 1975, p. 22.)

project to the other side, while nerve fibers that innervate the middle turn project to the middle of that sequence. Thus, an orderly mapping of the receptor surface of the cochlea spans the CN. This illustrates a principle of topographic organization, i.e., the orderly spatial representation in the CNS of peripheral receptor surfaces. In the auditory system, this topographical map is the tonotopic organization, or frequency map of the auditory pathways. The basal turn of the cochlea represents high frequencies and successively more apical regions correspond to progressively lower frequencies. In other words, the

CN has a frequency map of the cochlea. The auditory system thus preserves the frequency analysis of the cochlea, and it does so at all levels of the auditory system (see Chapter 4). The ascending pathways throughout the central auditory system are tonotopically organized according to the same principle—by an orderly spatial arrangement of afferent axons.

ASCENDING AUDITORY SYSTEM

The second-order neurons of the auditory pathways are located in the CN in the medulla oblongata. The second-order auditory axons cross the midline at the base of the pons in the trapezoid body (TB), enter the lateral lemniscus (LL), and ascend to the midbrain (Fig. 3-7, bottom). The lateral lemniscus is analogous to the other lemnisci of the somatic sensory system, e.g., the medial lemniscus, which contain second-order crossed axons. Many of the LL axons synapse in the inferior colliculus (IC). The IC is the auditory part of the caudal midbrain tectum and contains the third-order neurons in this chain. The third-order axons project through the brachium of the IC to the medial geniculate body (MGB), which is the auditory part of the thalamus, just as the lateral geniculate body is the visual part of the thalamus (see Chapter 14). The role of the thalamus is to relay different ascending pathways to the appropriate parts of the cerebral cortex. The MGB projects through the auditory radiation, or thalamocortical tract, to the auditory cortex. The auditory cortex is in the superior temporal gyrus of the temporal lobe, forming a transverse horizontal ridge, the transverse gyrus of Heschl (Brodmann's area 41).

The main ascending pathways represent the shortest route by which auditory signals can travel from the cochlea to the auditory cortex. Compared to most other sensory systems, it is a relatively long route, especially as related to the number of synapses that occur in the cochlea, the medulla, midbrain, thalamus, and auditory cortex. Since it is such a long pathway, it offers great potential for clinical neurology, i.e., the opportunity to localize lesions at various levels of the brain stem. It has been difficult, however, to study the function of the central auditory pathways. With the development of methods for surface-recorded potentials and audiological testing for CNS function, it has become possible to use the auditory system to localize pathology in the central pathways while gaining insight into their function (see Chapters 10-13).

INTERCALATED NUCLEI

The auditory system would be a relatively simple pathway if there were not a number of other nuclei intercalated within the TB as the superior olivary complex (SOC) and within the LL as the nuclei of the LL. For example, Figure 3-7 shows a tract that projects from the CN to the SOC; a neuron in the SOC projects to the nucleus of the LL, and that one in turn projects to the IC. Thus, there is a multisynaptic pathway running through these intercalated nuclei. The result is that any train of activity in the CN will produce a complex array of signals which are modified and dispersed in time when they reach the IC. This is one reason why it is difficult to assign individual waves of the BSER to specific structures. It is this complex array of synaptic interruptions, however, that provides an increase in the integrative capacity of the system. In this respect, the auditory system seems to have a greater integrative capacity than some of the other sensory systems. This, very likely, is related to the complex analyses of different aspects of sounds during acoustic communication—not only frequency and amplitude, but also timing, duration, onset, and offset patterns and rhythms. The intercalated nuclei increase the integrative capacity of the brain stem auditory system for several different functions.

One integrative function relates to reflexes. For example, the tensor tympani and stapedius muscles in the middle ear can attenuate the acoustic input to the cochlea. These muscles are innervated by the trigeminal and facial nerves, respectively. Thus, information from the auditory system has to reach the motor trigeminal and facial nuclei (Fig. 3-7). This pathway probably has bilateral connections within the SOC and interneurons in the reticular formation. There are other more complicated reflexes, such as the startle reflex. If an individual is startled by a noise, the head and eyes turn toward the source of the sound, the pupils dilate, the body assumes a position ready to flee in the opposite direction, the eyes blink, the heart beats faster, and there may be vocalization and fear. These are only some of the many changes in bodily functions during startle.

How does the CNS bring about these complicated adjustments? The reticular formation is probably involved in conveying information from the auditory system to a number of cranial nerve and motor nuclei—the ventral horns of the spinal cord to position the body and to the autonomic centers that control pupil size, increase heart rate, regulate functions in the medulla, etc. The startle surely depends on neurons in the reticular formation that are located throughout the brain stem between the main sensory and motor nuclei. They have axonal branches projecting to different motor and sensory nuclei. Intercalated nuclei and the IC, which connect with the reticular formation, may also be involved. Insofar as conscious perception contributes to the startle response, the cerebral cortex and the corticoreticular tract are also required.

The arrangement of the intercalated nuclei also provides for binaural fusion and interaction. In these functions information from both ears must be integrated by the same cells and at different levels of the system. The opportunity for this results from the following anatomical fact. There are a number of secondary auditory neurons in the CN, perhaps one-third of them, that do not cross in the TB but project to the ipsilateral SOC (Fig. 3-7). These neurons provide a route by which information from the ear can reach the same side of the brain and the ipsilateral cerebral cortex. In other words, there is a bilateral representation in the auditory system. Consequently, it is unusual for higher CNS lesions to produce total deafness. Destruction of the auditory cortex on one side, however, may result in some contralateral hearing loss since most of the pathway crosses in the TB. Also, there is a commissure of the IC and another one for the auditory cortex (corpus callosum). The commissures not only provide bilateral connections and binaural interactions, but also binaural fusion and a continuous representation of auditory space.

Auditory information has to travel from both sides of the auditory system to the same place, to the very same cells, if there is to be an integration of the acoustic environment. One place where this occurs is the medial superior olive (MSO) of the SOC (Fig. 3-8). Symmetrical sets of neurons in the CN send axons to the MSO on both sides of the TB. The MSO has a special arrangement of its neurons: bipolar dendrites extend to either side outwardly like antennae. The CN neurons of the left side project to the left-hand dendrites of the left MSO and to the left-hand dendrites of the right superior olive. The CN neurons of the right side have a symmetrical, complementary relationship to the right-hand dendrites of the MSO. In this way the axons from the two sides converge on opposite ends of the very same neurons. Thus the inputs from the two sides can interact. For example, some neurons may have an inhibitory input from one side and an excitatory input from the other side. The interaction of the two inputs may affect the neuronal discharge rate, depending on timing and intensity differences between the two sides. If the inhibitory input arrives first, the neuron is not as responsive to the excitatory input. On the other hand, if the excitatory input arrives first, the MSO neuron can fire vigorously and send a strong signal to higher levels. This type of analysis is probably related to sound lateralization.

DESCENDING AUDITORY SYSTEM

Some neurons of the SOC send axons to the cochlea that synapse on hair cells or on sensory fibers innervating hair cells. These neurons are the crossed and uncrossed olivocochlear tracts, and they have an inhibitory influence on the cochlea. There is a whole series of descending pathways known as the descending auditory system (Fig. 3-7, bottom right). It runs parallel to the ascending pathways but begins in the auditory cortex, projects to the IC, and is relayed to nuclei in the pons and the medulla. Several nuclei of the SOC form the olivocochlear tracts, which send axons to hair cells. Thus the olivocochlear tracts appear to be the last link in a descending system. The auditory system has to function over a tremendous range of stimulus energies. It might operate more efficiently if the brain could set the gain for the system appropriate to different stimulus intensities or other physiologic conditions. It may well be that the olivocochlear tracts provide a basis for automatic gain control or other regulatory functions.

IMPLICATIONS FOR BSER

A number of structural features could be expected to provide an anatomic basis for generation of the BSER. Detection of such responses at the surface of the head would require that a large number of individual neurons fire in synchrony. The most likely place for this is the cochlear nerve. In the CNS, fiber tracts are less likely to discharge with the necessary degree of synchrony, since they all consist of mixtures of second, third, fourth, or higher order pathways (Figs. 3-7 and 3-8), including the TB, LL, brachium of the IC, and auditory radiation. An exception to this might be the dorsal acoustic stria, which consists mostly of the axons of fusiform and giant cells projecting to the IC from the dorsal CN (Fig. 3-8, DAS). The fibers of the dorsal acoustic stria, however, spread out in a fanlike arrangement as they sweep across the medulla and therefore may be less effective in providing a concentrated source of potentials for detection at a distance.

Since relatively larger potentials could be generated in the regions containing nerve cell bodies and synapses, the most likely sources are the auditory nuclei containing the largest numbers of cells, such as the CN, SOC, nuclei of the LL, IC, and MGB. The intercalated nuclei are in a region where large numbers of fibers and cells intermingle. One special arrangement of neurons favoring surface detection is that in which a dipole generator might appear. Such an arrangement is seen in the MSO, where inputs from both sides of the auditory system converge on a single layer of neurons. Depth recordings have shown a strong dipole generator in this nucleus (see Chapter 7). The number of neurons located here, however, is relatively small compared to the cell groups ordinarily considered as possible generators of the BSER. Other cell groups where binaural convergence may play a role in the generation of BSER occur in the LL, IC, and MGB. In these regions the lack of an obvious geometrical basis of cellular arrangement for dipole generators may be overcome by the very large numbers of cells involved. Particularly overlooked in this regard are the nuclei of the LL, which probably provide the largest input to the IC. Recent evidence that these nuclei may make a major contribution to the BSER has been provided by Møller and Janetta (1982).

Another factor that should be considered in the generation of a synchronized discharge of sufficient magnitude for a BSER is the size of the neurons and their fibers. Not only do larger cells generate larger potentials, as a rule, but their fibers tend to be thicker. The thicker fibers have faster conduction velocities and thus could provide for the generation of larger responses at minimum latencies. Information about large-fiber pathways, as distinct from small-fiber systems, is lacking. One example of a large-fiber projection in the dorsal CN is that of the fusiform and giant cells which project to the IC via the dorsal acoustic stria (Brawer, Morest, and Kane, 1974). Another example is provided by the bushy cells of the interstitial nucleus of the CN complex. These neurons have the thickest fibers in the CNS, and they project through the TB to the contralateral nucleus of the TB (Fig. 3-8) (Tolbert, Morest, and Yurgelun-Todd, in press).

Finally, at all levels of the auditory pathways there are specific morphological types of neurons, which differ in the arrangement of their synaptic connections and in their electrophysiologic response properties (Morest, 1975b). It is likely that the processing of acoustic information by the central auditory nervous system depends on the organization of these different types of neurons (Morest, Kiang, and Kane, et al., 1973; Morest, 1975a). Unfortunately, it is not clear how these specific populations of neurons contribute to the BSER (see Chapter 4). When this is clarified, it may be possible to use the BSER as a more powerful investigative tool. Meanwhile, as our understanding of the anatomical sources of the BSER progresses, it will become an even more useful diagnostic device.

Chiyeko Tsuchitani

4 Physiology of the Auditory System

There are at least three types of neuroelectric phenomena represented in the auditory brain-stem evoked response (BSER) or potential recorded from the head surface: the receptor potential, the somatodendritic field potential, and the spike potential. This chapter will examine the possible contributions of single-unit spike potentials to the auditory BSER. To avoid conflicting or confusing results related to species differences, this review will concentrate upon single-unit data from the cat, as it is the most commonly studied species. Neuroanatomical differences between the cat and human auditory systems will be described where applicable.

We see in the previous chapter that the auditory system is an information-processing system that can be subdivided into subsystems or functional components (Fig. 4-1). The peripheral auditory system includes the mechanical stages of the outer, middle, and inner ears, the transducer or receptor elements, and the first-order afferents of the auditory nervous system. The central auditory system consists of various tracts and cell groups located within the central nervous system. As it is the objective of this chapter to describe the neurophysiology of the auditory system, the functions of the mechanical and transducer stages will not be described in any detail.

In brief, the acoustic input to the ear is acoustically and mechanically transferred through the outer- and middle-ears, respectively, and is applied to

The preparation of this chapter was supported in part by grant R01 NS11218-07 from the National Institute of Neurological and Communicative Disorders and Stroke. The assistance of Gary Hazelwood and Gail Denny in preparing this manuscript is greatly appreciated.

67

Chiyeko Tsuchitani

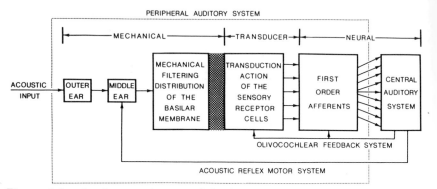

Figure 4-1. A schematic drawing of the functional components of the auditory system. (Redrawn from Weiss, T. J. A model of the peripheral auditory system. *Kybernetik*, 1966, 3:153-175.)

the inner ear in the form of stapes footplate displacement at the oval window. The pressure applied to the cochlear fluid by the movement of the stapes footplate results in a longitudinal wave of displacement of the basilar membrane that travels from the cochlea base towards the apex. Within the inner ear, the spectral components of the acoustic signal are analyzed and spatially represented along the basilar membrane. At the base of the cochlea, the basilar membrane vibrates maximally to high-frequency energy; at the apex, it vibrates maximally to low frequencies. The two basic characteristics of an

---

Figure 4-2. Schematic diagram of the principal ascending connections of the auditory system indicating the flow of acoustic information originating from the left ear. Solid lines, major input into the structure; dotted lines, minor input or size of input unknown; ?, evidence for input incomplete. Key: *receptor cells:* inner hair cells (IHC), outer hair cells (OHC). *First-order afferents:* auditory nerve (AN), spiral ganglion cells (SGC)—type I spiral ganglion cell (SGC-1), type II spiral ganglion cell (SGC-2). *Cochlear nuclear complex (CNC):* anteroventral cochlear nucleus (AVCN)—large spherical cell area (LSCA), small spherical cell area (SSCA), multipolar cell area (MCA), globular cell area (GCA); posteroventral cochlear nucleus (PVCN)—multipolar cell area (MCA), octopus cell area (OCA); dorsal cochlear nucleus (DCN)—granular cell layer (GCL), pyramidal cell layer (PCL), central nucleus (CN). *Superior olivary complex (SOC):* main olivary nuclei—medial superior olive (MSO), lateral superior olive (LSO), dorsal hilus of LSO (DH-LSO); nuclei of the trapezoid body (NTB)—medial nucleus (M), ventral nucleus (V), lateral nucleus (L); periolivary nuclei (PO)—anterolateral (AL), dorsomedial (DM), dorsolateral (DL), posterior (P), posteroventral (PV), ventromedial (VM), ventrolateral (VL). *Nuclei of the lateral lemniscus (NLL):* dorsal nucleus of the lateral lemniscus (DNLL), ventral nucleus of the lateral lemniscus (VNLL)—ventral (V), medial (M), dorsal (D), posteromedial (PM), dorsomedial (DM). *Inferior colliculus (IC):* central nucleus (CN), internuclear zone (IZ), external zone (EZ). *Medial geniculate body (MGB):* dorsal division (D), medial division (M), ventral division (V). *Principal auditory cortex (AC):* primary area (AI), secondary area (AII), posterior ectosylvian gyrus (EP).

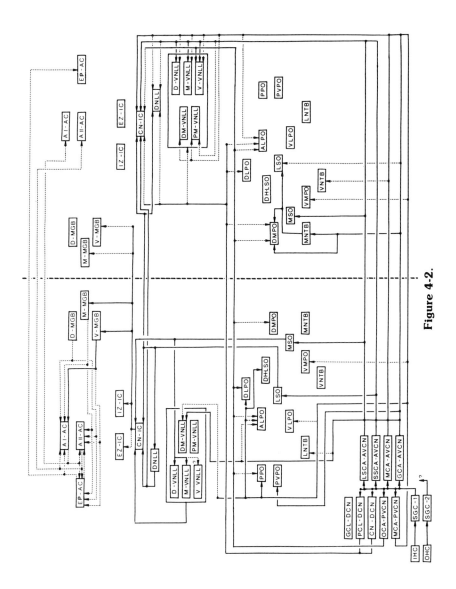

Figure 4-2.

69

acoustic stimulus, *frequency* and *amplitude*, are represented by the place of maximal vibration or location and the amplitude and spread of vibration along the basilar membrane. The displacement of the basilar membrane is assumed to result in the transfer of mechanical energy to the receptor cells. The receptor cells, in turn, transduce the applied mechanical energy into a form capable of exciting the auditory neurons which innervate them. The spectral properties of the acoustic stimulus are represented by the location and number of the receptor/first-order afferents activated and by the magnitude and time course of the elicited activity. Within each auditory neural structure, the stimulus also appears to be represented spatially in terms of the distribution of activity within the structure, and temporally, in the discharge patterns of the neural elements forming the structure.

As illustrated in Figure 4-2, the structure of the auditory nervous system is extremely complex even at levels as low as the cochlear nuclear complex. The structural complexity of this system, however, may reflect a simplification of its functional properties through its subdivision into specialized subsystems. For example, separate anatomic pathways exist for acoustic motor reflex systems, acoustic neural feedback systems, and ascending auditory systems (see Chapter 3). Anatomic studies have suggested the existence of a multiplicity of auditory pathways; neurophysiologic studies have also indicated that the auditory system consists of differentiated neurons, with different response characteristics. The correlation of neuroanatomic descriptions of neuron types and their connections with neurophysiologic data provide an indication of the functional properties of neurons within these separate anatomic pathways. The relative contributions of these different functional neuron groups to the BSER have not been fully described. It is highly probable, however, that not all neurons contribute equally to the BSER.

One approach to determining the contribution of neuron spike potentials to the BSER is the correlation of the temporal sequence of single-unit spike activity with the waveform of the auditory BSER (Antoli-Candela and Kiang, 1978). If the temporal sequence of spike activity corresponds with certain peaks in the auditory BSER, one might assume that neurons generating these spikes are responsible for producing the correlated peaks in the auditory BSER. Provided such an assumption is correct, the structures generating various components of the BSER may be identified and thus may provide an aid in the localization of auditory nervous system pathologies on the basis of alterations in the auditory BSER (see Chapters 10, 11, 12).

Assuming that certain peaks in the auditory BSER represent summed spike potentials (or gross potentials), the contribution of the individual spike potentials to the BSER would depend upon numerous factors. The amplitude of the BSER recorded from the head surface depends upon two factors: the distance and the electrical impedance between the spike generator and the electrode. The amplitude of a BSER resulting from the addition of individual spike potentials will depend upon the degree of similarity between the wave-forms of the individual potentials. The waveform of axon spike potentials, although smaller than the somatic spike, appears to be more uniform in shape, with small differences associated with axon diameter and myelin thickness. Given similar spike potential waveforms, the greater the degree of synchrony in the occurrence of the individual spike potentials of the activated units, the larger the amplitude of the summed potential.

Working with the hypothesis that certain components of the auditory BSER represent the summation of synchronized spike potentials, the responses of single auditory units will be examined, with special emphasis on describing unit characteristics that may be predictive of their ability to produce synchronized discharges to acoustic stimuli.

RESPONSE MEASURES

The measures commonly utilized to describe the response characteristics of single auditory units include the tuning curve, the intensity function, latency of response, post-stimulus onset time (PST) histogram, and period or post-zero crossing time (PZT) histogram. The *tuning curve* is a plot of the stimulus level required to elicit a threshold response as a function of stimulus frequency (Fig. 4-3). The characteristic frequency (CF) is the stimulus frequency to which a unit is most sensitive. The bandwidth of the frequencies capable of eliciting a response at a given stimulus level is often used to describe the tuning characteristics of an auditory unit. The *intensity function* is a plot of response output as a function of the stimulus level (Fig. 4-4). A monotonic intensity function is characterized by increases in the output with increases in stimulus level, up to some maximum value which is maintained with further increases in stimulus level. A systematic decline in the output with increases in stimulus level above that eliciting the maximum output describes the nonmonotonic intensity function. The dynamic range of the intensity function is the range of stimulus levels over which the response increases. The *latency* of the response is measured as the time elapsed from stimulus onset to the instant at which the first spike is elicited. The temporal pattern of spike discharges elicited by repetitive presentation of a stimulus is represented in the *PST histogram* (Fig. 4-5), which illustrates the time of occurrence of a spike relative to stimulus onset time. The PST histograms of discharges to short tone bursts of duration less than 300 msec will be called STB-PST histograms, while those produced by discharges to click stimuli will be referred to as click PST histograms. The *PZT histograms* illustrate the synchronization or phase-locking of spike discharges with the individual cycles of a low-frequency stimulus (Fig. 4-6). The time of occurrence of a spike potential is indicated as the time elapsed since the last negative zero-crossing of the sinusoidal stimulus.

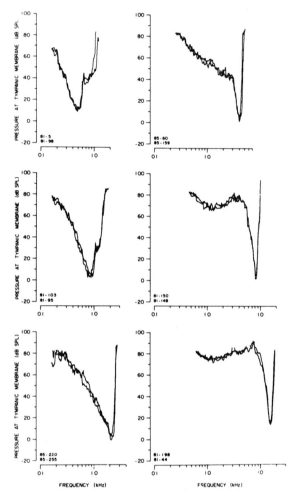

Figure 4-3. Examples of AN unit tuning curves. Tuning curves of two AN units with similar CFs are contained in each graph. The stimulus level required to elicit a discharge above the spontaneous rate is plotted as a function of stimulus frequency. Tone burst stimuli: 50 msec duration, 2.5 msec rise-fall times, and repetition rate of 10/sec. Abscissa, frequency in kHz; ordinate, threshold stimulus level in dB re 2×10^{-4} dynes/sq cm. (Reprinted with permission from Liberman, M. C. & Kiang, N. Y.-S. Acoustic trauma in cats: Cochlear pathology and auditory-nerve activity. *Acta Oto-Laryngologica* (Stockholm), 1978, *358*:1-63.)

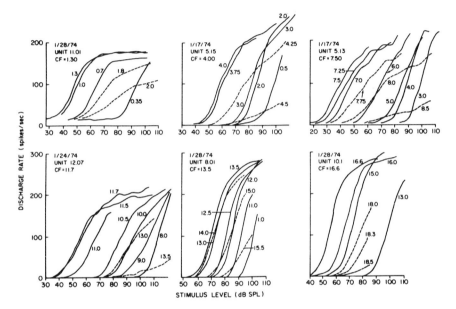

Figure 4-4. The intensity functions of AN units to tone bursts at unit CF and at lower (solid curves) and higher (dashed curves) frequencies. The intensity functions are illustrated for six units from three cats. The frequency of the tone is indicated next to each function in kHz. Tone burst stimuli: 400 msec duration, repetition rate 1/1.5 sec. Abscissa, stimulus level in dB re 2 × 10^{-4} dynes/sq cm; ordinate, discharge rate in spikes/sec. (Reprinted with permission from Sachs, M. B., & Abbas, R. J. Rate versus level functions for auditory-nerve fibers in cats: Tone burst stimuli. *Journal of the Acoustical Society of America*, 1974, *56*: 1835-1847.)

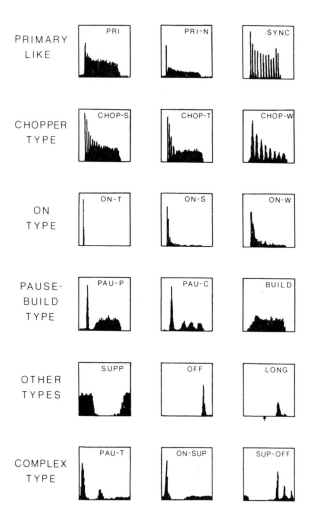

Figure 4-5. Illustrations of the types of post-stimulus onset time (PST) histograms produced by auditory neurons to short tone burst stimuli. See text for explanation of histogram classification scheme. Top 5 rows. Tone burst stimuli: 25 msec duration, 2.5 msec rise-fall times, repetition rate between 1/sec and 1/3 sec. Histogram: Bin width 0.2 msec; total analysis time 40 msec, with the exception of LONG, in which total analysis time is 80 msec, with the arrow indicating stimulus termination. Bottom row. Tone burst stimuli: 250 msec duration, 2.5 msec rise-fall times, repetition rate between 1/sec and 1/3 sec. Histogram: Bin width 2.5 msec; total analysis time 500 msec. Abscissa, the time after the onset of the electrical stimulus at the earphone; ordinate, number of spikes occurring at a particular time.

UNIT   M92   CF (kHz)

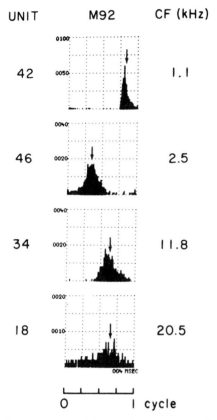

42   I. I

46   2.5

34   I I.8

I8   20.5

O   I cycle

Figure 4-6. Examples of the post-zero crossing time (PZT) histograms for four AN units to a 250 Hz tone. Zero time in each histogram is the time of the negative zero crossing of the pressure waveform at the tympanic membrane. The arrow indicates the calculated response phase. The unit identification number (left) and the unit CF (right) is indicated next to each histogram. Continuous tone stimulus: 10 sec duration, stimulus level at 83 dB-SPL. Histogram: Bin width, 20 μsec. Absicissa, the time and phase after negative zero crossing; ordinate, number of spikes produced at each particular time or phase. (Reprinted with permission from Kiang, N.Y.-S., & Moxon, E. C. Tails of tuning curves of auditory-nerve fibers. *Journal of the Acoustical Society of America*, 1974, 55:620-630.)

75

NEUROPHYSIOLOGY OF THE PERIPHERAL
AUDITORY SYSTEM

The Receptor Cell

Little information is available concerning the response characteristics of
mammalian auditory receptor cells. Single-unit intracellular recording and
marking studies of the organ of Corti in the lizard have demonstrated that
both the auditory receptor cells and the surrounding supporting cells produce
graded, analog potentials to acoustic stimuli and no spike potentials (Mulroy,
Altmann, and Weiss, et al., 1974). The potentials consist of a sustained DC
component and an oscillating AC component that resemble the gross summating potential and cochlear microphonic, respectively. According to
Russell and Sellick (1978), acoustically-evoked intracelluluar DC potentials
can be recorded from guinea pig inner hair cells identified by dye injection.
Both the AC and DC potentials could also be recorded from guinea pig cochlear units identified as "inner hair cells" on the basis of the amplitude of the
DC potentials generated to acoustic stimuli. It is probable that the cochlear
microphonic recorded with gross electrodes placed on outer- and middle-ear
structures represent, in part, the summed receptor cell, and possibly the supporting cell, AC potentials.

The First-Order Afferents

The first-order afferents of the auditory system are the spiral ganglion
cells whose central processes form the auditory branch of the VIIIth cranial
nerve. Auditory nerve (AN) units discharge spontaneously in the absence of
an experimenter-controlled stimulus. Since these discharges occur while the
animal is placed in a sound isolation chamber, it is assumed that the activity is
not acoustically driven (Kiang, Watanabe, and Thomas, et al., 1965). AN
units respond to acoustic stimuli of the proper frequency and level with an increase in discharge above the spontaneous rate. As described in anatomical
studies (Sando, 1965), AN units are arranged in a spiral manner with high-
CF units located external to the inner core of low-CF units. Most AN units exhibit narrowly distributed CF thresholds (between 10 and 25 dB of one
another, for units with similar CFs (Liberman and Kiang, 1978)). Although
cat AN units with CF between 1 and 15 kHz exhibit the lowest CF thresholds,
many with CF between 2 and 4 kHz have slightly higher thresholds.

The shapes of the AN tuning curves depend upon unit CF (Kiang, Liberman, and Baer, 1977). Those of high-CF units are characterized by a sharply
tuned, V-shaped "tip" region and a more broadly tuned, low frequency "tail"
segment (Fig. 4-3). The tuning curves of low-CF units may exhibit "tails" on
both the low and high sides of the tuning curve "tip." For units with CF above
2 kHz, tuning curve bandwidth is related to unit CF; high-CF units have the

widest tuning curves. The bandwidth of an AN tuning curve increases with stimulus level; typically, with the greatest spread in the low-frequency direction. As a consequence, as the stimulus level of a pure tone is increased, more units with CF greater than the stimulus frequency are activated as the stimulus exceeds the thresholds of their low frequency "tail" segments. The resulting distribution of the CFs of the responding units will be asymmetrical with respect to the stimulus frequency. This, among other factors, makes it difficult to obtain high-intensity frequency-specific audiograms using BSER (see Chapters 1, 9).

The vast majority of AN units produce monotonic intensity functions with dynamic range between 20 and 30 dB to tone burst and continuous tone stimuli (Fig. 4-4). For AN units with CF above 4 kHz, the maximum rate elicited with a CF tone increases with increasing CF (Liberman, 1978). The maximum discharge elicited from an AN unit is less to tones with frequency above the unit CF and is equal to or greater than that obtained at unit CF when the frequency is below CF (Sachs and Abbas, 1974). Increasing the stimulus level of a pure tone not only results in the activation of a greater proportion of units with CF above the stimulus frequency, it also elicits higher discharge rates from these units than from units with CF below the stimulus frequency.

The discharges of AN units to tones of frequency greater than 5 kHz appear to be irregular in temporal pattern (Fig. 4-5, Pri) and therefore asynchronous with one another. The discharges of AN units to tones of 5 kHz or less tend to be synchronized or locked to a particular phase (the response phase) of the sinusoid (Fig. 4-5, Sync). All AN units respond with phase-locked discharges to low-frequency stimuli of sufficient intensity (Fig. 4-6). Because of their tuning characteristics, the thresholds of high-CF units to low-frequency tones will be considerably higher than those of low-CF units tuned to the stimulus. The discharges of units with CF above 8 to 10 kHz tend to occur at the same response phase, whereas the response phase of AN units with lower CF depend upon the unit CF. As a consequence, while all AN units may be discharging in synchrony with an intense low-frequency tone, only those units with CF above 8 to 10 kHz will be discharging in synchrony with each other. The threshold level required to produce a phase-locked response is 10 to 20 dB below that required to produce a rate increase above spontaneous levels (Johnson, 1974). The degree of phase-locking increases as stimulus level is increased up to 10 to 30 dB above the phase-locking threshold.

The click-elicited discharges of AN units consist of one or more spikes that occur at preferred times, with respect to the click stimulus (Fig. 4-7). The discharges of units with CF above 3 to 4 kHz tend to occur in synchrony with similar latencies, regardless of unit CF. At most click levels, the latencies of units with CF below 3 to 4 kHz are progressively longer than units with higher CF. The systematic increase in latency with decreasing CF is believed to re-

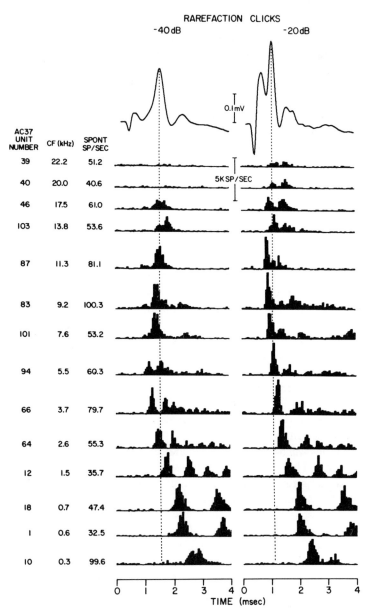

Figure 4-7. The PST histograms of 14 AN units from one cat to rarefaction clicks at two stimulus levels. The unit identification number, unit CF, and spontaneous activity rates are indicated to the left of each histogram. The gross round window responses for the two click levels are illustrated at the top. The dotted lines indicate the N_1 peaks. Click stimuli: 100 μsec pulse; repetition rate 10/sec; stimulus level expressed in dB re a 100 V pulse generating a 108 dB peak SPL. Histogram: Bin width, 50 μsec. Abscis-

flect the time required for the click stimulus to travel along the basilar membrane from the base of the cochlea to the more apical (low-frequency-sensitive) regions of the basilar membrane. Units with lower CF also tend to produce multiple discharges that occur at regularly spaced time intervals equal to the reciprocal of unit CF. Reversing the polarity of the click, e.g., from rarefaction to condensation, shifts the temporal sequence of the discharges of low-CF units but not the intervals between the spikes (Fig. 4-8). The discharges to the condensation clicks occur during the time the unit is silent to the rarefaction click, with the result that both types of clicks produce spikes separated by intervals related to 1/CF. As the latency to the rarefaction click is shorter than that to the condensation click at high click levels, it is believed that the rarefaction phase (stapes displacement out of the oval window) of the acoustic stimulus results in increased AN activity. The multiple discharges produced by low-CF units are believed to result from the oscillation of the low-frequency segments of the basilar membrane and organ of Corti at their resonant frequencies.

Units with CF above 5 kHz may produce click PST histograms with single or multiple peaks (Fig. 4-7). The period between the peaks of the multipeaked PST histograms of the high-CF units are unrelated to their CFs. The single-peaked PST histograms are produced by high-CF units to low-level clicks. Increasing the click level produces discharges of shorter latency, and early peaks often appear in the PST histograms of both low- and high-CF units. A rarefaction click with a level at least 30 dB above the thresholds of the most sensitive units produces a small, early peak in the PST histograms of units with CF between 4 and 14 kHz. Higher click levels are required to produce the early peak from other AN units. As the stimulus level is further increased, the early peak grows larger, until it becomes larger than the earliest peak of PST histograms generated at the lower click levels. At high click levels the latencies of the early peaks of units with CF between 1 to 3 kHz are comparable to those of units with higher CF.

AN Unit Responses and the Click-Evoked Potential

The temporal patterns of the peaks in the click PST histograms of AN units resemble the N_1 component of the click ECochG response and Wave I of the BSER (Fig. 4-7) (Antoli-Candela and Kiang, 1978). At low stimulus

---

sa, the time after the electrical pulses are delivered to the earphone; ordinate, normalized to instantaneous discharge rate expressed in spikes/sec. Gross response: The average of the responses recorded near the round window. Upward deflection indicates negativity at the round window electrode relative to the headholder. The gross response zero time is delayed by 0.2 msec with respect to the PST histogram zero time to compensate for the conduction time of the spike discharges from the site of spike origin in the cochlea to the microelectrode recording site in the AN. (Reprinted with permission from Antoli-Candela, F., & Kiang, N. Y.-S. Unit activity underlying the N_1 potential. In R. F. Naunton & C. Fernandez (Eds.), *Evoked electrical activity in the auditory nervous system*. New York: Academic Press, 1978, pp. 165-191.)

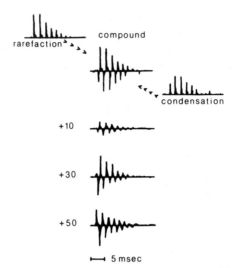

Figure 4-8. Illustrations of the PST histograms of low-CF AN unit discharges to rarefaction (left) and condensation (right) clicks. The middle column consists of the compound click PST histograms that are formed by the histogram of the condensation click responses, inverted and placed beneath the histogram of the rarefaction click responses. The lower three compound PST histograms illustrate the effects of stimulus level on discharge pattern. Click stimuli: Pulse width 100 μsec; repetition rates from 10 to 40 clicks/sec; stimulus level expressed as dB re threshold. Histogram: Bin width, 96 μsec. (Upper 3 histograms redrawn from Goblick, T. J., & Pfeiffer, R. R. Time-domain measurements of cochlear nonlinearities using combination click stimuli. *Journal of the Acoustical Society of America*, 1969, *46*:924-938.)

levels, the N_1 appears as a single peak, with latency similar to the latency of the single peak of the click PST histograms of AN units with CF between 4 and 10 kHz. Units with CF below about 4 kHz do not contribute as much to the N_1 and Wave I response at low click levels because their activity is not synchronized with that of units with higher CF. Units with CF greater than 10 kHz contribute less because the spectrum of the 100 μsec click and the poor transfer of high frequency acoustic energy through the earphone (see Chapters 1, 8) and the middle ear results in a lower sensitivity of these units to click stimuli. At click levels approximately 30 dB above the threshold of the most sensitive units, the early peak appears in the click PST histogram of units with CF between 4 and 14 kHz and the N_1 peak begins to divide into two peaks separated by 0.2 msec. At higher click levels the early peak in the click PST histogram becomes more prominent than the later peak and the N_1 appears as a single, shorter-latency peak. At very high click levels, the range of CFs of units producing early peaks is extended to below 3 kHz and above 20 kHz. At these high stimulus levels the latency of the early peak of the PST histograms of units with CF between 1 and 4 kHz will begin to correspond with that of units with higher CF.

The early peak of the click PST histograms (and the early N_1 potential, and Wave I) occur at click levels that produce low-frequency components in the acoustic signal of sufficient amplitude to exceed the thresholds of the low frequency "tails" of the most sensitive AN unit tuning curves. There is considerable evidence that the cochlear mechanisms generating the neural activity to frequencies within the "tips" of the AN unit tuning curves behave differently from those generating the neural activity to frequencies within the tuning curve "tails" (Kiang and Moxon, 1974). For example, a low-frequency masker has greater effect on the responses to tones with frequencies in the "tips" of AN-unit tuning curves than on the responses to tones with frequencies in the "tails." In contrast, a masker with a center frequency near the unit CF will nearly equally elevate the thresholds to tones with frequency in the "tips" and "tails" of AN unit tuning curves. Kemp, Coppée, and Robinson (1937) reported that the early component of the AN evoked potential is masked by higher frequencies and the later component by lower frequencies. The electrical stimulation of the crossed olivocochlear bundle (COCB), which provides neural efferent input to the cochlea, is more effective in reducing the discharges of AN units to tones with frequency in the "tips" than in the "tails" of their tuning curves (Wiederhold, 1970). The AN units with CF between 4 and 10 kHz are more sensitive to COCB stimulation than units with higher and lower CFs. Electrical stimulation of the COCB is most effective in reducing the amplitude of the N_1 peak of the evoked potential at low click levels, where the late N_1 peak is most prominent; electrically stimulating the COCB becomes less effective at high click levels, where the early N_1 peak dominates (Wiederhold and Peake, 1966).

The Human Auditory Nerve

The number of myelinated axons in the cat AN is approximately 50,000; the majority have diameters between 3 to 6 μm (Gacek and Rasmussen, 1961). The human AN contains approximately 31,000 myelinated nerve fibers, with the vast majority 5 to 7 μm thick (Rasmussen, 1940). According to von Békésy (1960), the propagation time of a high-level click along the human cochlear partition becomes greater than 0.1 msec at 20 to 21 mm from the stapes (CF of approximately 1 kHz), and increases progressively with distance from the stapes. Thus in both the human and the cat, AN units with CF above 1 kHz probably fire in synchrony to high-level click stimuli. If all AN units with CF between 1 and 32 kHz were discharging in synchrony to a high-level click, approximately 30,000 AN fibers in the cat (Schuknecht,

1960) and 20,000 AN fibers in the human (Guild, Crowe, and Bunch, et al., 1931) would contribute to the click BSER.

NEUROPHYSIOLOGY OF BRAIN-STEM AUDITORY STRUCTURES

The Cochlear Nuclear Complex

The cochlear nuclear complex (CNC) is the second stage of the auditory neural pathway, or the first stage of the central auditory system to receive auditory information from the periphery (Fig. 4-2). The major subdivisions of the CNC are the dorsal and ventral cochlear nuclear groups (DCN and VCN). The VCN is further subdivided by the entering auditory nerve into an anterior group (AVCN) and a posterior group (PVCN). The CNC neurons receive considerable nonprimary input from other CNC neurons, the superior olivary complex, and the nuclei of the lateral lemniscus. The DCN receives additional input from the inferior colliculus. The axons of CNC neurons form three main ascending tracts, the trapezoid body (from the VCN), the intermediate acoustic stria (from the PVCN), and the dorsal acoustic stria (from the DCN). They terminate in auditory structures up to and including the inferior colliculus.

Most CNC units are excited by stimulation of the ipsilateral ear only, although some DCN units are also affected by stimulation of the contralateral ear (Mast, 1973). All three divisions of the CNC are tonotopically organized with low-CF units located ventral to the higher CF units (Rose, Galambos, and Hughes, 1959). Neurophysiologic studies have demonstrated that CNC units with specific response characteristics occur in CNC cell groups containing certain morphologic cell types (Kiang, Pfeiffer, and Warr, et al., 1965; Godfrey, Kiang, and Norris, 1975a, 1975b; Bourk, 1976).

Primary-like Units

Many AVCN units respond similarly to AN units; they produce spontaneous activity with an irregular temporal pattern and a sustained discharge to continuous tones. The tuning characteristics and tone burst elicited discharge patterns of these AVCN units (Fig. 4-5, Primary-like) are nearly identical to those of AN units. While the STB-PST histograms of the rostral AVCN units resemble those of AN units (Fig. 4-5, Pri), those of caudal AVCN units tend to exhibit a short period (<3 msec) of reduced activity that follows the initial peak of activity (Fig. 4-5, Pri-N). This decrease in discharge rate is best observed at stimulus levels 20 dB above threshold, and becomes more prominent and longer-lasting at even higher stimulus levels. The ability of the discharges of Primary-like units to synchronize with low-frequency tones (<5 kHz) appears to be similar to that of AN units. Although the intensity functions of Pri units resemble those of AN units, those of Pri-N units are more variable in shape and may be nonmonotonic in form.

The Primary-like units with high CF tend to produce single-peaked click PST histograms. The range of latencies to click stimuli of the high-CF Pri and Pri-N units overlap (1.7 to 2.7 msec), although the shortest latencies are exhibited by Pri-N units. Units with low CF tend to produce multipeaked click PST histograms, with interpeak intervals equal to 1/CF. The latency of the first spike of the Pri-N click elicited discharges tends to be more tightly time-locked to the clicks than those of the AN and Pri units.

Chopper Units

Other AVCN units produce discharge patterns similar to those of PVCN units. The discharges of these CNC units to short tone bursts occur at regular intervals that are unrelated to unit CF, for units with CF above 2 kHz. Their STB-PST histograms consist of regularly spaced peaks that are most prominent at stimulus levels greater than 15 dB re threshold (Fig. 4-5, Chopper-type). Many of the Chopper units do not spontaneously discharge, but do discharge continuously to a maintained stimulus. There is greater variability in the tuning characteristics of Chopper units, with a slight tendency toward wider tuning in comparison to Primary-like units. Unlike AN and Primary-like units, the spontaneous activity of Chopper units can be inhibited by tones bordering the "excitatory" tuning curve (inhibitory sidebands).

The Chopper pattern is most prominent at the beginning of a STB-PST histogram; it becomes more prominent and usually lasts longer with increases in stimulus level. The peak widths and interpeak intervals of the STB-PST histograms of some Chopper units in the DCN tend to be greater (Fig. 4-5, Chop-W) than those of most VCN Chopper units. The initial discharges of most VCN Chopper units consist of a "fast" Chopper pattern characterized by STB-PST histograms, with narrow initial peaks separated by short (< 3 msec) interpeak intervals (Fig. 4-5, Chop-T and Chop-S). The discharges of Chopper units are incapable of synchronizing with tones of frequency above 1.5 to 2 kHz (Bourk, 1977). Their ability to synchronize their discharges with tones of frequency below 800 Hz is similar to that of AN units and Primary-like units, but that ability decreases significantly above 800 Hz. The STB and continuous tone intensity functions of most Chopper units are monotonic; the Chop-S units produce the highest output of all CNC units.

The Chopper units tend to exhibit higher thresholds to click stimuli and a wider range of click latencies (1.75 to 5.75 msec) than do the Primary-like units. The click latencies of the PVCN Chopper units tend to be shorter (1.75 to 2.75 msec) than the majority of the AVCN Chopper units (2.5 to 3.1 msec). The Chop-W units respond to clicks with a one-spike discharge of long and variable latency. The click PST histograms of the "fast" Chopper units may consist of from one to three narrow peaks regardless of the unit CF, with initial peak width as narrow as that of AN unit click PST histograms. For most AVCN Chopper units, the peaks of the click PST histograms are separated by short intervals (1.1 to 2 msec) that may be related to the refractory period of these units.

On Units

The majority of units in the central area of the PVCN and a few units in the other CNC areas display little or no spontaneous activity and a brief, transient discharge to a continuous CF tone (Fig. 4-5, On-type). The CF thresholds of the On units tend to be higher than those of other CNC units, with the tendency for CF thresholds to be the highest for On units with very brief (one spike) responses. Although the tuning curves of many On units appear to have a sharp tip, they tend to be wider than the tuning curves of AN units and other CNC units at stimulus levels of 20 dB or greater than CF threshold.

The tone burst elicited responses of On units with high CF are characterized by a brief discharge that is often sharply time-locked to stimulus onset. This initial onset discharge may be followed by a markedly lower discharge rate that becomes noticeable at stimulus levels at least 15 dB above threshold. The On units producing the most transient response (Fig. 4-5, On-T) tend to be located within the central PVCN, while those producing a more sustained discharge are more rostrally located in the VCN (Fig. 4-5, On-S) and in the DCN (Fig. 4-5, On-W). The On-S units produce an initial short high-frequency spike burst that is followed by a very low rate of discharge that may last the duration of the stimulus. The On-W units typically produce a more sustained, slower discharge during the initial 25 msec of the stimulus that gradually declines to zero or to a lower rate that is maintained for the stimulus duration. The initial spike of the tone burst response of VCN On-S units may not be as sharply time-locked to stimulus onset as that of the On-T units and may occur with a slightly longer latency. The DCN On-W units tend to produce a broad range of response latencies; the initial spike of some units is poorly time-locked to stimulus onset. At high stimulus levels many of the VCN On-S units appear to produce Chopper-type discharges with short (<2 msec) initial interpeak intervals. The discharge patterns of these On-S units may represent an extreme form of the Chop-T discharge pattern. The discharges of DCN On-W units display a varying degree of regularity, with most producing a pattern intermediate between Primary-like and Chopper-type. The On-T units respond to each cycle of a low frequency sinusoid as a separate stimulus. They synchronize best to tones with frequency below 700 Hz and exhibit an upper synchronization limit of 2 kHz. A few of the On-S units may synchronize with sinusoids as well as the Primary-like units of AVCN; others may be similar in their behavior to the Chopper units. By definition, the On units produce low maximum discharge rates to continuous CF tones. The lowest maxima are produced by the On-T units (one spike/ stimulus). The On-S units produce monotonic STB and continuous tone intensity functions, whereas those of DCN On-W units are nonmonotonic.

Although the On units tend to exhibit high thresholds to tonal stimuli, the thresholds of VCN On units to rarefaction clicks tend to be as low as those of AN units. Some of the DCN On-W units do not respond to click stimuli;

others exhibit higher thresholds to clicks than to tonal stimuli. The On-T units tend to produce single-peaked click PST histograms, often with the shortest latencies (1.5 to 2.5 msec) of all CNC units and with a peak narrower than the first peak of the AN unit click PST histograms. The PVCN On-S units tend to exhibit shorter click latencies (1.7 to 2.25 msec) than the AVCN On-S units (1.9 to 3 msec). The DCN On-W units responsive to click stimuli often exhibit the longest click latencies (2.65 to 5.75 msec) of all On units.

Pause Units

The tone burst elicited discharge of many DCN units and a few VCN units can be characterized as including a "silent" period of reduced activity that follows the initial burst of activity to stimulus onset (Fig. 4-5, Pause- and Build-type). Most Pause units are spontaneously active and produce maintained activity to continuous tones. The tuning curves of these units resemble those of AN units, although some may exhibit unusual shapes or inhibitory sidebands.

The STB-PST histograms of some Pause units (Fig. 4-5, Pau-P) resemble those of Pri-N units, except that the initial peak of the Pau-P histogram is often wider and the silent period is always longer (> 5 msec) than that of Pri-N units. Other Pause units produce Chopper STB-PST histograms (Fig. 4-5, Pau-C) in which the first or second interpeak interval is longer than subsequent interpeak intervals. In many cases, the silent period is not obvious at stimulus levels less than 20 dB re threshold. While the Pause discharge is the most typical pattern produced by many DCN units to a CF tone burst at 20 dB above threshold, the discharge pattern of some of these units varies with changes either in tone frequency or level (Goldberg and Brownell, 1973). In some cases, the silent period of the discharge increases such that only the initial response may remain when short tone bursts are used as stimuli. In other cases, the initial discharge may be entirely suppressed and only the sustained, longer-latency portion of the response remains (Fig. 4-5, Build). The spontaneous activity of Pause units may also be suppressed when the frequency of the tone burst is within the inhibitory sideband of the unit's tuning curve. There is some indication that the DCN Pause units may produce discharges that synchronize well with sinusoids of frequency less than 500 Hz, synchronize poorly as frequency is increased to 1 kHz, and fail to synchronize at frequencies above 1.5 kHz.

As the stimulus level of a short tone burst is increased from threshold to 30 dB above threshold, the output of a Pause unit may increase above, decrease below, or remain at spontaneous levels. Further increases in stimulus level may not change the output reached at 30 dB re threshold. In contrast, their continuous CF tone intensity functions are monotonic and reach maxima between 40 and 120 spikes/sec.

The click thresholds of Pause units are often much higher than their thresholds to CF tone bursts. These units display a wide range of click latencies (2.75 to 8.75 msec); some exhibit an increase in latency to an increase in click level. The click-elicited discharges of some do not appear to be as securely time-locked to the click as those of other CNC units.

Build Units

Other DCN units respond to tone bursts with a very gradual rise in discharge to a steady rate that lasts the duration of the stimulus (Fig. 4-5, Build). The STB-PST histograms of the DCN Build-type units resemble those of DCN Pause-type units with the initial response removed. Most of the response characteristics of the DCN Build units are similar to those of DCN Pause units, with the exception that the latter tend to produce higher maximum output to short tone bursts and to continuous tone stimuli.

Suppressed Units

Few units in the DCN exhibit a decrease of spontaneous discharge rate to tone burst stimuli (Fig. 4-5, Supp).

Morphological Correlates of CNC Unit Types

The frequency of occurrence of unit types within the CNC appears to be correlated with the distribution of morphological cell types within the CNC. The Pri units occur most frequently in the AVCN where large and small spherical cells with cell bodies enveloped by one or two large calyx terminals predominate [the large spherical cell area (LSCA) and the small spherical cell area (SSCA)]. The Pri units tend to produce spike potentials of complex waveform, which includes a small positive potential precedent to the unit spike potential. This positive prepotential is believed to be the extracellular recording of the presynaptic potential generated by the large calyx terminals. The spherical cells of the AVCN give rise to medium-sized axons that terminate (Fig. 4-2) ipsilaterally in the superior olivary complex, or decussate in the dorsal component of the trapezoid body, to end in the contralateral superior olivary complex, ventral nucleus of the lateral lemniscus, and (to a minor degree) in the inferior colliculus. The Pri-N units are more frequently encountered in the GCA (globular call area)-AVCN, where the globular cells that receive three to four smaller, modified calyx terminals on their cell bodies are found. These units also generate spike potentials with a complex waveform, but signal-averaging of the spike potential is often required to detect the smaller positive prepotentials. The thick axons of the AVCN globular cells decussate in the trapezoid body to end primarily within the contralateral superior olivary complex.

The Chopper units most frequently occur in areas where multipolar neurons predominate [multipolar cell area (MCA)]. Multipolar neurons and Chopper units are also found in the AVCN, where they are intermingled with spherical and globular cells and Primary-like units. They are frequently encountered in the MCA-PVCN and number slightly less than the Pri-N units in the GCA-AVCN. Thin fibers believed to arise from the multipolar and small cells of the PVCN travel in the middle and ventral zones of the trapezoid body and terminate bilaterally, in the superior olivary complex, and contralaterally, in the nuclei of the lateral lemniscus and inferior colliculus.

The central PVCN [octopus cell area (OCA)] consists almost exclusively of large octopus cells and On-T units. The octopus cells give rise to coarse axons that leave the CNC dorsally in the intermediate acoustic stria. These axons are believed to terminate in the ipsilateral superior olivary complex and the contralateral ventral nucleus of the lateral lemniscus.

Within the DCN pyramidal cell layer (PCL-DCN) pyramidal neurons predominate, as do the Pause and Build units. The On-W units occur almost exclusively in the DCN central nucleus (CN-DCN) where giant cells and other types of neurons are also located. A large proportion of the CN-DCN units are difficult to classify but do exhibit the response characteristics of Pause and Chopper units. The innervation of DCN neurons and their response characteristics indicate that their behavior may not be as strongly influenced by their AN inputs as that of VCN units. The AN input to DCN neurons does not appear to be as great as the inputs arising from the VCN and other brain-stem structures, especially in the CN-DCN (Kane, 1977). Section of the AN produces very light to almost negligible degeneration of terminal processes in the DCN, while producing massive degeneration in the VCN. Many of the CN-DCN units produce more complex and variable discharge patterns than VCN units. The spontaneous discharges of DCN units are not as strongly in-fluenced by AN inputs as are those of VCN units (Koeber, Pfeiffer, and Warr, et al., 1966). Many DCN units appear to be more strongly affected by anesthesia than VCN units (Evans and Nelson, 1973); some are responsive to binaural stimuli. The output of most DCN neurons appear to be confined to the CNC, with only the pyramidal cells of the PCL-DCN and the few giant cells of the CN-DCN sending thin axons in the dorsal acoustic stria to higher auditory structures.

CNC Unit Responses and the Click BSER

The click latencies of all CNC units with CF below 3 to 4 kHz are related to unit CF, as are those of AN units, and therefore tend not to fire in syn-chrony with higher CF units to all but high-level click stimuli. The CNC units capable of producing short latency discharges synchronized to click stimuli are confined to the VCN, and include the On-T units of the PVCN, the Primary-like units of the AVCN and some of the On-S units of the VCN. The VCN Chopper units tend to require slightly higher click levels to elicit a discharge and exhibit slightly longer latencies. The DCN units tend, as a group, to have high click thresholds and, in many cases, long and variable click latencies.

The Human Cochlear Nuclear Complex

The cytoarchitecture of the human cochlear nuclear complex (CNC) is not identical to that of the cat CNC (Moore and Osen, 1979). The neurons that produce short-latency synchronized discharges to click stimuli in the cat CNC (the spherical, globular, and octopus cells) appear to be less numerous in humans. Multipolar and small-cell areas form the greater mass of the human VCN. Although the VCN is larger than the DCN in both the human and the cat, the DCN is proportionally larger in the human than in the cat. In the human DCN there are fewer granular and giant cells; pyramidal cells are randomly oriented and intermingle with other DCN neurons in an area ana- logous to the cat CN-DCN. The dorsal and intermediate acoustic striae, which in cat contain the ascending axons of and the efferent fibers to the DCN and the central and caudal areas of PVCN, are much reduced in size in humans. The axons of the human VCN neurons form a large trapezoid body that lies deep in the brainstem covered by the fibers of the middle cerebellar peduncle. In the cat, the trapezoid body is located near the ventral surface of the brainstem, caudal to the middle cerebellar peduncle.

The Superior Olivary Complex

The superior olivary complex (SOC) is considered the second stage of the central auditory pathway, or the third stage of the auditory neural path- way. It consists of a number of cell groups (Fig. 4-2), some of which receive inputs from both the ipsilateral and contralateral CNC. The CNC inputs to the major SOC nuclei—the medial superior olive (MSO), the lateral superior olive (LSO) and the medial nucleus of the trapezoid body (MNTB)—arise from the AVCN, whereas the periolivary nuclei and the ventral and lateral nuclei of the trapezoid body (VNTB and LNTB, respectively) receive input primarily from the PVCN (Warr, 1966, 1969, 1972; van Noort, 1969). The DCN input to the SOC is minor compared to the VCN input. The SOC cell groups receiving PVCN input also appear to be the major termination sites of descending inputs to the SOC (Rasmussen, 1953). These same SOC cell groups contain the cells of origin of efferent axons, the olivocochlear bundle, that end in the CNC and the cochlea. The majority of the SOC axons ascend- ing in the lateral lemniscus take origin in the LSO and MSO (Elverland, 1978; Adams, 1979). The MSO and LSO are the first stages in the ascending auditory pathway believed to be involved in the processing of binaural infor- mation. Because of the diffuse nature and small size of most SOC cell groups, neurophysiologic descriptions of the unit types in most of the SOC nuclei are lacking. In general, the SOC units located ventromedial to the MSO are ex- cited by stimulation of the contralateral ear; those located dorsolaterally are excited by stimulation of the ipsilateral ear. The discharge characteristics of most SOC units resemble those of the CNC units, except that fewer On, Pause, and Build-type units are encountered in the SOC (Guinan, Guinan, and Norris, 1972; Guinan, Norris, and Guinan, 1972; Tsuchitani, 1977).

Units with extremely long latencies and units that discharge selectively to stimulus offset are also found in the SOC.

Primary-Like Units

Units with Primary-like response characteristics occur within the cat
SOC. Approximately two thirds of these units produce Pri-N type STB-PST
histograms and one third the Pri type. The units with CF above 3 kHz produce relatively uniform click latencies of approximately 3 msec. The majority
of SOC units producing Primary-like discharges are located within the MNTB.
These units also produce spike potentials of complex waveform that resemble
those produced by the Pri units of the AVCN, i.e., a positive potential pre-
cedes the unit spike potential by approximately 0.5 msec. The MNTB Primary-like units are excited by stimulation of the contralateral ear and are unaffected by stimulation of the ipsilateral ear (monaural, contralaterally
excited). They exhibit short latencies to tone burst stimuli ($\cong 5.6$ msec). Very
small numbers of Primary-like units are found in the VNTB and LNTB, and in
and around the LSO.

Chopper Units

Units with Chopper discharge patterns are found throughout the SOC.
All types of Chopper patterns are produced by SOC units; the type of pattern
produced is related to the location of the unit within the SOC. The click-
elicited discharges of the Chopper units have not been described in any detail.
It has been reported that SOC Chop-W units tend to exhibit higher thresholds
to clicks than do other SOC Chopper and Primary-like units. The majority of
units in the LSO are of the "fast" Chopper type, while those located in surrounding nuclei tend to be the Chop-W type. Although all LSO units are excited by stimulation of the ipsilateral ear, the ipsilaterally elicited discharges of
those units with CF above 1 to 2 kHz are inhibited by simultaneous stimulation of the contralateral ear (binaural, contralaterally inhibited). The LSO
Chopper units tend to produce monotonic STB intensity functions with
higher maximum output and shorter response latencies ($\cong 5.8$ msec) than do
the Chopper units located around the LSO. The STB-PST histograms of
LSO units typically contain a narrow initial peak that is securely time-locked
to a stimulus with a 1.0 or 2.5 msec rise time. The click latencies of the few
LSO units tested appear to be slightly greater (> 3.2 msec) than those of
Primary-like MNTB units.

SOC units producing Chop-W discharge patterns are located around the
LSO, and medial to the MSO within the VNTB, MNTB, and dorsomedial
periolivary nucleus (DMPO). All of the medially located Chop-W units are excited by stimulation of the contralateral ear; a few are also either excited or inhibited by stimulation of the ipsilateral ear. Most units located along the
caudal margin of the LSO and in the dorsolateral periolivary (DLPO) nucleus
produce Chop-W type STB-PST histograms. Many of the caudal LSO units
and the majority of the DLPO units are only excited by stimulation of the

ipsilateral ear (monaural, ipsilaterally excited). These laterally located Chop-W units also produce monotonic STB intensity functions. While the MNTB Primary-like units and the LSO Chopper units exhibit small changes in the latency of the first spike with increases in tone burst stimulus level, large shifts in latency are exhibited by the lateral Chop-W units. Decreasing the duration of a short tone burst (from 200 msec to 20 msec) has a small effect on the thresholds of LSO units, but results in large increases in Chop-W unit thresholds. It appears that the time required by the Chop-W units to integrate their synaptic inputs is greater than the time required by the LSO "fast" Chopper units. The long-time constant of the Chop-W units suggest that they will either be unresponsive or will exhibit high thresholds to clicks, because of the click's very brief nature.

On Units

Very few On units appear to occur in the cat SOC, even within the DLPO, which reportedly receives a large input from the PVCN via the intermediate acoustic stria (Warr, 1966). However, some of the LSO Chop-T units do not appear to be capable of maintaining discharges to tones of long (>30 sec) duration; these might be classified as On-S units.

Pause and Build Units

Although few Pause units are observed in the cat SOC, some of the STB-PST histograms of SOC Chop-W units do exhibit an initial interpeak interval that is slightly longer than the subsequent interpeak intervals. The Pau-P and Build units are infrequently found in the SOC.

Off Units

Some of the SOC units either do not respond or may exhibit inhibition of spontaneous activity during a short tone or white noise burst, and produce discharges after the stimulus is terminated (Fig. 4-5, Off). The tuning curves of many of these units do not resemble those of AN units and tend to be wider than those of SOC Primary-like units. Although some of the Off units produce a transient discharge 5 msec or more after the stimulus is terminated, others produce multiple discharges that last several hundred msec, with latencies of 15 msec or longer after the stimulus offset. Very few of the Off units respond with click latencies comparable to those of the SOC Primary units. Many of the Off units are located medial to the MSO and are influenced by stimulation of the contralateral ear.

Long-Latency Units

Very few of the SOC units respond with latencies of at least 40 msec (Fig. 4-5, Long). Their discharges are transient to 25 msec duration tone bursts and produce one or two peaks in their STB-PST histograms.

Morphological Correlates of SOC Unit Types

Except for the MNTB (Morest, 1968), little is known of the cytoarchitecture of the cat SOC nuclei. The Primary-like units of the MNTB are believed to be the MNTB globular (principal) cells, each of which receives a single, large calyx terminal arising from the thick axon of an AVCN globular cell of the contralateral CNC (Tolbert and Morest, 1977). The Primary-like units of MNTB are tonotopically organized; low-CF units are located lateral to the higher CF units. The MNTB also contains multipolar and elongate neurons and units that produce Off and Chop-W discharges. The MNTB globular cells are believed to provide input to the ipsilateral LSO. The large multipolar cells of the MNTB have been demonstrated to contribute to the crossed olivocochlear bundle (Warr, 1975).

The vast majority of LSO units are the "fast" Chopper-type; many of the LSO neurons are fusiform cells with disc-shaped dendritic fields (Scheibel and Scheibel, 1974). Although it has been reported that the cat LSO receives ipsilateral input from the AVCN small spherical cell area (SSCA) (Osen, 1970), it is not known whether the input arises from the spherical, multipolar, and/or small cells. The contralateral ear is believed to provide input to the LSO through the globular cells of the contralateral AVCN and ipsilateral MNTB. The LSO is tonotopically organized with low CF units located at the dorsal tip of the lateral limb of the S-shaped structure. Unit CF increases progressively along the curvature of the S; high-CF units are located in the ventral tip of the medial limb of the S. The representation of the two ears in the LSO appears to be matched in terms of CFs and tuning curves. The output of LSO units with CF above 1 to 2 kHz is related to the spectral content of the stimuli at the two ears and to interaural spectral/intensity differences. Most of the LSO neurons send their axons into either the ipsilateral or contralateral lateral lemniscus and provide bilateral input to the dorsal nuclei of the lateral lemniscus and the inferior colliculi.

The MSO neurons are reportedly similar to, but larger than, the LSO neurons (Ramón y Cajal, 1899; Scheibel and Scheibel, 1974). They receive terminals from the ipsilateral and contralateral AVCN large spherical cell area (LSCA) (Osen, 1970). Most MSO units appear to be excited by stimulation of either ear (binaurally excited); others are of the binaural, ipsilaterally inhibited type. They are tonotopically organized with dorsally located low-CF units and ventrally located high-CF units. A seemingly disproportionate amount of the MSO appears to represent frequencies lower than 10 kHz. The CFs of the binaural units appear to be matched for stimulation of either ear. The discharge patterns of MSO units to tone bursts have not been described in sufficient detail to provide a basis for their classification. They discharge in a sustained manner with high rates and irregular temporal patterns to continuous tones. The few canine MSO units examined were capable of producing discharges synchronized with low CF (< 1 kHz) tones and were also sensitive to variations in interaural phase differences of low-frequency tones (Goldberg and Brown, 1969). The high-CF (> 1 kHz), binaurally excited units produced higher maximum output when both ears were stimulated than when either ear was stimulated alone. These high-CF units are thus able to convey binaural intensity information. The axons of MSO neurons ascend uncrossed in the lateral lemniscus to terminate ipsilaterally in the ventral nucleus of the lateral lemniscus and the inferior colliculus.

The cell types and synaptic organization of the dorsolateral periolivary nucleus (DLPO) have not been described in any detail. The intermediate acoustic stria (a major input to the DLPO) appears to contain the axons of the multipolar and small cells of the PVCN, as well as the axons of the octopus cells (Adams and Warr, 1976). The DLPO also receives input from the ipsilateral PVCN multipolar cell area (MCA) by way of the thin fiber ventral component of the trapezoid body. A small contralateral input from the DCN may reach the DLPO by way of the dorsal acoustic stria. The DLPO units appear to be as narrowly tuned as MNTB and LSO units, and are tonotopically organized with low-CF units located laterally, and higher CF units more medially located. The most common type of DLPO unit produces Chop-W type STB-PST histograms, has longer latency, and lower maximum output to tone bursts than the LSO Chopper units. The DLPO is believed to be part of an efferent system that sends axons back to the cochlea in the uncrossed olivocochlear bundle and to the CNC. Its contributions to the ascending auditory pathway are considered to be minor.

SOC Unit Responses and the Click Gross Potential

The large amplitude of the click gross potential generated by the SOC has impeded the study of SOC unit discharges to click stimuli. The click latencies of most SOC units with CF below 2 to 3 kHz relate to unit CF. The SOC units with CF above 10 kHz tend to exhibit higher thresholds to rarefaction clicks produced by a 100 μsec electric pulse. As the SOC Primary-like units with CF > 3 kHz exhibit short, uniform click latencies (2.7 to 3.8 msec), stimulation of the contralateral ear should produce a well synchronized discharge from the MNTB. The behavior of MSO units cannot be predicted as their response characteristics have not yet been described in any detail. The early studies of "MSO unit" responses to click stimuli (Moushegian, Rupert, and Whitcomb, 1964) utilized methods that were insufficient for localizing units with any confidence within the specific cell groups of the SOC. An ipsilateral click stimulus may produce a slightly longer latency but a well synchronized discharge from the LSO, as the first spike of the discharges to stimuli with fast rise-time is securely time-locked to the stimulus onset.

The Human Superior Olivary Complex

The relative size and configuration of the SOC nuclei differ among species (Moore and Moore, 1971). In most mammals, the number of neurons in the MNTB matches that of the LSO: the ratio of LSO neurons to MSO neurons appears to depend on the species. In the cat, the neurons in the LSO appear to slightly outnumber those in the MSO, while in the human LSO neurons are only one third the number of the MSO (Strominger and Hurwitz, 1976). The number of LSO neurons in the cat is reportedly almost twice that found in the human. The LSO forms a conspicuous S-shaped structure in the cat but only a series of small cell clusters in the human. The general shape of the MSO is similar in both cats and humans, as is the orientation of the polar dendrites within it. The MNTB in humans is a poorly defined cell group.

The Nuclei of the Lateral Lemniscus

The nuclei of the lateral lemniscus (NLL) form an ill-defined and infrequently studied nuclear complex located within the fibers of the lateral lemniscus (LL). The NLL is subdivided into a loosely organized ventral nucleus (VNLL) and a smaller, more circumscribed dorsal nucleus (DNLL). NLL neurons receive ascending acoustic input from the CNC and the SOC (Fig. 4-2). The input from the CNC is primarily contralateral and may be greater in the VNLL than in the DNLL. The VNLL receives additional input from the ipsilateral MSO; the DNLL receives a bilateral LSO input. The NLL also receives descending inputs from higher auditory structures (Powell and Hatton, 1969), and sends descending axons to lower auditory structures (Rasmussen, 1960). The NLL provides a major input to the inferior colliculus that appears to have a distribution similar to those of the CNC and SOC.

The few studies of the response characteristics of NLL units were limited to small samples of units from different areas of this diffusely distributed nuclear complex (Aitkin, Anderson, and Brugge, 1970; Guinan, Norris, and Guinan, 1972). The available descriptions of NLL unit response characteristics are sketchy; the following summary should be considered tentative: The majority of NLL units appear to be excited by stimulation of the contralateral ear. While most DNLL units may be influenced by stimulation of the ipsilateral ear, there is some question as to which, if any, VNLL units are also affected by ipsilateral stimulation. Most NLL units appear to exhibit little or no spontaneous activity; many produce a maintained discharge to continuous tones. The limited data describing NLL unit discharge patterns suggest that NLL units most commonly produce "sustained" or Pause-type STB-PST histograms to moderate-level CF tones. A few produce On-type histograms. In some cases, the discharge patterns of the "sustained" or Pause units may be modified to the On, Build, or Suppressed type, with changes in tone fre-

quency or level. The only response of the few NLL units exhibiting very regu
lar spontaneous activity appears to be suppression of this activity.

Morphologic Correlates of NLL Unit Types

Although the NLL provides a major input to the inferior colliculus, little is
known about this structure. VNLL neurons are scattered along the length of
the LL. The initial report of tonotopic organization in the VNLL (Aitkin,
Anderson, and Brugge, 1970) has not been supported by a second single-
unit study of the VNLL (Guinan, Norris, and Guinan, 1972), or by anatomic
studies of the topographic projections of CNC and MSO terminals onto the
VNLL (van Noort, 1969; Elverland, 1978), or of the VNLL terminals onto
the inferior colliculus (Roth, Aitkin, and Andersen et al., 1978; Adams,
1979). The VNLL reportedly consists exclusively of monaural, contralaterally
excited units that produce "sustained," Pause, or On discharges (Aitkin,
Anderson, and Brugge, 1970), or "sustained" discharges only (Aitkin and
Boyd, 1978). Binaural units are dorsally located in an "interstitial region" between the VNLL and DNLL (Aitkin, Anderson, and Brugge, 1970). According to Guinan, Norris, and Guinan (1972), the binaural units are intermingled
with the monaural units within the VNLL and produce either Chopper or On
discharges. Aitkin and Boyd (1978) suggest that, given their experience of
difficulties in differentiating VNLL units from those in surrounding structures,
the conflicting results may be due to unit localization errors in VNLL studies. It
is more probable, however, that the results conflict because the small samples
of units in each of the studies were collected from different areas of the
VNLL. Anatomical studies of the VNLL indicate that it consists of from three
to five cell groups (Fig. 4-2) that differ in morphology and connectivity (Warr,
1969; Adams, 1979). The VNLL was approached from different angles in
each of the three studies cited.

Studies confined to the ventral division of the VNLL (V-VNLL) indicate
that most of the V-VNLL units produce Chopper discharges in response to
tone bursts, with many of the remaining units producing On discharges
(Guinan, Norris, and Guinan, 1972). Some of the V-VNLL On units resemble the On-T units of OCA-PVCN, and also produce spike potentials
with prepotentials (Adams, 1978). These V-VNLL units may correspond to
the globular cells of the V-VNLL that receive large calciform endings believed
to arise from OCA-PVCN axons. The Chopper units may correspond to the
V-VNLL elongate neurons that resemble the VCN multipolar cells in receiving few terminals on their cell bodies.

The DNLL is a smaller, more compact, and more clearly delineated cell
group than the VNLL, except at its rostral and caudal extremities. The DNLL
units are tonotopically organized with low CF units located dorsal to higher
CF units (Aitkin, Anderson, and Brugge, 1970). The topographic projection
of the DNLL axons to the IC has been reported to be somewhat discrete

(Adams, 1979), but the reverse of the single unit tonotopic organization (Roth, Aitkin, and Andersen, et al., 1978). While the topographic projections of the CNC and LSO to the inferior colliculus have been demonstrated, none has been demonstrated for the projection of CNC or LSO to the DNLL (Elverland, 1978). The predominant effect of an ipsilateral stimulus is the suppression of contralaterally evoked activity (binaural, ipsilaterally suppressed), but under certain conditions increased activity may result. Most of the DNLL neurons are multipolar and most DNLL units produce "sustained," Pause, or On discharge patterns to moderate levels of CF tone burst stimuli. The discharges of some DNLL units with low CF can synchronize with tones of frequency below 1 kHz presented either monaurally or binaurally (Brugge, Anderson, and Aitkin, 1970). Others, incapable of synchronizing with low-frequency tones, do produce an output (spike counts) that is a function of the interaural phase difference of low-frequency tones. The binaural, ipsilaterally suppressed DNLL units are similar to most LSO units and produce a spike count related to interaural intensity differences.

NLL Unit Responses and the Click BSER

While few NLL units are known to be capable of producing well synchronized discharges to click stimuli, too little is known of the response characteristics of the majority of the NLL units to predict their behavior to click stimuli.

The Human Nuclei of the Lateral Lemniscus

The human lateral lemniscus has been described to contain three cell groups; an olivary remnant, the VNLL, and the DNLL (Ferraro and Minckler, 1977). The olivary remnant is a loosely organized group of cells that extends dorsally from the rostral pole of the SOC and may correspond to the VNLL posteromedial group (PM) of the cat. The VNLL is a large, scattered cell group containing predominantly oval and spindle shaped cells apparently multipolar in nature. The DNLL neurons are reportedly similar in appearance and size to those in the VNLL and have been described in the Golgi studies of Geniec and Morest (1971).

Inferior Colliculus

The inferior colliculus (IC) is a prominent midbrain structure that receives ascending and descending inputs from auditory and nonauditory structures. The core of the IC, the central nucleus (CN-IC), is surrounded by a capsule of neurons that form the internuclear or pericentral zone (IZ-IC) dorsally and caudally, and the external or lateral zone (EZ-IC) laterally and ventrally. The main input to the CN-IC is from lower auditory neurons that send their axons into the lateral lemniscus (Fig. 4-2). The IZ-IC receives input from auditory cortex; the EZ-IC receives ascending fibers of the somatosensory system. There are also considerable intrinsic connections between IC neurons. As the CN-IC is the main source of acoustic input to the thalamus, it is considered to be of primary importance in the perception of acoustic stimuli. The projection of IZ-IC axons to the pontine nuclei and the cerebellum (Rasmussen, 1964; Powell and Hatton, 1969) suggest it may play a role in eliciting or coordinating motor responses to acoustic stimuli. The IC also sends axons to midbrain and brain stem structures involved in acoustic reflexes, to the lateral tegmental system, and to lower auditory cell groups.

The response characteristics of the units in the major subdivisions of the IC differ considerably from one another (Aitkin, Webster, and Veale, et al., 1975). Although most CN-IC units produce a fairly stable response to acoustic stimuli, the units within the IZ-IC often fail to respond to repeated acoustic stimuli. Many EZ-IC units respond to acoustic stimuli and/or to stimulation of the spinal somatosensory system (Aitkin, Dickhaus, and Schult, et al., 1978). Most units in the CN-IC and EZ-IC are influenced by stimulation of both ears, while auditory units in the IZ-IC tend to be responsive only to contralateral stimulation.

The majority of IC units that are affected by acoustic stimuli respond to tone bursts with an initial burst of spikes that may or may not be followed by a silent period and a sustained discharge (Rose, Greenwood, and Goldberg, et al., 1963). The initial spike burst is the only stable feature of the IC On unit response under all stimulus conditions. The IC units producing a sustained discharge with a Pause pattern under certain stimulus conditions might produce Build On, Suppressed, or Off patterns under other stimulus conditions. Some IC units with low CF appear to be capable of synchronizing their discharges with low-frequency sinusoids (Rose, Gross, and Geisler, et al., 1966). The IC units that produce a stable initial burst of discharges to tones respond with uniform latencies at all but near threshold levels of click stimuli (Hind, Goldberg, and Greenwood, et al., 1963). Variable and usually longer click latencies are exhibited by IC units that do not respond with a stable initial spike burst to CF tone bursts.

Morphologic Correlates of IC Unit Types

The description of the cell groups forming the IC is still in a state of flux, as is the terminology used to designate the cell groups and cell types of the IC (Geniec and Morest, 1971; Rockel and Jones, 1973a). The specifications of the cell areas and cell types providing LL input to the IC are also still in dispute (Roth, Aitkin, and Andersen, et al., 1978; Adams, 1979). There are very little single-unit data useful for correlating unit type to cell morphology other than for relating response characteristics to unit location within the major IC divisions.

The CN-IC is the primary receiving area of the ascending lateral lemniscal fibers; it also receives corticofugal and intrinsic inputs. Fibers from the contralateral CNC, the ipsilateral MSO and VNLL, and from the ipsilateral and contralateral LSO and DNLL end within the CN-IC. The majority of CN-IC units are excited by stimulation of the contralateral ear and are affected by stimulation of both ears. Approximately one-third of the binaural units are excited by stimulation of either ear and exhibit a wide CF range. Many produce a spike output to binaural stimuli that is greater than the output to stimulation of either ear alone. Many of the low-CF (< 3 kHz) binaural units exhibit a relationship between spike output and interaural time or phase differences. The binaural, ipsilaterally suppressed units have CF between 1 and 21 kHz and comprise half of the binaural CN-IC units. These units are sensitive to interaural intensity differences. The CN-IC monaural units are excited by stimulation of the contralateral ear and appear to be concentrated in caudal areas of the nucleus. A few CN-IC units are monaural and ipsilaterally excited, or binaural and contralaterally suppressed.

The tuning curves of the CN-IC units resemble those of AN units, although some are reported to lack a low frequency "tail" segment. The CN-IC is tonotopically organized; low-CF units are located dorsolateral to the higher CF units, in agreement with anatomical studies (Osen, 1972; Elverland, 1978). Merzenich and Reid (1974) report that most CN-IC units produce a phasic onset discharge to monaural tone bursts. The data of Rose and coworkers (1963) suggest that both Pause and On units occur within the CN-IC. The CN-IC units sensitive to interaural time delays are equally divided into those with short (4 to 5 msec) and long (15 msec) latencies to monaural clicks (Benevento, Coleman, and Loe, 1970).

The CN-IC is the major source of acoustic input to the next stage of the central auditory system, i.e., the medial geniculate body of the thalamus. Some of the axons of the CN-IC neurons decussate and join the uncrossed CN-IC axons contralaterally to form the brachium of the inferior colliculus. Most of the CN-IC axons are binaurally responsive and carry information concerning binaural intensity level or interaural time, phase, or intensity differences.

Corticofugal fibers arising from auditory cortex and intrinsic IC axons end in the IZ-IC. Lateral lemniscal fibers, perhaps from the DNLL, may terminate in the deeper, large-cell layer of the IZ-IC. The IZ-IC units are excited by stimulation of the contralateral ear, with the ipsilateral ear often ineffective when stimulated alone or simultaneously with the contralateral ear. The few binaural units appear to be more narrowly tuned than the monaural units. The inability of the IZ-IC units to reliably respond to repetitive tone bursts is related to the repetition rate of the burst. Changing the frequency of the tone will result in resumption of the response as long as the frequency is varied with each burst presentation. The failure of IZ-IC units to respond to repetitive stimuli prevents the characterization of their discharge patterns. The contribution of the IZ-IC to the ascending auditory pathway appears to be minor.

The EZ-IC receives input from the ascending somatosensory system, the cerebral cortex, and from other IC neurons. Approximately half of the EZ-IC units exhibit bimodality and are influenced by acoustic and somatosensory stimulation. The remaining units are almost equally divided into those influenced by acoustic or somatosensory stimuli. The majority of the units responsive to acoustic stimuli are binaural with the contralateral ear having an excitatory effect. Low rates of tone burst repetition (1 burst/2 sec) are required to elicit reliable responses from EZ-IC units. Their tuning curves are wider and more irregular than those of CN-IC units. The EZ-IC appears to be tonotopically organized (high-CF units located laterally to the low-CF units). Their discharge patterns to tone bursts are divided equally into "sustained" and On-type. While the majority of the bimodal units are excited by acoustic stimuli and inhibited by somatosensory stimuli, a small group are excited by both. The EZ-IC may contribute to the lateral tegmental system which provides an ascending input to regions of the medial geniculate body that do not receive input from the CN-IC.

IC Unit Responses and the Click-Evoked Potential

A few of the binaural CN-IC units have been demonstrated to be capable of discharging to clicks with relatively short (3 to 5 msec) uniform latencies. However, the click-elicited discharges of most IC units have not yet been fully described.

The Human Inferior Colliculus

The IC of the human and the cat share numerous common features (Geniec and Morest, 1971). The cell types observed in the cat IC are homologous to those observed in the human IC and are similarly organized. Within the cat and human CN-IC the laminar arrangement of the bipolar neurons occur parallel to the lateral lemniscal fibers. However, the large bipolar neurons tend to be located in the lateral regions of the cat CN-IC and are more widely distributed in the human CN-IC. The IZ-IC of the cat and human occupies a large portion of the IC and, according to Geniec and Morest (1971), can be distinguished from the other areas of the IC by their cortical architecture. The neurons within the EZ-IC of the cat correspond to those within the EZ-IC of the human.

NEUROPHYSIOLOGY OF HIGHER AUDITORY STRUCTURES

The Medial Geniculate Body of the Thalamus

The medial geniculate body (MGB) is a complex neural structure that receives ascending multisensory input and descending corticofugal input. The major subdivisions of the MGB include the ventral (V-MGB), medial

(M-MGB), and dorsal (D-MGB) cell groups (Fig. 4-2). The V-MGB is the chief thalamic receiving area for acoustic information arising from the IC. The M-MGB receives multimodal sensory input via the lemniscal and ascending thalamic and tegmental tracts. The D-MGB may receive polysensory input from the lateral tegmental system.

While few of the D-MGB units are responsive to acoustic stimuli, the vast majority of M-MGB and V-MGB units respond to tone bursts and clicks (Aitkin and Webster, 1972; Aitkin, 1973). Most of the acoustically responsive MGB units are excited by stimulation of the contralateral ear and are either binaurally excited or binaural and ipsilaterally suppressed. MGB units discharge spontaneously, even under barbiturate anesthesia (Galambos, Rose, and Bromiley, et al., 1952). The discharges elicited from most MGB units by a monaural tone burst are described as extremely complex and difficult to classify (Galambos, 1952). A long period (50 to 400 msec) of decreased spontaneous activity appears to be a typical feature of the response, with the degree and duration of the suppression related to stimulus level. According to Galambos (1952), a Pause pattern consisting of an initial discharge followed by a silent period of decreased spontaneous activity and a later sustained discharge may be characteristic of MGB discharge patterns. Others (Aitkin and Webster, 1972; Aitkin, 1973) report that most MGB units are incapable of producing a sustained discharge and typically produce an initial burst of spikes succeeded by a suppression of spontaneous activity that may be followed by a late transient discharge (Fig. 4-5, Pau-T). The complex discharge patterns described by Dunlop, Itzkowic, and Aitkin (1969) were elicited with binaural stimuli and may or may not be typical of the monaural responses of MGB units. The responses to monaural tone bursts appear to be extremely variable with the repetition of the same stimulus eliciting On-suppressed, Pause, Suppressed-long-latency, or Suppress-off discharge patterns in an unpredictable manner (Galambos, 1952) (Fig. 4-5, Complex Type). The discharge pattern elicited from an MGB unit also depends upon stimulus conditions (e.g., tone frequency and level, stimulus repetition rate and duration, and interaural differences). Low-CF MGB units do not appear to discharge in synchrony with low-frequency stimuli.

The responses of MGB units to monaural clicks have been described to be of three types (Aitkin, Dunlop, and Webster, 1966). Almost half of the units may or may not produce an initial discharge (latency between 8 and 16 msec), which is succeeded by a silent period of suppressed spontaneous activity that lasts from 50 to 200 msec, in turn followed by a Chopper-type discharge that may last from 1 to 2 sec. Clicks presented at repetition rates greater than 1 click/sec or at moderate to high levels may fail to elicit the initial onset discharge and produce an initial silent period with latency between 10 and 20 msec. The initial response of approximately one third of the MGB units to clicks is the suppression of spontaneous activity with a latency that varies from 8 to 40 msec. This initial silent period lasts from 40 to 200 msec and is immediately followed by a transient discharge of variable duration. Over one fifth of the units may respond with a pure onset discharge character- ized by an initial short burst of spikes with latencies between 7 and 25 msec (Aitkin and Dunlop, 1968). Some of these units respond within 7 to 10 msec of the click with a very uniform latency. Others, with longer latencies (11 to 25 msec), respond more variably and are also unable to follow click rates much above 3 clicks/sec; the units with shorter latencies may follow rates in excess of 20 clicks/sec.

Morphologic Correlates of MGB Unit Types

Although the response characteristics of individual MGB units are com- plex and difficult to specify, MGB morphology appears to be fairly simple when compared to the CNC and SOC (Morest, 1964). The complexity of the responses of the MGB units may result from the integration of acoustic infor- mation already processed at lower levels of the auditory system, from the in- fluence of corticofugal and intrinsic connections within the MGB, and from the polysensory inputs to the MGB.

The tufted neurons of the V-MGB receive acoustic information from the CN-IC, as well as receiving corticofugal input and intrinsic MGB input. The V-MGB projects to the principal auditory cortex; it is considered to be the primary auditory nucleus of the thalamus. The majority of the V-MGB units are responsive to binaural stimulation, with over half excited by stimu- lation of both ears. Less than one third of these binaurally excited units pro- duce an output related to binaural intensity level. Approximately one fifth of the units are binaural and ipsilaterally suppressed, tend to have CF above 6 kHz, and are sensitive to interaural intensity differences. Those binaural units that are tuned to lower frequencies tend to be sensitive to interaural time dif- ferences. The tuning curves of the V-MGB units vary in shape, even for units with similar CFs, and tend to be broader than those of AN units. Although binaural units appear to be influenced by a similar range of frequencies de- livered to the two ears, the tuning curves for the two ears may be dissimilar in shape and in CF. Most of the units produce monaural STB discharge patterns characterized by an initial burst of spikes and a silent period that may or may not be followed by a later discharge. Less than one fifth of the units produce an Off response; even fewer produce a "sustained" response. The initial dis- charges of the V-MGB units can be abolished and a late discharge exhibited to tones with frequency in the upper and lower extremes of a unit's tuning curve. Units producing a variety of discharge patterns to clicks are encoun- tered within the V-MGB.

As in the EZ-IC, neurons in the M-MGB receive polysensory input, are broadly tuned, and exhibit an inability to respond to acoustic stimuli pre- sented at repetition rates much above 1/sec. The M-MGB receives acoustic input from the CN-IC and the lateral tegmental system, and sends its axons to areas in and around the auditory cortex. Although all regions of the M-MGB reportedly receive CN-IC input, units located in the rostral M-MGB have been found to be unresponsive to click stimuli (Love and Scott, 1969). Most rostral M-MGB units respond to vestibular and/or somatosensory stimuli, whereas units in the more caudal areas of M-MGB only respond to acoustic stimuli (Wepsic, 1966; Love and Scott, 1969). Many of the units sensitive to acoustic stimuli are binaural and ipsilaterally suppressed, and tend to have CFs greater than 6 kHz. Irregularly shaped tuning curves much wider than those of V-MGB units are characteristic of M-MGB units. An On discharge consisting of an initial spike burst followed by a very low level of activity is typical of many M-MGB unit responses to monaural tone bursts. Others produce a Pause discharge with a silent period lasting 200 to 300 msec, irrespective of the tone burst duration. Very few produce "Sustained," Off, or Long-latency discharges. Units with long and short click latencies appear to be found in the M-MGB, with the long-click-latency type forming over three quarters of the population (Love and Scott, 1969).

The multipolar cells of the D-MGB may receive multisensory input from the lateral tegmental system and send their axons to auditory cortical areas. Very few (if any) D-MGB units are responsive to acoustic stimuli.

MGB Units and the Click Evoked Potential

The first spike of an MGB unit discharge may occur within 7 to 125 msec of the click. Units producing a well synchronized, short-latency (7 to 10 msec) discharge appear to occur infrequently in the MGB. The vast majority of the click-driven MGB units appear to respond with a poorly synchronized first spike whose latency may shorten or lengthen with changes in click level or click repetition rate.

The Human Medial Geniculate Body

Comparing the MGB of the human and the cat is made difficult by the use of different terms and criteria to specify its subdivisions. Hassler (1959), using Nissl and myelin stains, subdivided the human MGB into four nuclear groups. The human MGB nucleus fibrosus appears to correspond to the cat V-MGB in containing fibers arranged in parallel horizontal layers. Compact multipolar cells are densely and regularly arranged within these fibers. The laminated arrangement of the fibers and cells within the nucleus fibrosus suggests that the human homolog of the cat V-MGB may also be tonotopically organized. Intrinsic MGB neurons occur infrequently in this area. In contrast, many larger intrinsic neurons are observed in the human MGB nucleus fasciculosus, which probably corresponds to the cat D-MGB. Medium-sized multipolar cells, smaller than those in the nucleus fibrosus, are irregularly and sparsely situated within a light feltwork of fibers. Large neurons with broad processes predominate in the human MGB nucleus magnocellularis. They are randomly organized along with medium and small cells and a few intrinsic cells within a dense fibrous plexus. The human MGB nucleus limitans may partially correspond to the cat suprageniculate nucleus, which Morest (1964) includes as part of the cat D-MGB. The nucleus limitans contains few myelinated fibers and elongated neurons with long dendritic processes. The nucleus fibrosus is the largest nucleus in the human MGB, while the D-MGB appears to occupy a larger area than the V-MGB in the cat.

The Auditory Cortex

The cortical areas responsive to acoustic stimuli have been subdivided on the basis of cytoarchitecture, connectivity and the appearance of auditory evoked potentials into a number of auditory cortical areas or fields (Woolsey, 1960). However, the cytoarchitectural boundaries and thalamic projection patterns are not clearly delimited, and the subdivisions of the acoustically responsive cortex may well be redefined on the basis of single-unit studies (Knight, 1977). For the present discussion, the principal auditory cortex (AC) includes the primary auditory cortex (AI), the secondary auditory cortex (AII), and the posterior ectosylvian gyrus (EP) (Fig. 4-2). While the V-MGB may project to all areas of the AC, its main termination site is area AI. The AC receives multimodal input from the D-MGB and the M-MGB, which also send fibers to cortical areas surrounding the AC. Association fibers interconnect the subdivisions of the AC to the AC, and the AC to surrounding cortex. Commissural fibers provide interhemispheric connections between symmetrical AC areas.

Most single unit studies of the AC have concentrated upon the area AI. The surface landmarks used to define the boundaries of the subdivisions of the AC are subject to great individual variability (Merzenich, Knight, and Roth, 1975; Brugge and Merzenich, 1973). Differences in the definition of AI and other experimental factors have led to some confusion over the response characteristics of AI units. The responses of AC units may also be affected by a number of nonauditory variables. Anesthetic agents may reduce the responsiveness of AC units to acoustic stimuli (Erulkar, Rose, and Davies, 1956). Surgical procedures (e.g., pressure on the cortex) may alter the discharge pattern or the responsiveness of certain types of AC units (Evans and Whitfield, 1964). In unanesthetized animals, the states of wakefulness and sleep modulate the excitability of AC units; even small body movements may have a dramatic effect on AC unit responses (Brugge and Merzenich, 1973). Chemicals used to immobilize unanesthetized animals may also alter the discharge patterns of AC units to acoustic stimuli (Goldstein, Hall, and Butterfield, 1968). The responsiveness of units located within the superficial layers of AI and in surrounding cortical areas appear to be more affected than that of units in the middle layers of AI. As a variety of experimental conditions have been used to study AC units, the abbreviations UA for unanesthetized, P for paralyzed, and R for restrained will be used herein to describe the type of preparation studied. As many studies have been carried out in monkey AI, data from these animals will be included.

Most AC units are binaurally responsive, with contralateral stimulation more effective than ipsilateral stimulation. The majority of AI units are binaurally excited; the response to binaural stimulation is greater than the response to monaural stimulation of either ear (Hall and Goldstein, 1968). However, for some binaurally excited units, simultaneous stimulation of both ears results in an output similar to that elicited by the more effective monaural stimulus. A small proportion of binaural units are sensitive to interaural intensity differences, while others with low CF (< 2.4 kHz) are sensitive to interaural time differences (Brugge, Dubrovsky, and Aitkin, et al., 1969).

Although many AI units in UA-P cats are spontaneously active, they tend to discharge at very low rates (< 1 spike/sec), with the vast majority firing at rates below 35 spikes/sec (Goldstein, Hall, and Butterfield, 1968). A large proportion of the AI units isolated on the basis of the occurrence of spontaneous activity respond to tone burst stimuli. Their tuning curves may be narrow and lack a low frequency "tail" segment, broader than AN unit tuning curves, or may exhibit two or more low threshold "tip" regions. Approximately half (Abeles and Goldstein, 1970) or most (Evan's comments in Merzenich, Roth, and Andersen, et al., 1977) AI units in UA cats are so widely tuned, multitipped, or so poorly responsive to tone bursts that unit CF is impossible to define. In anesthetized cats and monkeys, the majority of units in the middle layers of AI exhibit clearly defined CFs and precise tonotopic organization (Merzenich and Brugge, 1973; Merzenich, Knight, and Roth, 1975). However, the definition of unit "CF" in these and other studies describing precise tonotopic organization of AI is unclear, as it is not evident whether or how tuning curves were obtained from the units. Many AII units of anesthetized cats are sensitive to tonal stimuli but are so broadly tuned that their CFs cannot be defined.

The discharge patterns of AI units are extremely labile and may differ with repetition of the same stimulus, especially in UA animals. For many AI units, the discharge pattern elicited depends upon the stimulus frequency and level, and upon interaural stimulus differences. For the binaurally excited units, similar discharge patterns are not necessarily elicited by identical stimuli delivered to either ear or by binaural stimuli. Stimulus duration and repetition rate will also have an effect on discharge patterns. Although Erulkar and coworkers (1956) report that some acoustically responsive AC units in the lightly anesthetized cat produce "sustained" discharges to binaural continuous tones, nearly all AI units in the anesthetized cat and monkey produce an On discharge of 1 to 5 spikes to monaural and binaural tone bursts (Brugge and Merzenich, 1973). In a few cases, a late discharge may occur after a silent

period of 50 to 100 msec. Very few units produce a "sustained" or Off discharge. According to Evans and Whitfield (1964), who used binaural continuous tones, most AC units in the UA cat respond with an initial discharge,
followed by a silent period lasting 100 msec and a late discharge that is maintained for a variable period of time. In the UA-R monkey, the majority of AI
units produce a "sustained" response and nonmonotonic intensity functions
to 100 to 500 msec monaural tone bursts (Brugge and Merzenich, 1973). AI
units producing Suppression-off responses are not uncommon in the UA-R
monkey, while those producing On discharges are rarely encountered. In the
UA-P cat, most AI units discharge in a sustained manner to 100 msec
monaural tone bursts when stimulus level is near threshold, and produce a
transient On discharge at higher stimulus levels (Abeles and Goldstein,
1972). At high stimulus levels, the On discharge is followed by a silent period
and, in some cases, by a transient or long-lasting Off discharge. It is not clear
whether experimental conditions (e.g., the use of Flaxedil to paralyze cats),
species differences, and/or the different stimulus conditions are responsible
for producing conflicting results.

      In the UA-P cat, half of the AI units are unresponsive to monaural clicks
(Goldstein, Hall, and Butterfield, 1968). Other units may produce a time-
locked onset discharge, a discharge of long and variable latency, or a reduction of spontaneous activity to monaural clicks. Some units produce a short
latency (9 to 11 msec) On discharge of one or more spikes to binaural clicks
(de Ribaupierre, Goldstein, and Yeni-Komshian, 1972). These units are
more responsive to binaural than monaural clicks, respond with fairly fixed
latencies, and are capable of following rates up to 100 clicks/sec. Many of
them are broadly tuned and respond to monaural tone bursts with an On discharge. The click-suppressed units respond with a decrease in spontaneous
activity lasting 50 msec that may be followed by a transient increase in discharge. The tone burst responses of these units are a variety of types and are
not necessarily the Suppressed type.

Morphologic Correlates of AC Unit Activity

      The auditory cortex encompasses a large area of the cerebral cortex. In
the cat, it includes the anterior, middle, and posterior ectosylvian gyri, and
parts of the anterior sylvian gyrus, insular, and temporal cortex. Evoked-
potential and single unit responses to acoustic stimuli can be recorded also
from areas of the suprasylvian and anterolateral gyri, sensorimotor cortex,
and the second visual area. Area AI consists of the dorsal regions of the
middle ectosylvian gyrus, described cytoarchitecturally as koniocortex (Rose,
1949). It has a laminated structure, with thalamic inputs concentrated in the
middle layers (deep III and IV) and cortical inputs in the more superficial
layers. Large- and medium-sized cells are concentrated in and around layers
IV and VI. Within layer V, a thin, discontinuous band of large cells is situated

superficial to a thicker band of small-sized cells. Pyramidal cells of various sizes are found in layers II through VI, while medium-sized multipolar cells appear to be concentrated in layer IV (Wong, 1967). In anesthetized cats, acoustically driven units are most frequently encountered in the middle layers of AI (Merzenich, Knight, and Roth, 1975). Acoustically responsive units are encountered throughout the depth of AI of UA-P cats (Abeles and Goldstein, 1970). There appears to be little relationship between the depth of a unit and its tuning characteristics, CF, and the representation of the two ears. AI units are organized in vertical columns with similar CF and similar binaural representation in UA-P and anesthetized cats (Abeles and Goldstein, 1970; Imig and Adrián, 1977).

AC Units and the Click-Evoked Potential

AC units producing short latency (9 to 11 msec, perhaps wave VI or VII) discharges that are securely time-locked to binaural clicks appear to be located within AI in cats. They represent a small proportion of all acoustically responsive cortical units. Arousal states and body movement of unanesthetized subjects appear to have marked effects on the responsiveness of AI units and will therefore greatly effect their click-elicited discharges.

The Human Auditory Cortex

The auditory koniocortex of humans (area TC of von Economo, 1929) is located in a small patch of the dorsal surface of the superior temporal gyrus within the depths of the lateral fissure. The cellular architecture of the human temporal lobe has been described in great detail by von Economo (1929). According to Rose (1949), if the granular nature of the human TC is not stressed, the previous description of the cat AI is applicable to the human TC.

DISCUSSION

Single-unit studies of auditory units provide some insight into the possible contributions of unit spike potentials to the auditory BSER. The hypothesis that synchronized single-unit discharges may summate to produce specific components of the BSER is supported by the work of Antoli-Candela and Kiang (1978). Anatomic and neurophysiologic studies indicate that there are numerous spatially distributed central auditory cell groups and fiber tracts that may contribute to the BSER. The spike potentials generated in the cell soma, axon, or terminal endings, as well as the somatodendritic field potentials, may each contribute to the BSER. The complexity of the problem of specifying the locations of the generators of the various components of the BSER is obvious even at levels as low as the CNC. However, the data at hand suggest that not all auditory cell groups are capable of producing synchronized discharges and that the further removed a cell group is from the periphery the less synchronized are the discharges of its units.

Single-unit AN studies have elucidated the role of the tuning characteristics of auditory units in determining their responsiveness to click stimuli. The influence of the types and configurations of synapses on the response characteristics of central auditory neurons are exemplified by the synaptology and the behavior of CNC units. Most of the CNC units that are strongly influenced by their AN input (Primary-like, fast Chopper-type, On-T, and On-S types) respond reliably with stable latency and reproducible discharge patterns. They do not markedly alter their discharge patterns with changes in stimulus frequency or level. They also produce click-elicited discharges that are securely time-locked to clicks and synchronized with the click-elicited discharges of similar CNC units. In contrast, the responses of CNC units receiving a large nonprimary or nonascending input are often nonstationary, exhibit variable latencies, and are more influenced by anesthetic agents. They tend to produce Pause or On-W type discharge patterns and often modify discharge pattern with changes in stimulus frequency and level. The click-elicited discharge patterns of many of these units depend upon the spectral properties of the acoustic click, the tuning characteristics of the unit, and upon the interaction of the factors determining the discharge pattern that each of the spectral components of the acoustic click would elicit when presented alone.

The further removed an auditory unit is from the periphery the greater the nonascending input to the unit, and the more variable and complex the discharge patterns elicited from it (Fig. 4-9). Binaurally responsive units predominate, and the effects of stimulating the two ears may vary, depending upon a number of stimulus variables. Units producing "sustained" discharges occur less frequently, and the Pause and "Onset" type discharge patterns become more common. The response characteristics of these units resemble those of CNC units that receive a large nonprimary input. Fewer of these units appear to respond to click stimuli, and the discharge patterns elicited by clicks are difficult to predict from the tone-burst-elicited discharges. The number of units capable of producing time-locked discharges to clicks decreases, and the dispersion of first spike latencies appears to increase at each level of the auditory system.

One might predict that the spike potentials of few units above the level of the NLL contribute to the fast components of the click BSER. However, neither the tone-burst- nor the click-elicited auditory unit discharges above the level of the SOC have been studied in sufficient detail to support this prediction. There is considerable confusion and disagreement in the descriptions of the response characteristics of units above the level of the SOC. The effects of various stimulus parameters on discharge pattern, especially stimulus duration and repetition rate, have not been systematically explored, and more importantly, have not been controlled to minimize their effects on discharge

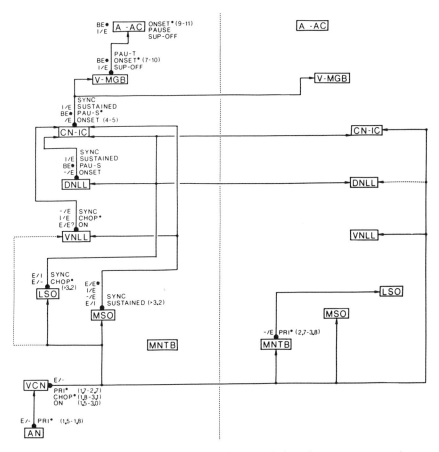

Figure 4-9. The main connections of cell groups believed to participate in the cat ascending auditory system. The DCN connections are not included, as the distribution of its axons have not yet been described in detail. The effects of stimulating the two ears are indicated to the left of the output of each cell group. The effects are ordered with the most frequently encountered type at the top of the list. The effect of stimulating the ear ipsilateral to the structure is indicated to the left of the slash; that of stimulating the contralateral ear is indicated to the right. An increase in discharge is excitatory (E) and a decrease is inhibitory (I). The binaurally excited (BE) units may be (1) excited by stimulation of either or both ears, (2) excited by stimulation of one ear and facilitated by the simultaneous stimulation of the opposite ear, or (3) may be excited and inhibited by binaural stimulation. The asterisk indicates that some of the low-CF units are sensitive to interaural phase or time of arrival differences. The major types of monaural STB-PST histograms generated are indicated to the right of the cell group output. The STB-PST histograms for units described to produce the "onset" or "sustained" types are unavailable for classification. The dot indicates the typical type of discharge elicited from the cell group. The range of the shortest click latencies obtained for each cell group is indicated in msec where the data are available for high-CF (> 3 kHz) units producing sharply time-locked discharges. It should be kept in mind that the proportion of units producing discharges synchronized to clicks and low-frequency tones decreases considerably from the auditory nerve to the primary area of auditory cortex.

pattern. Binaural stimuli are often used without first examining the monaural response and the effects of binaural stimulation on discharge pattern. While the use of anesthetic agents undoubtedly has some effect on the responses of central auditory units, most studies involving unanesthetized animals have confused matters by failing to control other experimental and stimulus variables acknowledged to influence the behavior of these units.

Our ability to predict the contributions of the single-unit spike potentials of a given central auditory cell group to the auditory evoked potential is limited by the lack of single-unit data. More systematic studies relating single unit responses to tonal and click stimuli, to cell group membership, and to the gross BSER are required. The importance of studying the responses to click *and* tonal stimuli, and of identifying cell group membership, cannot be overstressed. Because of the complexity and nonlinear behavior of the auditory system, the click cannot be considered an ideal stimulus for studying central auditory units. Some may be unresponsive to clicks (e.g., in AI-AC), and properties of a unit, as tones appear to be the most effective stimulus for central auditory units. Some may be unresponsive to clicks (e.g., in AI-IC), and awareness of this fact is relevant to the assessment of the value of the click BSER in localizing central auditory lesion sites. Knowledge of the unit location is required both to identify the cell groups producing synchronized click-evoked discharges and to provide a basis for determining the type of subsystem (reflex, feedback control, sensory, etc.) in which the unit functions. The correlation of the single-unit click responses of identified unit-neuron types with the auditory BSER may then be used to help identify the possible generators of components within the gross potential. A substantial treatment of these possibilities can be found in Chapter 7.

Michael M. Paparella
Timothy T. K. Jung

5 Disorders of the Auditory System

In order to successfully carry out ECochG and/or BSER testing, knowledge of the disorders of the auditory system is essential. In this chapter, these disorders will be reviewed, since most, if not all, auditory system disorders cause impairment of hearing, and as such may influence the resultant ECochG or BSER data. From Chapters 3 and 4, we know that the auditory system is anatomically divided into an external, middle, and inner ear, as well as central connections. It follows that the several disorders can best be considered along this continuum. While several evoked potentials do overlap in time, it is unclear whether the underlying anatomical regions functionally overlap. The logical sequel to this reasoning would suppose that disorders of the system may or may not overlap in causing aberrant evoked responses.

The first question to answer in diagnosing hearing loss with ECochG and BSER testing is, Was the hearing loss congenital or delayed in onset? Congenital deafness is usually not progressive, whereas delayed deafness may be progressive. Second, Is the deafness genetic or nongenetic? Approximately half of all profound deafness in children is genetic in origin. However, the ECochG/BSERs are certainly not pathognomonic for hereditary transmission. The third question in diagnosis concerns whether other anomalies accompany the hearing loss, which may alert the clinician to the possibility of involvement of more than one segment of the auditory system. A fourth question concerns whether the hearing loss will manifest itself in some atypical way via ECochG and BSER potentials.

DISORDERS OF THE EXTERNAL EAR

The external ear is composed of the auricle and the external auditory canal. Most of the disorders of the external ear are acquired and nongenetic. As it turns out, disorders of the external ear result in a conductive hearing loss and cause a latency delay as well as a dimunition of BSER amplitude.

Congenital: Genetic

Congenital Aural Atresia

Aural atresia may be uni- or bilateral, membraneous or osseous, appear as an independent entity or be associated with other malformations. The majority of atresias are inherited as an autosomal dominant mode with variable penetrance. Aural artresia or a nonpatent external auditory meatus will impede the sound from reaching the tympanic membrane. In practice, this causes a dimunition in the amplitude of the evoked potential. If certain waves are present, especially wave V, a corresponding prolongation of latency, or a displaced intensity-latency curve to the right on the abscissa occurs (Berlin, Gondra, and Casey, et al., 1978; Finitzo-Hieber, Hecox, and Cone, 1979; Mokotoff, Schulman-Galambos, and Galambos, 1977; Moore, 1978; Picton, 1978).

The associated malformation syndromes include Crouzon's disease and Treacher Collins syndrome (Nadol, 1979). They are classified as minor, moderate, or severe, depending on the degree of malformation. The middle-ear anomalies include deformed or absent stapes head and crura; absent, fused, or malformed malleus and incus; lack of incudostapedial connection; absence or reduction of tympanic cavity; and replacement of the tympanic membrane by a bony plate. Audiometric tests will show a nonprogressive conductive hearing loss, and a variable degree of sensorineural hearing loss. ECochG or BSER may show amplitude reduction and prolonged latency, since most of these conditions interfere with the adequate conduction of intensity to the cochlea (Finitzo-Hieber, Hecox, and Cone, 1979). Different wave patterns and clearly delineated amplitude and latency characteristics for each of the above conditions have not yet been documented. In bilateral aural atresia, surgical correction is recommended when the child is 5 years of age; in unilateral atresia, not until the patient reaches adolescence. BSER results can help make a decision about surgical correction (Finitzo-Hieber, Hecox, and Cone, 1979).

Acquired: Genetic

Cerumen Impaction

Perhaps the most common cause of hearing loss from within the external auditory canal is cerumen impaction, preventing sound waves from reaching the drum. Ear wax is the product of sebaceous, apocrine, and ceruminous glands, which are located in the cartilaginous portion of the external auditory canal. There are two types of ear wax: the wet, sticky type, which is dominant (Caucasian), and the dry type (Mongolian) (Matsunga, 1962). Removal of cerumen by the physician is commonly done with a curette or by water irrigation prior to performing either ECochG or BSER procedures.

Acquired: Nongenetic

Otitis Externa

Infection in the skin of the external auditory canal may occur as a result of certain predisposing factors, such as change of pH of the canal skin from normal acid to alkaline, hot and wet climate changes, and mild trauma (e.g., cleaning the ear, or excessive swimming). The spectrum of infections and inflammations include bacterial, fungal, and viral agents or dermatoses. The prominent symptoms are pain and small drainage from the ear. Under typical testing conditions when this condition is present, pressure from the earphone placed on the ear may exacerbate the pain. Testing with a remotely located speaker will allow testing to proceed, but one should be cautious in interpretation of the evoked potentials (described in Chapter 8). There usually is no lasting hearing loss unless the swelling of the skin completely closes the ear canal.

Furunculosis

This condition is an infection of pilosebaceous follicles of the fibrocartilaginous portion of the external auditory canal usually caused by *Staphylococcus aureus* or *S. albus*. Pain is quite marked because of limited room for the swelling or edema. The precautionary measures in testing noted above are certainly applicable to this condition.

Diffuse Otitis Externa

This infection is known as "swimmer's ear," and is predominantly caused by the *Pseudomonas* group. Severe pain and canal edema usually requires wick placement. It can certainly be argued that if the edema completely blocks the external auditory meatus, a prolonged latency and amplitude reduction of evoked potentials will be noted. At times, it may be useful to resort to the use of bone conduction ECochG/BSER testing (Berlin, et al., 1978; Moore and Harris, in preparation).

Herpes Zoster Oticus (Ramsey Hunt Syndrome)

Virus inflammation of the geniculate ganglion is accompanied by facial paralysis, otalgia, and a herpetic eruption of the external ear. The vestibular and acoustic fibers of the VIIIth cranial nerve may be involved. Alterations in the potentials can be observed due to the conductive as well as sensorineural components. In practice, one should exercise extreme caution in interpreting the resultant evoked potentials.

Malignant External Otitis

This refers to external otitis in elderly diabetics caused by *Pseudomonas* that results in osteomyelitis of the temporal bone and skull base, with palsies of facial and other cranial nerves, and even death. Treatment may involve long-term intravenous carbenicillin, gentamycin, and surgery (Chandler, 1977). Our literature search failed to turn up any evoked potential testing done on patients exhibiting this condition.

Relapsing Polychondritis

This rare disease of unknown etiology is characterized by recurrent, painful involvement of multiple cartilaginous structures including auricles, nasal cartilages, larynx, trachea, bronchi, eustachian tubes, peripheral joints, and costal cartilages. The common presenting signs and symptoms are recurrent auricular chondritis, arthralgia, nasal chondritis, ocular inflammation, chondritis of respiratory tract, and cochlear and vestibular changes. With recurrent auricular inflammation, the ear may assume a cauliflower appearance and the external canal may become stenotic.

Cochlear and vestibular involvement with accompanying sensorineural hearing loss, tinnitus, and vertigo may be encountered in approximately 50 percent of the cases. Histology reveals chondritis and perichondritis with lacunar breakdown and neutrophil infiltration. The sedimentation rate may be elevated and the antinuclear factor may be positive. No correlative data exist for evoked potential findings.

Steroids and immunosuppressive drugs have been used with some success in order to treat such cases; Dapsone has been used with encouraging results (Barrance, et al., 1976; Diamiani and Levine, 1979).

Neoplasms

The external ear may be the site of any benign or malignant tumor. This discussion will be limited to those lesions in the external auditory canal which may affect hearing and thus affect ECochG and BSER waves.

Benign Tumors

Exostosis and Osteoma

Exostosis is more common than osteoma; it consists of rounded nodules of compact bone. The nodules rarely occur during childhood and are usually bilateral. While their exact etiology is unknown, they most frequently occur in people who do a great deal of swimming in cold salt water. The individuals are usually asymptomatic and require no treatment. The nodules may occasionally become large enough to cause obstruction and impair hearing; surgical excision may then be advisable.

Osteoma is a relatively rare, single, cancellous bony tumor. Osteomas tend to enlarge and eventually occlude the meatus, resulting in hearing loss and discomfort. Surgical removal should be universally advised.

Keratosis Obturans

This is a rare condition, in which a desquamating pearly white epithelial squamous mass develops deep in the canal. It is probably related to faulty migration of squamous epithelial cells from the tympanic membrane surface and adjacent canal. This lesion is frequently associated with bronchiectasis and sinusitis. Pain is a common presenting symptom; deafness and otorrhea may be present. Treatment consists of periodic removal of the accumulated debris.

Adenoma

Adenomas are rare tumors that originate from sebaceous glands in the fibrocartilaginous portion of the external auditory canal. They usually are small, soft, painless swellings at the entrance of the meatus. They can become large enough to cause obstruction of the canal, resulting in a reduced sound input to the cochlea, thereby affecting the resultant evoked potential. Treatment is complete surgical excision followed by electrocauterization of the tumor bed.

Ceruminoma

This tumor, originating from the ceruminous glands, is uncommon; it presents as a smooth, intraverted, polypoid swelling in the outer end of the meatus. The presenting symptom is usually a blocked feeling in the ear. Regular follow-up is necessary after surgical excision because of common local recurrence and potential for malignancy.

Malignant Tumors

Though malignancies of the external auditory canal are rare (Tabb, et al., 1964), early diagnosis is imperative if good results are to be expected (Nelms and Paparella, 1968).

Common symptoms include pain, otorrhea, bleeding, fullness, and decrease of hearing. (Such cases have not been documented in the ECochG/BSER literature.) Pain usually occurs in the early stage and may be intense and "out of proportion" to the physical findings. Occasionally, deafness may initially occur, with facial nerve paralysis as a later development. It is important to biopsy any suspicious growth in the canal.

Squamous cell carcinoma is the most common malignancy of the canal (70 percent). The remainder are adenocarcinoma and basal cell carcinoma (Fig. 5-1), with rare cases of adenoid cystic carcinoma, mucoepidemoid carcinoma, melanoma, and various sarcomas.

Recommended treatment consists of wide surgical excision combined with radiation therapy. It is essential to distinguish the location of the origin of tumors. Anterior canal lesions spread through lymphatics in the fissures of

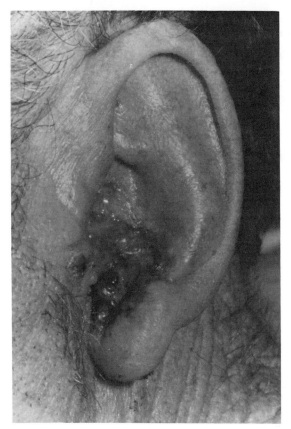

Figure 5-1. Basal cell carcinoma of the auricle and external
auditory canal.

Santorini. Adequate surgery includes removal of the drumhead, anterior
wall, condyle, and parotid gland for isolated anterior canal lesions. One should
consider total removal of the temporal bone in instances of middle-ear or
mastoid involvement.

Foreign Bodies

Foreign bodies in the external auditory canal are commonly seen in children or in institutions for the mentally retarded and mentally ill (Moore,
Baker, and McCoy, 1969). Various objects may be encountered, including
cotton, beans, corn, rosary beads, small stones, etc. Symptoms of irritation,
pain, and hearing loss may result. Foreign bodies of a vegetable substance will
expand and may become painful if the ear is irrigated. It is safest to remove
foreign bodies under direct visualization with instruments such as an alligator-
type forceps, fine hooks, or cerumen loops. The first attempt of removal has
the best chance. General anesthesia and careful removal under an operating
microscope may be called for; it should not be delayed. Fundamental to these
procedures are their use prior to ECochG/BSER testing.

Acquired Atresia

Canal atresia can follow surgery, trauma, or intractable canal infection. Surgery will help restore patency and hearing (Paparella and Meyerhoff, 1978). It can be argued, within limits, that ECochG/BSER testing in cases such as these would rarely require masking of the contralateral ear, since crossover is confined to certain stimulus configurations (Finitzo-Hieber, et al., 1979).

DISEASES OF THE MIDDLE EAR

The tympanic membrane, ossicles, and air chamber of the middle ear conduct sound from the air in the external ear to the fluid in the inner ear. Diseases of the middle ear may involve one or more of these components, thus producing conductive hearing loss. We already know that interference with the air-conducting component diminishes the size of the evoked potentials. Such conductive hearing losses will show a characteristic lengthening of the latency of BSER waves (e.g., waves I and V) and the ECochG (N_1) response. A true conductive component, on the other hand, will still exhibit normal interwave latencies (e.g., wave I vs wave V) (Berlin, et al., 1978).

Inflammation of the middle ear (otitis media) is one of the most common health problems, especially in the pediatric age group. Since the widespread use of antibiotics, the rates of mortality and serious complications resulting from acute otitis media have been lowered. However, chronic and insidious forms of otitis media and ensuing morbidity with hearing loss remain common. Because otitis media causes a hearing loss, with perhaps a resultant language impairment and speech delay in children, recent attention to the several consequences of otitis media has appeared in the results of the literature (Hanson and Ulvestad, 1979).

Congenital and genetic disorders of the middle ear with conductive hearing loss, though less common, may be remedied through microscopic reconstructive surgery of the middle ear.

Congenital Diseases

Hearing loss in this category may occur alone or as a part of many syndromes. Treatment is usually accomplished via surgery or mechanical amplification.

Genetic Diseases

Middle-Ear Anomalies with Branchial Arch Anomalies

Congenital aural atresia. This hereditary disorder of autosomal dominance is frequently accompanied by middle ear anomalies (discussed before).

Mandibulofacial dysostosis (Treacher Collins syndrome). Middle-ear abnormalities in this hereditary disorder of dominant inheritance include deformities of malleus, incus, stapes, absence of the tensor tympani muscle, stapedial muscle and tendon, and pyramidal eminence. There may be canal atresia. The tympanic membrane and mastoid antrum may be absent.

Other associated anomalies include antimongolian slant of the eyes with colobomas of the lower lids, absence of medial eyelashes, micrognathia, short palate, and hypoplasia of the malar bone. The audiogram shows a nonprogressive conductive hearing loss. A sensorineural component may coexist. The logical sequel to these conditions is a myriad of ECochG/BSER findings that affect latency, amplitude, and the form of the electrical potentials (Nadol, 1979).

Middle-Ear Anomalies with Skeletal Anomalies

Acrocephalosyndactylia (Apert's syndrome). This autosomal dominant disorder, with craniofacial dysostosis, syndactylia, brachiocephaly, hypertelorism, saddle nose, high arched palate, and spina bifida may in addition have congenital stapedial footplate fixation. The clinician should remember the possible conductive and/or sensorineural nature of such a condition.

Klippel-Feil syndrome. This is a rare recessive hereditary disorder with deformity of the cervical spine, short immobile neck, low hairline of the neck, spina bifida, and Spregel's scapular deformity; it predominately affects females. The middle-ear anomalies include an elongated stapes with the anterior crus fused to the cochleariform process, absent lenticular process, fused short process of the incus to the floor of the attic, and a slit-like incudomalleal joint. The clinical caution noted above is also in order here.

Craniofacial dysostosis (Crouzon's disease). This rare autosomal dominant disorder includes craniosynostosis, exophthalmos, hypoplastic maxilla and mandible, hypertelorism, parrot-beaked nose, and mandibular prognathism. The middle-ear anomalies include stapes malformation with bony fusion, malleus ankylosis, and narrowing of the middle ear space. Stenosis or atresia of the external auditory canal may also be present.

Craniometaphysical dysplasia (Pyle's disease). This is a rare hereditary autosomal dominant disorder with hypertelorism, saddle nose, prognathism, posterior choanal atresa and obliteration of paranasal sinuses. The middle-ear anomalies include encasement of the malleus in bone, deformed and fixed incus, and obliteration of mastoid air cells.

Oral-facial-digital syndrome (Mohr's syndrome). This is a hereditary, autosomal recessive disorder with widely spaced medial canthi, flat nasal ridge, high arched palate, hypoplastic body of the mandible, lobuled tongue, and digital abnormalities. The middle-ear anomalies include blunting of the long process of the incus and absence of the incudostapedial joint.

Otopalatodigital syndrome. This is a hereditary autosomal recessive disorder with frontal and occipital bossing, hypertelorism, small mandible, cleft palate and digital anomalies. Middle-ear anomalies include fetal forms of the ossicles.

Middle-Ear Anomalies with Connective Tissue Anomalies

Achondroplasia. This is a hereditary dominant disorder with dwarfism and shortened extremities. The middle-ear deformities include fusion of ossicles to the surrounding bony structures. There are also inner-ear deformities, including a deformed cochlea and thickened intercochlear partitions.

Middle-Ear Anomalies with Eye Anomalies

Congenital facial diplegia (Moebius syndrome). This rare autosomal disorder (dominant or recessive) manifests ophthalmoplegia facial diplegia, involvement of cranial nerves III, V, VII, XII, and malformation of extremities. The middle-ear anomalies include an ossicular mass without clear-cut identification of the stapes and oval or round window deformities. Also associated are auricular malformation and atresia of the external auditory canal.

Nongenetic Diseases

Intrauterine factors (such as viral infection or ototoxicity) may be associated with nongenetic middle-ear abnormalities and conductive or mixed hearing loss.

Congenital cholesteatoma of the middle ear. Cholesteatoma is usually acquired; the exception is a rare congenital form. The middle-ear findings include an epidermoid mass with or without bony resorption. A conductive hearing loss may result from involvement of ossicles or tympanic membrane. Sound transmission to the cochlea is affected in this instance.

Turner's syndrome. The middle-ear anomalies in this disorder (caused by chromosomal aberration) include malformation of stapes, poor development of the mastoid air cells, and low-set ears.

Chromosomal abnormalities. Both trisomy 13-15 and trisomy 18 syndromes have multiple middle-ear anomalies, such as canal atresia and ossicular deformities. (Associated anomalies will be described later in this chapter.)

Others.   The congenital rubella syndrome and thalidomide ototoxicity are known to produce multiple middle-ear anomalies; these will be described later in this chapter.

Acquired or Delayed Onset Diseases

Genetic

Otosclerosis.   This primary disease of the labyrinthine capsule is transmitted by autosomal dominant genes. It is most common in Caucasians and much less common in Orientals and Afro-Americans. The clinical onset is usually post-pubertal, most often occurring in the third or fourth decade. Otosclerosis is usually bilateral.

The main surgical findings are bony fixation of the stapedial footplate to the otic capsule resulting in a conductive or mixed hearing loss (Fig. 5-2). Stapedectomy is the treatment of choice (Fig. 5-3).

Osteogenesis imperfecta (Van der Hoeve's disease).   Osteogenesis imperfecta is an hereditary autosomal dominant disorder with fragile bones, large skull, blue sclera, triangular facies, and hemorrhagic tendencies. The hearing loss is clinically evident by the patient's third decade and is usually conductive, due to stapes fixation, or of the mixed type. Stapedectomy may be considered.

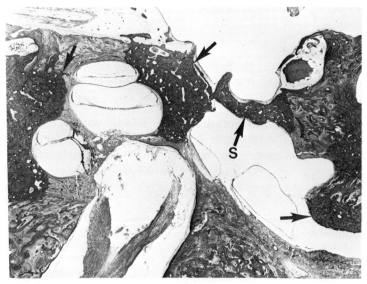

Figure 5-2.   Extensive otosclerosis. Large areas of otosclerotic bone (arrows) are seen surrounding the cochlea and semicircular canals. The stapes footplate is involved and fixed (Stapes (S)).

Paget's disease. This hereditary autosomal dominant disease of os-
teitis deformans with deformities of the skull and long bones primarily affects
elderly males. Middle-ear anomalies include pagetic bone growth in the
epitympanum with fixation of the malleus head, incus body, and stapes. Associated anomalies of the external are seen, and inner ear anomalies include
narrowing of the organ of Corti. The hearing loss is either mixed or purely
sensorineural. Stapedectomy may be considered.

Albers-Schönberg disease. This is a recessive disorder of osteope-
trosis, with brittle sclerotic bones, cranial neuropathies, large skull and man-

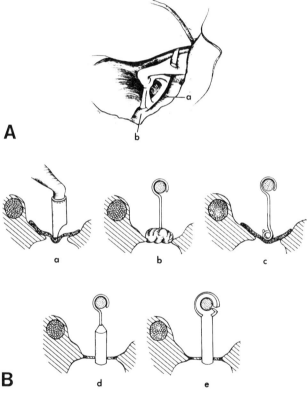

Figure 5-3. Stapedectomy. A. The otologist's microscopic
view, showing adequate footplate exposure achieved when
facial canal (a) and pyramidal process (b) are seen. B. Stapedectomy prostheses: a. vein-polyethylene strut (Shea); b. wire
fat (Schuknecht); c. wire on compressed Gelfoam (House); d.
wire Teflon piston; e. Teflon piston (Shea). (Reprinted with permission from Paparella, M. M., & Shumrick, D. A. (Eds.). *Otolaryngology. Vol. 2.* Philadelphia: W.B. Saunders, 1980, p.
1650.)

dible, absence of paranasal sinuses, choanal atresia, and facial paralysis. Middle-ear anomalies include the fetal form of the stapes, abnormal malleus and incus, and a small middle-ear space. The hearing loss is primarily conductive.

Nongenetic

Disease of the tympanic membrane. Diseases of the tympanic membrane usually are associated with pathologic changes of the middle ear and mastoid. The tympanic membrane may become thickened due to inflammation, or may contain white plaques due to deposition of hyalinized collagen in its middle layer (tympanosclerosis). The tympanic membrane may be retracted due to negative pressure in the middle ear, or may bulge when fluid, infection, or a mass is present in the middle ear. Perforation of the tympanic membrane may result from trauma or from acute or chronic otitis media. Myringitis, primarily an inflammation of the tympanic membrane, may accompany middle-ear inflammation. In hemorrhagic or bullous myringitis, the most notable finding is bleb formation on the tympanic membrane.

Disorders of the eustachian tube. The eustachian tube ventilates and drains the middle ear. Obstruction of the eustachian tube from whatever cause induces fluid in the middle ear and results in a conductive hearing loss.

Nonsuppurative Middle-Ear Inflammatory Disease

Aerotitis. Aerotitis is caused by relative negative pressure in the middle ear with rapid loss of altitude, during flying or underwater diving. Transudate type of fluid accumulates in the middle ear and results in a conductive hearing loss. This may be treated with decongestants and eustachian-tube exercise. If the problem persists, myringotomy can be considered.

Serous and mucoid otitis media. The middle-ear fluid problem is currently the most prevalent cause of hearing loss in school-age children. Serous otitis media is mainly caused by transudation of plasma from the blood vessels into the middle ear space due to hydrostatic pressure differences. Mucoid otitis media results from active secretion from glands that line the middle-ear cleft. Eustachian-tube dysfunction is a major underlying factor. Medical management includes antibiotics (if bacterial infection is present), antihistamines, decongestants, a combination of antihistamines/decongestants (although recently found to be of limited value), and eustachian-tube exercises. Surgical management, consisting of a myringotomy and insertion of a ventilation tube (Fig. 5-4), is reserved for those patients who are refractory to medical treatment.

Acute purulent otitis media. Normal middle-ear mucosa is protected by physiologic action of cilia, mucus-secreting enzymes, antibodies, and subepithelial cellular components. Acute otitis media is caused when the

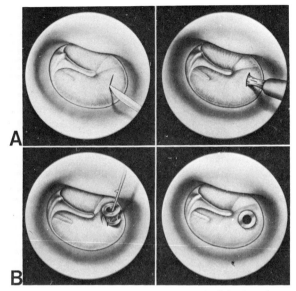

Figure 5-4. A (left). Myringotomy, A (right). Aspiration of fluid. B (left). Insertion of tympanostomy tube. B (right). Tympanostomy tube in place. (Reprinted with permission from Paparella, M. M., & Shumrick, D. A. (Eds.). *Otolaryngology. Vol. 2.* Philadelphia: W.B. Saunders, 1980, p. 1419.)

normal physiologic mechanism is somehow disrupted, e.g., obstruction or contamination of the eustachian tube. The most frequently recovered bacteria in children under 5 years of age is *Hemophilus influenzae*; in children five years or older, *Diplococcus pneumoniae* and betahemolytic streptococci are most often recovered. Symptoms include pain, fever, and malaise. The tympanic membrane typically is red and bulging. Medical treatment with antibiotics and decongestants is usually sufficient, but myringotomy may be required if there is no evidence of resolution (Søhoel, Mair, and Elverland, et al., 1979).

Chronic otitis media; mastoiditis. This refers to a permanent tympanic membrane perforation with (active) and without (inactive) otorrhea. Tympanic membrane perforations may be central, marginal, or attic. The otorrhea may be mucoid, from activity of secretory glands, or a foul-smelling discharge of grayish-yellow hue, suggesting the presence of a cholesteatoma. The hearing loss is usually conductive from osseous destruction; it may also be sensorineural. Pain is an uncommon symptom and its presence is a serious sign. Vertigo in a patient with chronic otitis media suggests the presence of a fistula of the labyrinth.

The frequent pathologic conditions are cholesteatoma (keratinizing squamous epithelium that becomes entrapped in the middle-ear space and mastoid (Fig. 5-10), or granulation tissue, which can cause bony resorption and severe changes throughout the middle ear and mastoid. Cholesterol granuloma is a special kind of granulation tissue with interspersed giant cells (Fig. 5-5). Treatment includes local cleaning, ear drops, and, frequently, surgery. Surgery is aimed at eradicating infection (mastoidectomy) and maintaining or improving hearing (tympanoplasty). In Figure 5-6, different tympanoplasty types are described. Possible complications of otitis media and mastoiditis are listed in Table 5-1.

ECochG/BSER results with most patients who exhibit otitis media, display longer latencies for wave V, but the input–output curve (Intensity-latency function) almost nearly parallels the normal curve (Fria and Sabo, 1980; Wiederhold, Martinez, and Paull, et al., 1978a; Wiederhold, Martinez, and Scott, et al., 1978b; Yamada, Yagi, and Yamane, et al., 1975). Interestingly, even when a middle-ear "pathology" is artificially created, the results can be quite similar to those of otitis media (Wiederhold, et al., 1978a, 1978b; Yamada, et al., 1975).

Tumors of the Middle Ear and Mastoid

A variety of benign and malignant tumors can originate from the middle ear and mastoid. These tumors can be primary, meaning their origin is in the temporal bone, or secondary, indicating that they have metastasized to the temporal bone from either a distant or adjacent site.

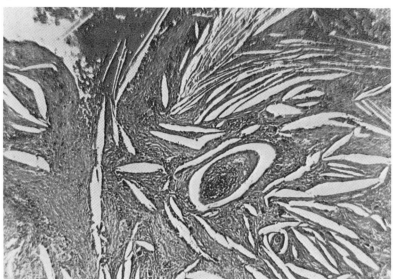

Figure 5-5. Cholesterol granuloma. Cholesterol clefts are seen in the dense fibrous granulation tissue bed with interspersed giant cells. (Reprinted with permission from Paparella, M. M., & Shumrick, D. A. (Eds.). *Otolaryngology. Vol. 2.* Philadelphia: W.B. Saunders Co., 1973, p. 109.)

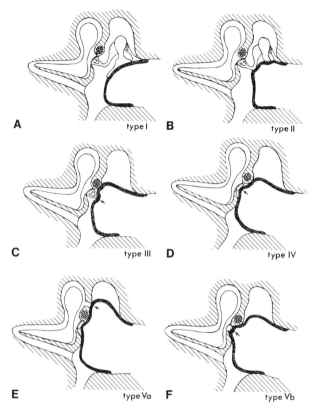

Figure 5-6. Tympanoplasty types. Middle-ear space decreases in size from type I to type IV. Assuming many other factors (the most common of which is good eustachian-tube function) to be stable and under control, hearing results are decreasingly good as one proceeds from type I through type IV tympanoplasty. A. Type I—graft rests on malleus. B. Type II—graft rests on incus. C. Type III—graft attaches to head of stapes. D. Type IV—graft attaches to footplate of stapes. E. Type Va—fenestration of lateral semicircular canal (arrow). F. Type Vb—stapedectomy (arrow). (Reprinted with permission from Paparella, M. M., & Shumrick, D. A. (Eds.). *Otolaryngology. Vol. 2.* Philadelphia: W.B. Saunders, 1980, p. 1525.)

Primary tumors. *Glomus jugulare* or *gloma tympanicum* is the most common and therefore most important primary middle-ear tumor. The tumor originates from glomus bodies which relate to the jugular bulb in the floor of the middle ear. This tumor can cause hearing loss, a sense of fullness, tinnitus, and even cranial-nerve and intracranial complications. It may present as a bulging purplish mass in the floor of the middle ear. Polytomography, angiography, and retrograde jugular venography may be necessary to

Table 5-1
Complications of Otitis Media and Mastoiditis

Middle ear	Extradural
Persistent perforation	Extradural abscess
Ossicular erosion with hearing loss	Lateral sinus thrombosis
Facial nerve paralysis	Petrositis (Gradenigo's syndrome)
Inner ear	Central nervous system
Fistula with	Meningitis
Vertigo	Brain abscess
Sensorineural hearing loss	Otitic hydrocephalus
Suppurative labyrinthitis	
Sensorineural hearing loss	

delineate the extent of the tumor (Fig. 5-7). To the best of our knowledge, ECochG/BSER testing has not been added to the battery of tests; surgery is the best primary modality of treatment. If the tumor is extensive, combined surgery and radiotherapy often are indicated.

Rhabdomyosarcoma occurs in young children. This disease was once considered fatal, however, recent cures have been reported from radical surgery with combined radio- and chemotherapy.

Squamous cell carcinoma may originate primarily from the ear canal, then secondarily invade the middle ear and mastoid. One should suspect any lesion in the external canal which does not spontaneously heal as a possible malignancy. Symptoms and signs include bloody drainage, pain, sense of fullness, hearing loss, and vertigo. Facial nerve paralysis develops late in the course of the disease. Other primary tumors include fibrosarcoma and neurofibroma of the facial nerve.

Secondary tumors. Tumors that arise from distant primary foci and metastasize to the middle ear, mastoid, and temporal bone include adenocarcinoma of the prostate, breast carcinoma, hypernephroma, renal carcinoma, adenoma, bronchogenic carcinoma, gastrointestinal carcinoma, and melanoma.

Tumors from adjacent structures, such as meningioma, acoustic neuroma, glioma, neurilemoma, cylindroma of the parotid gland, epidermoid carcinoma, melanoma of the external ear, and nasopharyngeal cancers, may also invade the middle ear and mastoid.

Malignant lymphoma and leukemia may involve the temporal bone, especially the bone marrow of the petrous apex, and can cause infiltration of the middle ear and eustachian tube, resulting in conductive hearing losses and effusions. In terminal leukemia, acute hemorrhage can occur in the inner ear, causing sudden and profound deafness as well as vestibular symptoms.

The effects that these conditions will have on the evoked potentials is far from obvious. In practice, many patients may not be tested with these

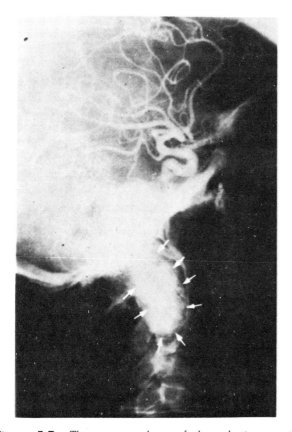

Figure 5-7. The venous phase of the selective carotid arteriogram outlines a dense vascular tumor stain as a filling defect in the internal jugular vein. (Reprinted with permission from Adams, G. L., Boies, L. R., & Paparella, M. M. *Fundamentals of otolaryngology. 5th ed.* Philadelphia: W.B. Saunders, 1978, p. 56.)

methods. On the other hand, as the use of ECochG/BSER testing increases, different pathologies will present to the clinical situation. Thus, an awareness of the attendant conditions associated with the various pathologies is of major importance.

Temporal bone trauma. Trauma to the temporal bone (from automobile accidents or other blows to the head) may cause temporal bone fracture, which is often accompanied by basilar skull fracture. Symptoms may include loss of consciousness, facial nerve paralysis, bleeding from the ear, spinal fluid leakage, vertigo, and hearing loss. The fracture may be longitudinal along the axis of the petrous pyramid, or transverse, crossing the

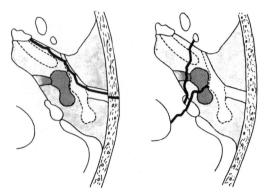

Figure 5-8. Diagramatic representation of a longitudinal (left) and transverse (right) fracture of the temporal bone. (Reprinted with permission from Gros, J. C.: The ear in skull trauma. *Southern Medical Journal*, 1967, *60*:705.)

petrous pyramid (Fig. 5-8). A longitudinal fracture is more common and may cause hemotympanum, facial nerve paralysis, and conductive hearing loss, whereas a transverse fracture produces complete loss of function and vertigo due to the fracture through the bony labyrinth.

Diagnosis can be made by clinical signs and polytomography. Audiology (tympanometry) is indispensable to determine whether the middle ear (conductive deafness), the inner ear (sensorineural deafness), or both (mixed deafness) are involved. An electrophysiologic test such as ECochG/BSER is also indispensable, since many of these patients cannot actively participate in the test situation (see Chapters 10 and 12).

After the patient has stabilized and cerebrospinal fluid drainage has stopped, the facial nerve may have to be surgically explored and decompressed. A perforated tympanic membrane or persistance of a conductive hearing loss can be corrected in later surgery.

DISEASES OF THE INNER EAR

The most important symptoms of inner-ear disease are sensorineural hearing loss, tinnitus, and vertigo. At times, an inner-ear conductive hearing loss may be evident (Schuknecht, 1978). Hearing loss only will be discussed in this section.

Hearing loss is an important medical problem; at least 13 million Americans (some estimate 20 million or more) have a significant hearing loss (Schein and Delk, 1974). Most have sensorineural hearing impairment, indicating inner-ear involvement. Since hearing loss is a symptom of an underlying disease process, proper management depends upon identification of the underlying disorder. The classification in Table 5-2 is useful in the differential diagnosis of sensorineural deafness.

Table 5-2

Etiologic Classification of Sensorineural Deafness

Congenital Sensorineural Deafness	Delayed or Acquired Sensorineural Deafness
GENETIC ETIOLOGIES	
• Deafness occurring alone	• Deafness occurring alone
Michel's aplasia	Familial progressive sensorineural
Mondini's aplasia	deafness
Scheibe's aplasia	Otosclerosis
Alexander's aplasia	Presbycusis
• Deafness occurring with other	• Deafness occurring with other
abnormalities	abnormalities
Waardenburg's syndrome	Alport's syndrome
(deafness may be delayed)	Hurler's syndrome
Albinism	(gargoylism)
Hyperpigmentation	Klippel-Feil syndrome
Onychodystrophy	Refsum's disease
Pendred's syndrome	Alstrom's disease
Jervell's syndrome	Paget's disease
Usher's symdrome	Richards-Rundel syndrome
	von Recklinghausen's disease
	Crouzon's disease
• Chromosomal abnormalities	
Trisomy 13-15	
Trisomy 18	
NONGENETIC ETIOLOGIES	
• Deafness occurring alone: ototoxic	• Inflammatory diseases
poisoning (streptomycin, quinine,	Bacterial (labyrinthitis and otitis
etc.)	media)
• Deafness occurring with other	Viral (measles, mumps, influenza,
abnormalities	labyrinthitis)
Viral infection (maternal rubella)	Spirochetal (congenital and acquired
Bacterial infection	syphilis)
Ototoxic poisoning (thalidomide)	• Ototoxic poisoning
Metabolic disorders (cretinism)	• Neoplastic disorders
Erythroblastosis fetalis	(leukemia, peripheral and
Radiation (first trimester)	central ear tumors)
Prematurity	• Traumatic injury (acoustic trauma,
Birth trauma, anoxia	temporal bone fractures)
	• Metabolic disorders (hypothyroidism,
	allergies, Ménière's disease)
	• Vascular insufficiency (sudden deafness,
	presbycusis)
	• Central nervous system disease
	(multiple sclerosis)

It can be argued that the various etiologic conditions may seriously alter the so-called normal evoked-potential patterns. Most of the conditions that have been clinically documented to date are mainly descriptive (e.g., see Aran, 1978; Brackman, 1977; Glasscock, Jackson, and Josey, et al., 1979; Selters and Brackman, 1977; Stockard and Rossiter, 1977). Attempts have been made to quantify the evoked-potential patterns of numerous peripheral ear disorders (see Chapter 11). In practice, however, a number of the congenital and delayed or acquired conditions have only been anecdotally reported, a usual precedent to quantitative studies in the clinical sciences. It follows that perhaps future studies will attempt to more clearly document BSER/ECochG findings for the subclassifications of this etiologic system (Table 5-2).

Congenital: Genetic

Deafness occurring alone.   *Michel's deafness* is characterized by a total lack of inner-ear development. This defect appears to be inherited by a Mendelian autosomal dominant transmission.

Mondini's deafness is characterized by a decrease in the number of turns in the bony labyrinth (from 2½ to about 1½), with the middle and apical turns occupying a common cloaca. The osseous vestibular labyrinth may also be malformed. This condition is genetically transmitted as an autosomal

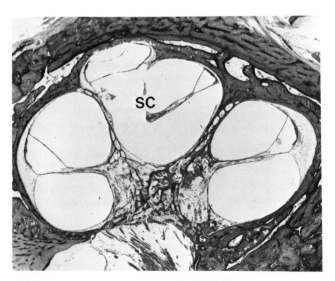

Figure 5-9. Mondini's deformity. The cochlea demonstrates 1½ instead of the usual 2½ cochlear turns. The bony interscaler septum which separates the middle from the apical cochlear turn was incomplete, with the formation of a scala communis (SC) or cloaca. The organ of Corti was flattened or diminished throughout. The number of spiral ganglion cells was markedly reduced, especially in the basal turn.

dominant trait (Fig. 5-9). Organ of Corti dysfunction will be present if sensori-neural hearing loss exists. In many cases, one or both windows in the middle ear are occluded.

Scheibe's deafness represents a membranous cochleosaccular hypoplasia in the presence of a normal bony labyrinth. This is the most common of all inherited congenital deafnesses and usually is transmitted as an autosomal recessive trait. There may be some residual hearing in the low frequencies.

Alexander's deafness is characterized by aplasia of the cochlear duct affecting the organ of Corti and adjacent ganglion cells of the basal coil of the cochlea. These patients manifest a high-frequency hearing loss and do well with amplification.

The above genetic conditions may preclude recording several of the brain-stem waves, since input to the cochlea is most likely impaired. Whether remnants of cochlear anatomy would portend altered evoked potentials remains to be tested.

Deafness associated with other abnormalities. Waardenburg's disease is transmitted as a dominant trait. The primary features include sensorineural hearing loss, lateral displacement of the medial canthi, white forelock, heterochromia of the irises, and hypoplasia of nasal alae.

Albinism may be autosomal dominant, recessive, or sex-linked. Deafness may be bilateral and severe.

Hyperpigmentation has been associated with severe sensorineural deafness. The pigmented defects may progress from small spots in childhood to larger lesions in adults.

Onychodystrophy is a recessive trait of congenital male dystrophy and congenital sensorineural hearing loss. Affected siblings have small, short fingernails and toenails, and severe high-frequency deafness.

Pendred's disease is characterized by severe hearing loss and abnormal iodine metabolism resulting in thyroid enlargement. This syndrome may account for 10 percent of the cases of recessive hereditary deafness.

Jervell and Lange-Nielsen disease is characterized by congenital bilateral severe hearing loss, prolongation of the Q-T intervals, and Stokes-Adams attacks. Children with this recessive trait suffer frequent episodes of syncope and risk sudden death.

Usher's disease is a recessive sensorineural hearing loss with progressive retinitis pigmentosa.

Chromosomal abnormalities. Chromosomal abnormalities account for some types of congenital deafness. They are not truly hereditary.

Trisomy 13-15 syndrome may include low-set ears, absence of external auditory canals or "missle ear," cleft lip and palate, microphthalmia, coloboma iridis, and aplasia of the optic nerve. Trisomy 13-15 victims usually die in early infancy.

Trisomy-18 syndrome may include low-set deformed ears, micrognathia, atretic external auditory canals, decreased spiral ganglion cells, and anomalies of the cochlea and vestibule.

Nongenetic

Deafness associated with other abnormalities. A child with con-genital rubella syndrome may show aplasia of the organ of Corti and of the saccule. Other associated anomalies occur, such as middle-ear deformities, mental retardation, microcephaly, retinitis, congenital cataracts, cardiovascular deformities, and limb malformations.

Kernicterus in the newborn may result from Rh blood incompatability. Erythroblastosis fetalis is characterized by a deposition of bilirubin in the central nervous system, jaundice, mental retardation, cerebral palsy, and deafness.

Thyroid disease may be associated with deafness, as it is in cretinism. It is generally accepted that iodine deficiency is responsible for the cretinism. The hearing loss is of a mixed type.

The ear anomalies due to the maternal use of thalidomide, namely thalidomide ototoxicity, include atresia of external auditory canal, Michel or Mondini deformities of the inner ear (described earlier), absence of VIIth and VIIIth nerves in the internal auditory canal, and middle-ear abnormalities. We have previously alluded to possible associated evoked potentials.

Other causes of nongenetic congenital hearing loss include premature birth, hypoxia, prolonged labor, or extensive irradiation during pregnancy. Here again, the astute clinician will want to employ the ECochG/BSER technique according to the assistance that such procedures can provide to diagnosis.

Delayed or Acquired Deafness: Genetic

Deafness occurring alone. Familial progressive sensorineural deafness is usually bilateral and considered to be autosomal dominant. It can appear in childhood or in early adulthood and will progress in severity. There may be absence of the organ of Corti and spiral ganglion cells in the basal turn, and irregular degeneration of the stria vascularis. Audiograms show flat or basin-shaped sensorineural configurations with fairly good speech discrimination.

Otosclerosis, as described earlier, is an autosomal dominant disorder causing a conductive hearing loss. This may be associated with a progressive sensorineural hearing loss, as well as vertigo in some cases.

Presbycusis refers to decreased sensitivity of hearing that occurs with advancing age. There are four major kinds of presbycusis based on pathological and physiologic observations: sensory, neural, central, and metabolic. Schuknecht (1967) described five types of presbycusis; he added an inner ear conductive type. The sensory type refers to a hearing loss, often a high-frequency sensorineural hearing loss (with good speech discrimination), due sometimes to atrophy of the organ of Corti in the basal end of the cochlea. Neural presby-cusis refers to certain conditions attendant to the auditory nerve. Discrimina-tion ability in this case may be very poor. Central presbycusis refers to a hear-ing loss whereby the patient may have fairly good hearing but has difficulty in understanding speech (phonemic regression), usually due to a loss of ganglion cells or physiologic dysfunction of the central auditory system. Metabolic presbycusis is characterized by a relatively flat audiometric pattern and fairly good discrimination; the main pathologic correlate seems to be degeneration of the stria vascularis. This latter type may be genetically in-duced. Attempts should be made to reach a specific diagnosis (Lowell and Paparella, 1977) and, if possible, use the evoked-potential method (Berg-holtz, Hooper, and Mehta, 1977) to chart the progression of changes longitu-dinally. The ECochG/BSER waves have not been followed in the same pop-ulation over a period of declining age, for obvious reasons. The waves have been documented in different age groups, and what one observes is an initial shortening of latency (see Hecox and Galambos, 1974), with a stabilization period, and prolongation of latency in advancing years. Whether this latter observation is due to true presbycusis remains to be verified.

Deafness associated with other abnormalities. *Alport's syn-drome*, a dominantly transmitted syndrome, is a progressive glomerulone-phritis and bilateral, high-frequency sensorineural hearing loss manifested by about the age of 10. Males are more frequently affected than females.

Hurler's syndrome begins in early childhood and results in skeletal de-formity, dwarfism, mental retardation, hepatosplenomegaly, blindness, and profound sensorineural hearing loss. It appears to be transmitted as a reces-sive trait and may be sex-linked.

Klippel-Feil syndrome consists of skeletal defects with fusion of cervical vertebrae, spina bifida, scoliosis, torticollis, and profound sensorineural deaf-ness. The disease is inherited as an autosomal recessive trait.

The primary features of *Alstrom's disease* are retinitis pigmentosa, dia-betes mellitus, obesity, and progressive deafness. Hearing loss appears at around 10 years of age. This syndrome is inherited through autosomal reces-sive traits.

Paget's disease, an autosomal dominant syndrome, is characterized by skeletal deformities of the skull and long bones, and sensorineural hearing loss.

Richards-Rundel syndrome, an autosomal recessive syndrome, includes mental deficiency, ataxia, hypogonadism, and severe deafness. All of these symptoms appear in childhood; hearing loss is total by the age of 5 or 6.

Von Recklinghausen's syndrome is an autosomal dominant syndrome and includes neurofibromatosis, bilateral acoustic tumors, café-au-lait spots, ataxia, visual loss, and sensorineural hearing loss.

As described earlier *Crouzon's disease* is characterized by atresia of the auditory meatus and a mixed hearing loss, as well as synotosis of the cranial suture, exophthalmos, parrot nose, and protruding lower lip.

Nongenetic

Labyrinthitis. Labyrinthitis is an inflammation or infection of the inner ear. There may be hearing loss as well as vertigo. Infection may spread into the inner ear from adjacent regions, such as the meninges, middle ear, or mastoid, or through the blood stream, often seen in viral inflammations.

Suppurative labyrinthitis is characterized by complete deafness due to permanent loss or destruction of sensory elements in the labyrinth (Fig. 5-10). It has been described according to three stages: (1) acute stage, characterized by invasion of pus cells; (2) chronic stage, characterized by fibroblastic proliferation within the inner ear space; and (3) healed stage, characterized by ossification (called labyrinthitis ossificans). Acute stage treatment consists of bed rest, antibiotics, and antivertiginous drugs. A complete mastoidectomy and a possible labyrinth drainage operation may be indicated for otogenic labyrinthitis. The chronic condition is managed with aural rehabilitation, including amplification as indicated.

Viral labyrinthitis is seen in mumps, influenza, and measles, in which viruses enter the endolymph apparently via the stria vascularis. Deafness develops quickly and persists. Treatment is symptomatic and supportive.

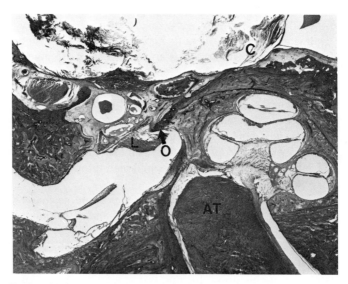

Figure 5-10. Multiple pathologies are seen in this one temporal bone specimen, including acoustic tumor (AT), otosclerosis (O), labyrinthitis (L), and cholesteatoma (C) in the middle ear and mastoid. This myriad of pathologies may cause a myriad of ECochG/BSER findings.

Table 5-3
Ototoxic Drugs and Chemicals

Chemicals	Antibiotics	Diuretics	Miscellaneous
Carbon monoxide	Streptomycin	Ethacrynic acid	Salicylates
Mercury	Neomycin	Furosemide	Quinine
Gold	Gentamycin		Nitrogen mustard
Lead	Viomycin		
Arsenic	Dihydrostreptomycin		
Alcohol	Vancomycin		
Aniline dyes	Polymixin B		
Tobacco			

Toxic (serous) labyrinthitis is characterized by the presence of inflammation within the inner-ear fluid spaces, but not profuse invasion of pus cells. This inflammation may be transient and may not be permanent. Endolymphatic hydrops may also be present. Treatment should be active and prompt to prevent suppurative labyrinthitis, and may consist of myringotomy for drainage, bed rest, antibiotics, and possibly mastoidectomy.

Ototoxicity
Hearing loss and tinnitus can result from ototoxicity of drugs and chemicals. Table 5-3 cites those agents that have been implicated.

Neoplasms
Malignant lymphoma and leukemia commonly involve the temporal bone, including the bone marrow of the petrous apex as well as infiltrations in the middle ear; these malignancies can result in mild conductive hearing losses. When leukemia becomes terminal, hemorrhage may occur in the inner ear, resulting in complete deafness. (*Acoustic neuromas* will be discussed under the *Central Diseases* section.)

Trauma
Noise-induced hearing loss represents a common cause of sensorineural hearing loss and has both social and economic implications. Noise-induced hearing loss may result either from prolonged exposure to loud continuous noise or brief exposure to loud impulse noise. Excessive noise results in decreased oxygen tension in the cochlear duct and progressive, irreversible changes in the outer hair cells and stria vascularis. In the majority of cases, noise-induced hearing loss originates around the region of 4000 Hz.

Explosive blasts may produce an injury resulting from severe impact noise.

Sudden pressure change in the environment or in the cerebrospinal fluid may result in rupture of the oval or round window membrane with subsequent sensorineural hearing loss and vertigo.

Fractures of the temporal bone have been described earlier.

Coats (Coats, 1978; Coats and Martin, 1977) warned us, and rightly so, of the pitfalls encountered in evoked-potential testing when cochlear damage is present. Numerous precautionary measures must be taken into account if such inner ear damage is present.

Metabolic Disorders

Hypothyroidism can produce sensorineural hearing loss in 25 percent of the patient population. Diabetes mellitus, adrenal insufficiency, hyperlipoproteinemia, and chronic renal disease are a few metabolic disorders which may accompany hearing loss.

Ménière's disease is described as idiopathic endolymphatic hydrops. Symptoms include tinnitus, intermittent vertigo, fluctuant hearing loss, loudness intolerance, fullness, and diplacusis. This disease should be conservatively managed. If necessary, surgery (endolymphatic sac procedures or vestibular nerve section) may be considered.

Sudden Hearing Loss

Sudden deafness is an abrupt, severe loss of sensorineural hearing. This is most likely due to viral agents or vascular occlusive phenomena. Other underlying diseases such as diabetes may be suspected. When sudden deafness develops, every attempt should be made to uncover an etiologic diagnosis. There is evidence to indicate some prognostic information in the ECochG response (Nishida, Kumagami, and Dohi, 1976). If the etiology is not determined, the treatment may be empirical, with bed rest, anticoagulants, steroids, and other medications. Exploratory tympanotomy may be indicated to seal an oval or round window leak of perilymph.

CENTRAL DISEASES

In this section retrocochlear and central lesions, including lesions of the acoustic nerve, brain stem, and cerebral cortex, which cause hearing impairment, will be briefly described.

Congenital: Nongenetic

Congenital cholesteatoma. This is a rare form of cholesteatoma which is neither associated with the middle-ear nor related to infections in the ear. It develops from embryonic ectodermal cells in the petrous portion of the temporal bone, and spreads around the labyrinth. It may extend to the middle-ear cleft or cranial cavity. Congenital cholesteatomas may present with facial nerve paralysis, hearing loss, vertigo, or intracranial complications (when infected). It may present clinically and audiologically as an acoustic tumor. The value of the ECochG/BSER technique in diagnosing acoustic tumor has been well documented (Brackman, 1977; Glasscock et al., 1979; Selters and Brackman, 1977; among others). (See also Chapters 10, 11, and 12.)

Congenital narrowing of the internal auditory canal.   The internal auditory canal (IAC) measures 3 mm or less in plain x-ray views. Stenosis of the internal auditory canal produces a compression of its contents with involvement of the auditory or facial nerve (Pulec, 1973). The usual symptoms are progressive hearing loss, instability, or symptoms of Ménière's disease. Decompression of the IAC by the middle fossa approach may relieve the symptoms. This rare condition requires further confirmation and hearing testing using evoked potentials may prove fruitful.

Acquired: Genetic

Von Recklinghausen's disease.   As discussed earlier, hearing loss can result secondary to acoustic neuroma formation (see Brackman, 1977) in this autosomal dominant syndrome.

Nongenetic: Inflammatory Diseases

Meningitis is the most common intracranial infection and is due to pyogenic organisms involving the pia arachnoid of the brain and spinal cord. It most commonly is the result of extension through previous fractures or defects from local sepsis in the middle ear and paranasal sinuses. It may further cause brain abscess, lateral sinus thrombosis, and otitic hydrocephalus.

Brain abscess is a localized collection of pus in a cavity surrounded by soft tissue, resulting from extension of the adjacent foci or from hematogenous spread. Otogenic sources account for 40-50 percent of all brain abscesses, and rhinogenic sources 10-15 percent (Tew, et al., 1980). The temporal lobe and the cerebellum are the most common sites of otogenic abscess. Temporal lobe abscess may produce aphasia, personality changes, and visual field defects; cerebellar abscess may result in an unsteady gait, nystagmus, and vertigo.

Encephalitis, from viral, bacterial, or spirachetal etiology, can cause hearing loss by direct extension via the modiolus and cochlear aqueduct into the perilymphatic spaces of the inner ear. An alternate strategy in these conditions would be to employ the late components (Chapter 13) and evoked potentials of other sensory systems (Chapter 14).

Neoplasm

Acoustic neuroma is a benign neoplasm which typically originates from the neurilemma sheath of the vestibular nerve within the internal auditory canal (vestibular schwannoma). The patient may present with vertigo, tinnitus, unilateral sensorineural hearing loss, absence or prolonged latency of BSER waves, a shorter interval between wave I and wave V, or facial paralysis. The diagnostic work-up should include a complete neuro-otologic examination, audiometric tests, ECochG/BSER testing, blood tests, and x-ray studies. Posterior fossa myelography is the most accurate diagnostic test. The new generation of computerized tomography (CT) scans, especially with air contrast, are just as accurate and may totally eliminate the need for posterior fossa myelography. Treatment when indicated is surgical.

Meningiomas may arise in the cerebellopontine angle. It is difficult to clinically distinguish a meningioma from an acoustic neuroma, but they may be recognized by an osteoblastic reaction in the petrous portion of the temporal bone or by an arteriographic stain. Other tumors involving the cerebellopontine angle include metastatic tumors, glomus jugulare tumors, arachnoid cysts, and neuromas of the trigeminal and glossopharyngeal nerves. The clinical literature has documented a number of cases using evoked-potential testing (see Chapter 12).

Trauma

Hearing loss may occur after concussion injury to the brain, even without skull fractures. Many centers utilize not only the auditory BSER, but also use visual and somatosensory potentials for diagnostic monitoring and prognostic indicators (see Chapter 14).

Degenerative Disorders

Multiple sclerosis (MS) is a common disorder of young adults and is characterized by remissions and exacerbations together with scattered neurological deficits. Presenting symptoms may include transient sensory disturbances, paresthesias, and sudden onset of hemiplegia. The cerebellar type of MS may mimic symptons of an acoustic tumor. Starr and co-workers (Starr, 1977, 1978; Starr and Achor, 1975; Starr and Hamilton, 1976), as well as others, have published a number of papers in this area that show predictable changes in amplitude and latency of brain-stem and cortical potentials (see Chapter 10).

Cerebrovascular Accidents

There are three types of cerebrovascular accidents (CVA): hemorrhage, thrombosis, and embolus. Any CVA involving the central pathway of hearing can of course affect audition.

Superior cerebellar artery thrombosis produces ipsilateral cerebellar asynergia, ipsilateral Horner's syndrome, contralateral loss of pain and temperature sensation of the face and body, and partial hearing loss.

Thrombosis of the lateral pontine branches produces ipsilateral cerebellar asynergia and signs of involvement of the Vth and VIIIth cranial nerves.

Thrombosis of the internal auditory artery will produce ipsilateral deafness and loss of vestibular function. They are also associated with syringobulbia, multiple sclerosis, trauma, and neoplasms.

DISCUSSION

In the space allotted, numerous hearing disorders have been addressed that the otologist, audiologist, and neurologist should be cognizant of in using the ECochG and BSER techniques. Certain of these disease states have been shown to directly affect the evoked-potential waves. In several of these categories, it is not certain whether a clearly definable evoked potential will be present, and if it is present, whether the latency and/or amplitude of the evoked potential will be altered. Within this frame of reference, the otologist, audiologist and neurologist must work closely together in making the appropriate diagnosis, determining the underlying etiology, and prescribing a course of treatment. Both ECochG and BSER can greatly assist in this task.

II FUNDAMENTALS

Terence W. Picton
Peter G. Fitzgerald

6   A General Description of the Human Auditory Evoked Potentials

"Event-related potentials" are the electrical changes that can be recorded in association with some external physical stimulus or some internal psychological process. They are usually classified as either *exogenous* or *endogenous* (Sutton, Tueting, and Zubin, et al., 1967; Donchin, Ritter, and McCallum, 1978). Exogenous components are mainly determined by the physical characteristics of the stimulus and are little affected by psychological processes. Endogenous components are largely determined by psychological rather than by physical parameters. The event-related potentials may be considered as either *evoked* or *emitted* (Weinberg, Walter, and Cooper, et al., 1974). Evoked potentials occur in response to a physical stimulus, and may be either exogenous or endogenous in nature. Emitted potentials occur in the absence of any physical stimulus, in relation to decision or preparatory processes, and they are always endogenous in nature.

    There are many different auditory evoked potentials that can be recorded from the human scalp in response to various acoustic stimuli (Picton, Woods, and Baribeau-Braun, et al., 1977). Figure 6-1 shows the evoked potentials to

The financial support of the Medical Research Council and of Tracor Northern Incorporated is gratefully appreciated. Gilles Hamel provided technical assistance. Barbara Reynolds was responsible for typing the manuscript.

141

a click stimulus.[1] The top section of the figure shows the response plotted using linear scales for amplitude and time. The major components that can be recognized on the 500 msec sweep are the waves of the slow vertex potential—P1, N1, P2, N2 (see Chapter 13). If the time scale is expanded, the middle latency components Na, Pa and Nb can be more easily distinguished, and the prominent wave V of the brain-stem response can be recognized. The use of a logarithmic time scale, as illustrated in the middle section of the figure, makes it easier to view the entire evoked potential waveform. A logarithmic amplitude scale further facilitates the evaluation of the low amplitude early components of the response. Using the logarithmic scales, the click-evoked potential can be easily divided into three time epochs: fast (0–10 msec), middle (10–50 msec), and slow (50–500 msec). This is the basis of the most commonly used classification system for the auditory evoked potentials (Picton, Hillyard, and Krausz, et al., 1974). As well as these three time epochs, one may consider the "first" evoked potentials that are generated in the cochlea, and the "late" or endogenous evoked potentials occurring after 250 msec (Davis, 1976b).

There are several nomenclatures (see Chapter 13) used to designate the components of the auditory evoked potential. One system uses the polarity and typical latency of the component (Donchin, Callaway, and Cooper, et al., 1977). In this system, the most prominent component of the auditory brain-stem response is termed P_6. Unfortunately, the latency of a component will vary with such parameters as stimulus intensity, frequency, and rise-time (see Chapter 9). The P_{15} response to a low-intensity 500 Hz tone pip is quite probably the same component as the P_6 response to a moderate-intensity click. The old sequential nomenclature—I–VII for the fast responses; No, Po, Na, Pa, Nb for the middle responses; and P1, N1, P2, N2 for the slow responses—although somewhat idiosyncratic, has the advantage of being able to refer appropriately to components with similar stimulus or brain relations but different latencies.

The auditory evoked potentials may also be classified by their relationships to stimulus continuation (Davis, 1976b; Picton and Smith, 1978; Hillyard, Picton, and Regan, 1978). A *transient* response is one that is evoked by a change in some stimulus parameter. The most commonly recorded transient responses are those to the onset or offset of a stimulus. A *sustained* response is one that continues throughout the stimulus duration. A *steady-state* response is a combination of the two. This is the response to a regularly repeating stimulus change; it is recorded after the repeating stimulus

---

[1]Editor's Note. The usual convention among most audiologists, otologists, neurologists and pediatricians is to plot negative-going potentials in the downward direction. Here, Picton and Fitzgerald prefer to plot negativity in the upward direction in order to conform to the practice in electroencephalography. We acquiesced to this practice in this chapter, since the reader is bound to encounter it in several writings. The meaning of the potentials certainly remains unchanged.

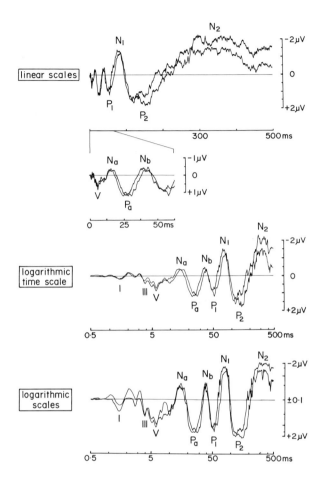

Figure 6-1. Human click-evoked potentials. This figure presents the scalp-recorded response to a 70 dB nHL 100 μsec click stimulus presented to the right ear at a rate of 1/sec. The response was recorded between vertex and right mastoid using a frequency band-pass of 1-3000 Hz. Relative negativity of the vertex electrode is represented by an upward deflection. Each tracing represents the average of 1000 individual responses. The upper section of the figure presents the response using linear time and amplitude scales. The slow components of the response are visible in the top tracings and the middle components (and wave V of the fast response) are more easily recognized on the expanded scale of the second set of tracings. The middle section of the figure presents the response using a logarithmic time scale. All the components of the response are now easily recognizable in the same tracing. The lower section of the figure uses a logarithmic amplitude as well as time scale. This makes the smaller, earlier components more easily distinguishable. The concept of presenting the auditory evoked potential on log-log scales derives from Picton, Hillyard, and Krausz, et al., 1974.

143

Table 6-1
Human Auditory Evoked Potentials

	Transient Responses	Sustained and Steady-State Responses
First	Cochlear nerve action potential (N1, N2)	Cochlear microphonic, summating potential
Fast	Auditory brain stem response (I-VII)	Frequency following response (FFR1, FFR2)
Middle	Middle latency response (No, Po, Na, Pa, Nb, Pb)	Sinusoidal response, 40 Hz potential
Slow	Slow vertex potential (P1, N1, P2, N2)	Sustained cortical potentials
Late	Late positive component (N2-P3 complex)	Negative waves relating to orientation and expectancy (O-wave, E-wave, CNV)

has been sufficiently presented so that any transient responses to its onset have ceased.

In this chapter, auditory evoked potentials will be considered according to their general latency and relationship to stimulus continuation. Table 6-1 lists the different evoked potential components that will be discussed. More extensive discussions of each of the components follow in Chapters 10 through 13.

FIRST RESPONSES

There are three evoked potential components that are generated within the human cochlea. The cochlear microphonic (CM) derives from the hair cells, the summating potential (SP) from the hair cell/dendrite junction, and the cochlear nerve action potential (AP) from the cochlear nerve fibers.

The human CM is best recorded from an electrode within or near the middle ear (Yoshie and Yamaura, 1969). It can be recorded from electrodes located on the auricle or mastoid but it is of much lower amplitude (Moore, 1971; Terkildsen, Osterhammel, and Huis in't Veld, 1974a; Sohmer and Pratt, 1976). Particular care must be exercised so as to differentiate this response from electrical artifact. Earphone shielding and acoustic delay lines are helpful in this regard (Moore, 1971) (see Chapter 8). The CM recorded from the external auditory meatus or mastoid is somewhat different from that recorded from the promontory in the middle ear. As well as being smaller in amplitude, it relates to a wider region of the cochlea than the more localized middle-ear recording (Elberling and Salomon, 1973).

The human cochlear SP is recorded as a negative potential lasting the duration of a stimulus (Eggermont, 1976c). It is extremely small in amplitude when recording is attempted at any distance away from the middle ear.

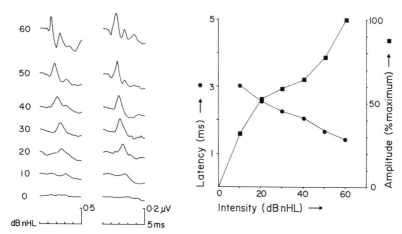

Figure 6-2. Cochlear nerve action potentials. The left side of the figure shows the cochlear nerve action potentials recorded in response to 10 μsec click stimuli presented at a rate of 5/sec and at the designated intensities (in dB nHL). Each tracing is the average of 512 individual responses, recorded using a band-pass of 10-3000 Hz from an electrode located in the external auditory meatus near the eardrum. A reference electrode was located on the ipsilateral earlobe; negativity of the active eardrum electrode is represented by an upward deflection. Responses are shown for two different subjects. At the higher intensities, two negative components, N1 and N2, are recognized; at the lower intensities, only one is distinguishable. On the right of the figure are shown the average amplitude (squares) and peak latency (circles) of the N1 component plotted against the stimulus intensity in dB nHL. There is a plateau in the amplitude-intensity function that occurs around 30-40 dB.

Pathological processes resulting in a loss of hair cells will cause marked attenuation of the SP.

The cochlear nerve AP to a click stimulus at high intensities consists of up to three negative waves—N1, N2, N3 (Yoshie and Ohashi, 1969; Portmann and Aran, 1971a; Eggermont, 1976). With decreasing stimulus intensity, the morphology of the response simplifies to a single negative peak, the amplitude decreases, and the latency increases (Fig. 6-2). Between 30 and 50 dB above threshold, there is often a plateau in the amplitude-intensity function and a change in latency. This is probably caused by the different areas of the cochlea each generating different components of the compound cochlear nerve AP (Elberling, 1973). As the intensity decreases, the response is generated more and more by the apical regions of the cochlea. Its latency becomes longer and, since the neural firing is less well synchronized, its morphology becomes broader. High-pass masking techniques can be used to demonstrate this compound nature of the cochlear nerve AP (Elberling, 1974; Eggermont, 1976b).

FAST RESPONSES

In the first 10 msec after a click stimulus, a series of small waves can be recorded between an electrode on the scalp or forehead and one on the ipsilateral mastoid or earlobe (Sohmer and Feinmesser, 1967; Jewett and Williston, 1971). These waves are designated using Roman numerals for the mastoid-negative or vertex-positive peaks. Wave I is mainly mastoid-negative in polarity and represents the surface-recorded cochlear nerve AP. The subsequent waves are recorded as positive waves from widespread areas of the scalp, maximally from the frontocentral regions. They reflect the transmission of the auditory impulse through the brain-stem auditory pathways (Starr, 1977). The most prominent and consistent components are waves III and V, which occur approximately 2 and 4 msec later than wave I. The morphology of the II–III waves varies somewhat between horizontal and vertical electrode montages, suggesting that there may be several underlying components to the scalp-recorded waves (Picton, Hillyard, and Krausz, et al., 1974). Waves III–IV–V are somewhat variable in shape between individuals. Wave III sometimes is double-peaked, and waves IV and V may overlap to a variable extent (Stockard, Stockard, and Sharbrough, 1978; Chiappa, Gladstone, and Young, 1979). The morphology of the brain-stem response may vary with the phase of the click stimulus (Stockard, Stockard, and Sharbrough, 1978; see Chapter 10). This variation in morphology can be a particular problem in patients with an abrupt high-frequency hearing loss (Coats and Martin, 1977; Coats, 1978). One of the most difficult problems in clinically evaluating the auditory brain-stem response is to determine how much of given abnormality is related to cochlear problems and how much to brain-stem dysfunction. The deconvolution of the recorded brain-stem response with the compound cochlear nerve AP can give the "compound impulse response" for the brain-stem, thereby allowing an assessment of brain-stem function independent of the cochlea (Elberling, 1978).

Wave V of the brain-stem response is the most prominent and consistent component. It is much less affected by increasing stimulus presentation rates than the earlier waves of the response (Terkildsen, Osterhammel, and Huis in't Veld, 1975; Don, Allen, and Starr, 1977). Wave V can be considered a compound response deriving from connections from different cochlear areas. High-pass noise-masking techniques can be used to separate these different subcomponents of the compound wave V (Don and Eggermont, 1978; Don, Eggermont, and Brackmann, 1979; Parker and Thornton, 1978a, 1978c).

Auditory brain-stem responses can be recorded using tonal stimuli as well as clicks (Suzuki, Hirai, and Horiuchi, 1977; Kodera, Yamane, and Yamada, et al., 1977). The response is less well defined than the click-evoked potential. Wave V remains with low-frequency tones, but the other response components are less prominent. For tones of 500 or 1000 Hz the electrical energy of the response contains relatively more low-frequency activity than does the click-evoked potential. The high-pass filter setting in the amplifier is, therefore, critical (Suzuki and Horiuchi, 1977; Elberling, 1979a). If the cutoff frequency is at 10 Hz or less, a normal positive-going wave V is recorded. If the cutoff is at 40 Hz, the response may be distorted by the filter (Stapells and Picton, 1981). The response then has a major negative component occurring 1–2 msec after the actual wave V peak. This negativity has been termed the "slow negative wave at about 10 msec" or SN_{10} (Davis and Hirsh, 1979). The effects of different filters on the response are shown in Figure 6-3.

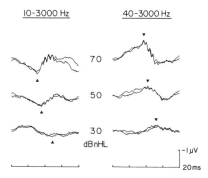

Figure 6-3.   The effects of filtering on the brain-stem response to low-frequency tone pips. Tone pips of 500 Hz frequency with rise and fall times of 4 msec and a plateau duration of 0.1 msec were presented to the right ear at a rate of 35/sec and at intensities of 70, 50, and 30 dB nHL. The responses recorded between vertex and right mastoid electrodes using a frequency band-pass of 1–10000 Hz were recorded on FM tape having a frequency bandpass of D.C. -5000 Hz. The responses were played back and averaged after filtering using two different frequency band-passes: 10–3000 and 40–3000 Hz. The filter settings were measured at the -3 dB points; the filter slope was 48 dB/octave. Each tracing represents the average of 2000 responses. Relative negativity at the vertex electrode is represented by an upward deflection. When the low-frequency cutoff is set at 10 Hz, the major component of the response is the positive wave-V peak, designated by the upward arrows. When the low-frequency cutoff is set at 40 Hz, the morphology of the response is quite different. The negative-going wave that follows wave V is now the most prominent peak in the response, as indicated by the downward triangle. This component—the slow negative wave at 10 msec or SN_{10}—occurs between 1 and 2 msec later than the wave V peak.

Tones with a relatively rapid rise-time of 5 msec or less are necessary to provide sufficient synchronization for recording the brain-stem response. There is a fairly broad range of frequencies in the acoustic energy during such a brief onset or offset (Brinkmann and Scherg, 1979). Such a frequency spread will result in activation of cochlear regions far beyond those specific to the nominal frequency of the tone. With low-frequency stimuli, this problem is further compounded by the asymmetry of the travelling wave in the cochlea. Another enemy of frequency-specificity is the nonlinear transmission (through the middle ear and cochlea) of abrupt, high-intensity stimuli. The frequency-specificity of the brain-stem response to tones can be enhanced by presenting the tone in notched noise, in order to mask out any response to the frequency spread of the stimulus (Picton, Ouellette, and Hamel, et al., 1979). This is illustrated in Figure 6-4.

As well as the onset response to a low-frequency tone of moderate or high intensity, there is also a frequency-following response (FFR) or potential (FFP) having the same basic frequency and waveform as the acoustic stimulus (Moushegian, Rupert, and Stillman, 1973; Marsh, Brown, and Smith, 1975). This response begins approximately 6 msec after stimulus onset and continues through its duration. It must be distinguished from the CM which can be recorded from the earlobe or mastoid ipsilateral to stimulation. The FFR is therefore best recorded using electrodes at the vertex and the ear or mastoid contralateral to stimulation. Unlike the CM, it is of greater amplitude for lower frequency tones. The FFR usually is not recordable at intensities below 40 dB nHL. There is very little binaural interaction in response generation—the FFR to binaural stimuli being essentially the same as the sum of the responses to the monaurally presented stimuli (Gerken, Moushegian, and Stillman, et al., 1975). The FFR to a continuous tone may be examined as a steady-state response (Galambos and Hecox, 1977; Michelson and Vincent, 1975). In this type of recording, great care must be taken to eliminate contamination by electrical artifact or cochlear microphonic. Human FFR recordings are illustrated in Figure 6-5.

High-pass masking studies and evaluations of patients with high-frequency hearing losses suggest that the FFR derives from the regions of the cochlea that are specific to frequencies below 2000 Hz (Moushegian, Rupert, and Stillman, 1978; Yamada, Kodera, and Hink, et al., 1978; Huis in 't Veld, Osterhammel, and Terkildsen, 1977). At high intensities in normally hearing subjects, however, there are quite possibly distinct FFRs deriving from connections with the basal end of the cochlea.

There appear to be at least two subcomponents of the brain-stem FFR (Stillman, Crow, and Moushegian, 1978). The first component occurs with an onset latency of about 4-5 msec and is best recorded using a horizontal electrode montage. The second component occurs some 1.5-2 msec later, and is best recorded with a vertical electrode montage. The two components

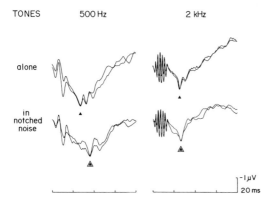

Figure 6-4. Brain-stem responses to tone pip stimuli. This figure presents the responses to tone pip stimuli of 95 dB peak SPL presented to the right ear at a rate of 45/sec. The tone pips had a frequency of either 500 or 2000 Hz, rise and fall times of 1 msec, and a plateau duration of 1 msec. The nHL threshold for the 500 Hz tone pips was 44 dB and for the 2000 Hz tone pips, 31 dB peak SPL. The responses were recorded using a frequency band-pass of 10-3000 Hz between vertex and low-neck electrodes. Relative negativity of the vertex is represented as an upward deflection. Each tracing represents the average of 2000 individual responses. The upper tracings represent the responses to the tone pips presented alone. There are prominent stimulus artifacts in the first 3 msec of the tracing. The wave-V component of the response is recognized as the most prominent positive peak in the tracing and is indicated by the single, solid triangles. The peak latency of this component is 6.8 msec for the 500 Hz tone pip and 6.4 msec for the 2000 Hz tone pip. This similarity in latency suggests that wave V to the 500 Hz tone pip derives from a similar region of the basilar membrane to the 2000 Hz response. The lower tracings show the responses to the tone pips presented in white noise of 70 dB SPL with a notch that was 48 dB down at the tone pip frequency. This noise masks out any neural response from a region of the basilar membrane that is not specific to the frequency of the tone pip. The wave V of the response to the 500 Hz tone pip, designated by the double triangles, is now recorded with a peak latency of 9.1 msec. The response to the 2000 Hz tone pip is little changed with wave V having a latency of 6.8 msec.

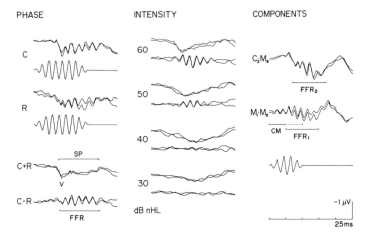

Figure 6-5. Human frequency-following responses (FFRs). The responses to 500 Hz tone bursts presented to the left ear at a rate of 23/sec using an acoustic delay line in order to prevent stimulus artifacts. Each tracing is the average of 2000 individual responses recorded using a frequency band-pass of 25-3000 Hz. In the left column are shown the effects of stimulus phase on the response. The top tracings (C) represent the response to a stimulus beginning with a condensation. The acoustic stimulus represented on the second line (with condensation shown as an upward deflection) had a total duration of 16 msec, with rise and fall times of 4 msec, and an intensity of 60 dB nHL. The response is recorded between vertex and right mastoid with relative negativity of the vertex showing as an upward deflection. The upper middle tracings (R) represent the response to a stimulus beginning on a rarefaction. At the bottom of the column are shown the results of adding (C+R) and subtracting (C−R) the two responses. Adding the two responses cancels the out-of-phase FFR and leaves the onset-response wave V and the suggestion of a sustained positivity (SP) underlying the FFR independently of its phase. Subtracting one response from the other leaves the FFR. The middle column of the figure shows the onset response and the FFR (recorded using the addition and subtraction techniques illustrated in the left column) at four different intensities. The FFR is not recognizable below 50 dB nHL, whereas a broad transient response persists. The right column shows the responses to a 70 dB nHL 500 Hz tone pip presented to the left ear with a total duration of 10 msec; rise and fall times of 4 msec. Two responses were simultaneously recorded—between vertex and right mastoid, and between the two mastoids. A small cochlear microphonic (CM) is just visible in the mastoid-mastoid recording. A somewhat larger FFR (FFR1) beginning at about 5 msec is also recorded from this electrode derivation. This response appears to be somewhat different from the FFR2, recorded from the vertex beginning at about 7 msec.

150

are best recognized at frequencies below 500 Hz, since at 500 Hz their latency difference causes them to synchronize. With 250-Hz stimuli, the two components may appear as a 500 Hz harmonic response (Krogh, Blegvad, and Stephens, 1977).

MIDDLE RESPONSES

In the 10-50 msec latency range there are various scalp muscle reflexes that can occur in response to loud acoustic stimuli (Bickford, 1972). The inion response in the neck muscles appears to depend upon vestibular rather than cochlear connections (Townsend and Cody, 1971). The postauricular muscle reflex, on the other hand, is initiated by cochlear stimulation. It is a bilateral reflex recorded from a localized region of the mastoid process at the level of the external auditory meatus (Yoshie and Okudaira, 1969; Douek, Gibson, and Humphries, 1973; Streletz, Katz, and Hohenberger, et al., 1977). The amplitude of the response varies with repetition rate, attention, head position, and muscle tension (Fig. 6-6). It usually has two major components—a mastoid-negative wave peaking at 12-15 msec followed by a positive wave at 18-25 msec. The threshold for eliciting this reflex is usually between 60 and 70 dB nHL. The response persists at rapid rates of stimulus presentation, being about 75 percent maximal amplitude at rates of 30/sec and about 25 percent at rates of 80/sec. The auditory brain-stem response to rapidly presented stimuli can thus be distorted when the reflex response to one stimulus overlaps with the succeeding brain-stem response. Other scalp muscle reflexes can also be elicited by loud auditory stimuli, particularly in the temporalis or frontalis muscles (Picton, Hillyard, and Krausz, et al., 1974). All of these muscle reflexes can distort the middle-latency brain responses. It is therefore best to record the middle responses during sleep, when reflex muscle activity is minimized.

The cerebral middle components of the auditory evoked potential consist mainly of a triphasic Na-Pa-Nb response (see Fig. 6-7 and Chapter 13). Earlier components No-Po have been reported (Mendel and Goldstein, 1969a), but it is difficult to determine their relationship either to the postauricular muscle response or to the brain-stem wave V delayed by filtering. Later components Pb-Nc-Pc have also been identified (McFarland, Vivion, and Goldstein, 1977), but because of the narrow filter band pass used to record them it is difficult to assess their relationship to the later slow components of the response.

The origin of the middle-latency components of the auditory evoked potential is not known. They are not recordable with barbiturate anesthesia, and therefore are not generated in the primary auditory cortex (Goff, Allison, and Lyons, et al., 1977). Nevertheless, they are audiometrically useful, since they can be recognized to within 10 or 20 dB of threshold (Mendel, Hosick, and

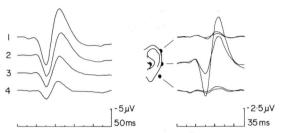

Figure 6-6. The postauricular muscle reflex. These recordings were taken between the vertex and the left mastoid area
using a frequency band-pass of 25-3000 Hz. Each tracing represents the average of 2000 individual responses with relative
negativity at the vertex (or relative positivity at the mastoid)
represented by an upward deflection. The stimulus was a 2 kHz
80 dB nHL tone pip with a total duration of 8 msec and rise/fall
times of 4 msec. On the left is shown the habituation of the
muscle reflex over four sequential averages when the stimulus
was presented at a rate of 11/sec. On the right are represented
three simultaneous recordings taken using reference electrodes
located at three different positions on the mastoid process. The
postauricular muscle reflex, consisting of a mastoid-negative
wave at 15 msec followed by a positive wave at 22 msec, is very
focal in distribution.

Windman, et al., 1975; Vivion, Wolf, and Goldstein, et al., 1979). This is illustrated in Figure 6-7.

Sinusoidal responses can be recorded using click stimuli presented at
rates of 10 to 200 Hz (Schimmel, Rapin, and Cohen, 1975). These responses
appear to be most prominent when the stimulus presentation rate is 40/sec
(Galambos, Makeig, and Talmachoff, 1981). Such middle-latency steady-
state response can be detected at intensities to less than 20 dB nHL.

SLOW RESPONSES

The most prominent peaks of the slow auditory response are P1, N1,
P2, and N2, occurring with peak latencies of approximately 50, 100, 170,
and 250 msec, respectively (see Chapter 13). The response is usually recorded
after the onset of an auditory stimulus, but other changes in the auditory stimulus may also elicit this transient response (Kohn, Lifshitz, and Litchfield,
1978). This complex of waves is maximally recorded from the vertex and
midfrontal regions of the scalp (Goff, Matsumiya, and Allison, et al., 1977;
Picton, Hillyard, and Krausz, et al., 1974).

Several subcomponents of the slow vertex potential have been identified
(see Chapter 13). An extra negative wave with a peak latency of between 125

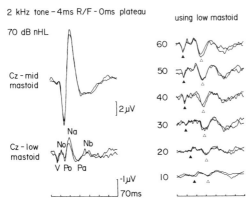

Figure 6-7. The middle-latency responses. The left side of this figure shows the middle-latency responses to an 8 msec 2 kHz tone burst of 70 dB nHL presented to the right ear at a rate of 11/sec. Two responses were simultaneously recorded—between the vertex and mid-mastoid region, and between the vertex and low-mastoid region. Each tracing represents the average of 2000 individual responses recorded using a bandpass of 25–3000 Hz with relative negativity of the vertex being represented by an upward deflection. A large postauricular muscle reflex is recorded from the mid-mastoid region. This consists of a mastoid negative wave peaking at 14 msec, followed by a positive wave at 20 msec, and a later broad negativity at around 35 msec. This is much less evident in the recording made using the lower mastoid reference. However, the Po wave is quite possibly equivalent to the initial component of the muscle reflex, and the Pa is possibly obscured by the tail end of the second component of the muscle reflex. On the right of the figure is represented a full intensity series for the fast and middle auditory responses. Both wave V (solid triangles) and wave Pa (open triangles) are recognizable down to 10 dB nHL.

and 175 msec has been identified in recordings from the temporal regions of the scalp (Wolpaw and Penry, 1975; Picton, Woods, and Stuss, et al., 1978; McCallum and Curry, 1980) (Fig. 6-8). Wolpaw and Penry have suggested that it is the second component of a positive-negative "T-complex."

The slow vertex potentials are quite variable to changes in the state of the patient. When stimuli are attended, the N1 component of the response may be increased in amplitude (Hillyard and Picton, 1979). There is some question as to whether this is an enhancement of the N1 wave or a superimposition of a "processing negativity" that indexes the attentional processing (Naatanen and Michie, 1979). During sleep, and particularly during the onset of sleep, there is a pronounced enhancement of the N2 component of the re-

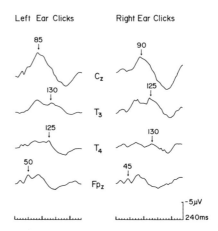

Figure 6-8. Slow components of the click-evoked potential. Simultaneous recordings were made from vertex (C_z), left and right temporal (T_3 and T_4) and frontal (Fp_z) electrodes each referred to a common balanced noncephalic reference. Relative negativity at the scalp is plotted as an upward deflection. The responses were evoked by click stimuli of 70 dB nHL presented to either ear at a rate of 1/sec. Each tracing represents the grand mean average over five different subjects. Each subject's waveform was the average of 200 individual responses. The overall frequency band-pass of the averaging system was 1-80 Hz; latency measurements are accurate to approximately 5 msec. At the vertex there is the usual N1 component, with a peak latency between 85 and 90 msec. In the temporal regions there is a later negative wave with a peak latency between 125 and 130 msec. This component varies in amplitude and latency with the ear of stimulation. In the frontal regions there is an earlier negative wave that occurs with a peak latency of 45-50 msec.

sponse (Ornitz, Ritvo, and Carr, et al., 1967a; Osterhammel, Davis, and Wier, et al., 1973).

There is a complex relationship between the slow vertex potential and the electroencephalogram (EEG). The background EEG is not just random noise; it can be affected both by the stimulus and by the state of the subject. An auditory stimulus will cause alterations in the rhythmic EEG activity (Pfurtscheller and Aranibar, 1977). The auditory response itself can be considered not so much as an additional event as a restructuring of the background EEG activities (Sayers, Beagley, and Riha, 1979). Salomon (1976) has shown how both the background EEG and the evoked potential may be affected by the state of the patient. Thus, selective averaging of the responses on the basis of different EEG patterns may improve response detection, since responses of different morphology will not be averaged together. Furthermore, the deconvolution of the stimulating event from the ongoing background activity may prove to be a more efficient means of detecting the evoked potential than simple averaging (Salomon and Barford, 1977).

Rapid stimulus presentation may elicit slow steady-state evoked potentials. These are best evoked at stimulus rates of around 10 Hz (Campbell, Atkinson, and Francis, et al., 1977). Steady-state responses have been most extensively studied in the visual system (Regan, 1977). Auditory steady-state responses are much more difficult to evaluate than the visual responses because of the lower signal-to-noise ratio.

Sustained negative potentials can be recorded from the vertex and frontal regions during a prolonged auditory stimulus (Keidel, 1971; Picton, Woods, and Proulx, 1978a, 1978b; Jarvilehto, Hari, and Sams, 1978) (Fig. 6-9). There are probably two different negative sustained potentials. One relates to general perceptual processing; another relates more specifically to auditory analysis.

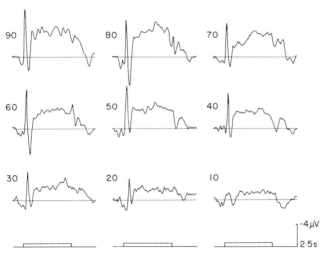

Figure 6-9. Human auditory sustained potentials. This figure presents the evoked potentials to a 1.4 sec tone burst of 1 kHz presented to the left ear at a rate of 1/3 sec. The responses were recorded between vertex and right mastoid electrodes using a frequency band-pass of 0-20 Hz. Each waveform represents the average of 128 individual responses. Negativity at the vertex electrode is represented by an upward deflection. The responses were obtained at different intensities (dB HL) of the toneburst. The response consists of an onset response (with N1-P2 components), followed by a sustained negativity lasting the duration of the stimulus. At times (e.g., at 60 dB), an offset response is distinguishable at the end of the tone burst; at other times, the sustained negativity just falls back down to baseline.

LATE RESPONSES

There is a great variety of evoked potentials that occur at latencies of greater than 150 msec (see Chapter 13), in keeping with the variety of ways in which auditory stimuli can be perceptually processed (Donchin, Ritter, and McCallum, 1978; Picton and Stuss, 1980). In response to informative signals, there occurs a sequence of waves P_{165}-N2-P3 that perhaps index different stages of information processing (Goodin, Squires, and Henderson, et al., 1978a). In response to rare and relevant auditory stimuli, there is a large slow negative wave recorded from the frontal regions (Rohrbaugh, Syndulko, and Lindsley, 1978, 1979). This component might relate in part to some general orientation to the stimulus. Such an "O-wave" might combine with the "expectancy" or "E-wave" preceding a motor act to form a large portion of the "contingent negative variation" (CNV)—a negative wave occurring after a warning stimulus and prior to an imperative stimulus that requires some motor or perceptual response (Walter, Cooper, Aldridge, et al., 1964).

CONCLUSION

At the present time it is difficult to do much more than list the components of the auditory evoked potential. Their exact site of generation and their functional significance to audition are not yet known. Ultimately we should be able to classify the auditory evoked potentials both by their source within the nervous system and by their purpose in auditory perception.

Jennifer S. Buchwald

7 Generators

Auditory brain-stem evoked responses (BSER) have been described for the adult cat (Jewett, 1970; Lev and Sohmer, 1972; Buchwald and Huang, 1975; Goldenberg and Derbyshire, 1975; Achor and Starr, 1980a); dog (Huang, 1980); mouse (Henry, 1979a, 1979b); rat (Jewett and Romano, 1972; Plantz, Williston, and Jewett, 1974); guinea pig (Dobie and Berlin, 1979b; Huang, 1980); monkey (Allen and Starr, 1978); and human (Jewett, Romano, and Williston, 1970; Sohmer and Feinmesser, 1970; Lev and Sohmer, 1972; Martin and Coats, 1973; Picton, Hillyard, and Krauz, et al., 1974; Terkildsen, Osterhammel, and Huis in't Veld, 1974b; Sohmer, Feinmesser, and Szabo, 1974; Starr and Achor, 1975; Starr and Hamilton, 1976; Stockard and Rossiter, 1977; Edwards, Buchwald, and Tanguay, et al., 1982); during development for the cat (Jewett and Romano, 1972; Shipley, Buchwald, and Norman, et al., 1980); rat (Jewett and Romano, 1972); mouse (Henry and Lepkowski, 1978); and human (Hecox and Galambos, 1974; Sohmer and Feinmesser, 1974; Jewett and Williston, 1971; Picton, Hillyard, and Krauz, et al., 1974; Hecox, 1975; Salamy and McKean, 1976; Starr, Amlie, and Martin, et al., 1977); during changes of stimulus intensity in the cat (Huang and Buchwald, 1978) and human (Jewett, Romano, and Williston, 1970; Hecox and Galambos, 1974; Starr and Achor, 1975; Stockard, Stockard and Sharbrough, 1978); of stimulus

Preparation of this chapter was supported in part by USPHS grants HD 05958 and HD 04612. The author wishes to thank Ms. Le Nae Boddie for invaluable help in manuscript typing and Ms. Mary Jacobsen for photographic assistance.

157

rate in the cat (Huang and Buchwald, 1978; Buchwald, Hinman, and Norman, et al., 1981); monkey (Allen and Starr, 1978) and human (Jewett and Williston, 1971; Picton, Hillyard, and Krauz, et al., 1974; Don, Allen, and Starr, 1977; Squires, Aine, and Buchwald, et al., 1980; Harkins, McEvoy, and Scott, 1979); and of stimulus frequency in the mouse (Henry, 1979a) and human (Suzuki, Hirai, and Horicuchi, 1977; Don and Eggermont, 1978).

There is general agreement among investigators of both human and animal BSER upon the following points:

1. The BSER are a series of volume-conducted neural potentials recordable from the scalp which originate from the primary auditory pathway of the brain stem (up to, and possibly including, the inferior colliculus);
2. The BSER show (positive) peaks and (negative) troughs when the scalp electrode registers positivity against a second noncephalic or cephalic reference electrode;
3. The peaks and troughs occur with latencies of less than 10 msec following an intense auditory stimulus;
4. The intervals between positive peaks are approximately 1 msec;
5. Peak latencies for any given subject are unchanging over successive trial blocks or recording sessions; and
6. BSER latencies and amplitudes are little affected by changes in arousal level or by sleep.

Insofar as the BSER peak positivities are almost exclusively addressed in the current literature, with little data available relative to the negative troughs, the subsequent discussion will focus on the positive components.

With regard to the problem of BSER generators, a number of relevant reviews have appeared (Terkildsen, Osterhammel, and Huis in't Veld, 1974a; Thornton, 1974; Goff, Allison, and Lyons, et al., 1977; Picton, Woods, and Baribeau-Braun, et al., 1977; Skinner and Glatke, 1977; Stockard, Stockard, and Sharbrough, 1978; Starr and Achor, 1978; Goff, 1979). Issues that have been extensively covered elsewhere, i.e., discussions of dipole generators (Schlag, 1973; Goff, 1979) and the effects of electrode configuration (Stockard, Stockard, and Sharbrough, 1978; Terkildsen, Osterhammel, and Huis in't Veld, 1974a; Jewett, 1970; Plantz, Williston, and Jewett, 1974; Martin and Coats, 1973; Streletz, Katz, and Hohenberger, et al., 1977; Allen and Starr, 1978; Martin and Moore, 1978) will not be emphasized here. Rather, an attempt has been made in the present chapter to integrate relevant data so as to suggest possible sources of BSER generation without making premature conclusions. To this end, a number of hypotheses are proposed. First, a set of general hypotheses, with supporting data derived from general electrophysiologic and specific BSER studies, will be presented in order to suggest a basic conceptual framework for the complex problem of BSER generation. Subsequently, specific hypotheses will be developed relevant to the generation of each BSER component with supporting data derived largely from the experimental animal literature. Little attempt has been made to incorporate clinical data, partly because that information is covered separately in this volume (Chapters 10, 11, and 12), and partly because of the difficulty in identifying the exact neuropathology present in many clinical cases.

When considering BSER generators, there is general agreement that the BSER reflect neural events. (The possible role of glia in field potential generation has been discussed, but the time constants of glial activation are too long to be directly relevant to the BSER (Speckmann, 1979). However, in the BSER literature, the term *generator* has been almost exclusively used in an anatomic sense. This tradition was initiated with the earliest descriptions of the BSER (Jewett, 1970; Lev and Sohmer, 1972), in which generators were discussed in terms of the acoustic nerve (wave I), the cochlear nucleus (wave II), the superior olivary complex (wave III), and the area around and within the inferior colliculus (waves IV and V). Numerous experimental approaches have subsequently been utilized to identify BSER generators, but the emphasis and interpretation of these remains anatomic.

Considerations of anatomy, however, cannot be totally separated from physiology. In the brain-stem auditory pathway, as elsewhere, graded post-synaptic potentials (PSPs) are initiated on the dendrites or soma and electrotonically spread over portions of the post-synaptic cell. PSPs are relatively localized in comparison with all-or-none action potentials (APs), which are generated at the cell body and transmitted along the axon to its termination. This contrast is particularly striking when AP transmission in long tracts, such as the trapezoid body and lateral lemniscus, is considered. Thus, PSPs and APs have distinctly different intracellular origins, time constants, current fields and spatial distributions. And, as pointed out by Tsuchitani in Chapter 4, the extent to which one or both of these forms of neuronal activation contributes to the BSER has been largely unexplored. Since PSPs are topographically fixed while APs are transmitted as traveling waves through the brain, any generator interpretation based upon a physiologic substrate has, of course, an immediate anatomic implication.

GENERAL HYPOTHESES

BSERs reflect graded post-synaptic potentials rather than all-or-none action potentials discharged at the cell soma or transmitted along the axonal projection. A number of excellent reviews have considered the general problems inherent in the analysis of evoked-potential generation; the reader is referred to these for discussions of this complex topic (MacKay, Evans, and Hammond, et al., 1969; Schlag, 1973; Speckmann, 1979). The spectrum of variables that may relate to the genesis of any evoked field potential is summarized in Figure 7-1. In the present section, the possible contributions of PSPs versus APs to evoked-field potentials will be discussed.

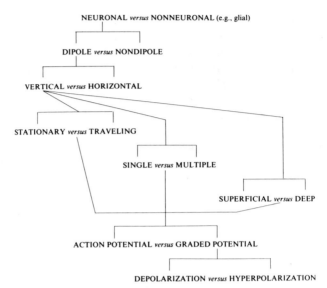

Figure 7-1. Summary of variables that may relate to evoked potential genesis. (Reprinted with permission from Schlag, J. Generation of brain evoked potentials. In R. F. Thompson and N. M. Patterson (Eds.), *Bioelectric recording techniques. Part A. Cellular processes and brain potentials.* New York: Academic Press, 1973.)

The major importance of PSPs and the relatively minor contribution of APs to evoked-potential phenomena was an argument advanced by Eccles in 1951 and amplified by Purpura in 1959. The elegant study of Humphrey (1968) provided both direct experimental data and a theoretical model regarding the effects of distance on PSP and AP fields. Based on theories of electrotonic and volume conduction, extracellular potentials generated by APs and PSPs in a model neuron were calculated. Humphrey postulated that (1) the distances between current sources (outward membrane current) and sinks (inward membrane current) are greater during peak PSP than peak AP activation, and these distances are as important as current magnitudes in determining value of voltage at a distant point; (2) the distribution of membrane current and the resultant external potential field is a function of the rise time and duration of the intracellular voltage transient; and (3) a rapid-voltage transient may reduce not only the probability of temporal summation but also of spatial summation of extracellular fields. Application of these predictions to the model neuron indicated that in generating a potential at a distant extracellular point (more than 150–200 μ from the active membrane regions), an intracellular PSP may give rise to a greater external voltage than a short-duration AP transient, even of greater amplitude.

Direct intracellular recordings of PSP and AP activity with adjacent extracellular recordings of field potential activity supported these theoretical results. Intracellular recordings from a pyramidal tract neuron were compared with simultaneous extracellular recordings from a site 0.4 mm distant (Fig. 7-2). The intracellular APs produced by antidromic stimulation were absent in the extracellular record, while the intracellular PSP showed a clear temporal correlation with the large-amplitude extracellular field potential. On the basis of both theoretical and empirical data, Humphrey concluded that APs generated at the cell soma contributed negligibly to evoked field potentials, whereas PSPs were causally related to them. Similar conclusions, reached by other electrophysiologists, have been discussed in detail elsewhere (Amassian, Waller, and Macy, 1964; Purpura, 1959; Schlag, 1973).

While the above data indicate that APs recorded within the cell soma probably contribute little to evoked field potentials recorded at a distance, the possible contributions of APs transmitted along axons must be separately considered insofar as the spatial distribution of membrane current in an axon can be markedly different than that in the cell body. Conductance changes related to cell discharge are confined to a relatively small area of the soma and axon hillock, which brings the current sources and sinks close together and thereby produces a restricted extracellular potential field. In contrast, peak inward and outward currents of an axonal AP may be separated by relatively large internodal distances, (e.g., up to a millimeter [Schlag, 1973]), so that a somewhat larger extracellular potential field can be produced. In this regard, it has been shown that a brief electrical stimulus applied to a thalamic sensory nucleus produces a short latency, small-amplitude surface potential, interpreted as the synchronous discharge of afferent fibers (Bishop and Clare, 1953; Perl and Whitlock 1955). However, when visual or somatosensory (rather than thalamic) stimulation was utilized, there were no afferent fiber field potentials but only the primary cortical response, attributed to cellular PSPs (Bishop and Clare, 1953, Perl and Whitlock, 1955; Amassian, Waller, and Macy, 1964). The cited literature suggests that the extreme synchrony induced by electrical stimulation of tracts within the brain is necessary to yield a fiber tract field potential. Under conditions of peripheral sensory stimulation, the resultant increase in temporal and spatial AP dispersion effectively precludes the appearance of such fiber tract fields.

Taken together, the preceding studies strongly support the concept that extracellular field potentials evoked by natural stimuli are caused by PSPs. There appears to be little support for a causal relationship between these field potentials and APs generated either at cell somas or travelling along axonal projection tracts.

BSER latencies and amplitudes reflect interactive but different physiologic processes. In a variety of situations, BSER latencies and amplitudes have been shown to vary independently. For example, demyelinating diseases, such as multiple sclerosis (see Chapters 12, 14) or central pontine myelinoly-

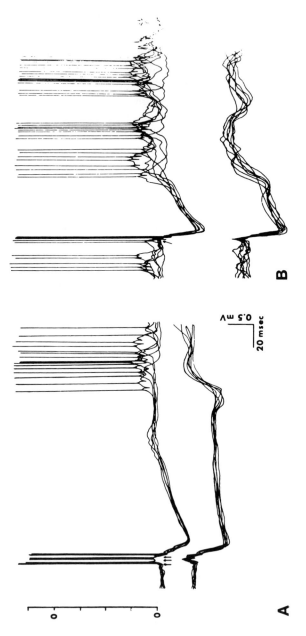

Figure 7-2. Antidromic responses in motor cortex to stimulation of the pyramidal tract (PT). A. Six consecutive responses recorded within a PT cell (upper traces) and simultaneously from a point at the same depth (1.5 mm) but 0.4 mm laterally; tip diameter of extracellular pipette approximately 15 μ. Stimuli: three 0.2 msec 100μ-A pulses delivered between two adjacent tips of PT stimulating electrodes. Note correlation between IPSP and extracellularly recorded positive wave, and almost complete absence of potentials related to cell discharge in extracellular record. B. Same situnation as in A., but records obtained subsequently and on a slower sweep. (Reprinted with permission from Humphrey, D. R. Re-analysis of the antidromic cortical response. II. On the contribution of cell discharge and PSPs to the evoked potentials. *Electroencephalography and Clinical Neurophysiology*, 1968, 25:421-442.)

162

sis, may produce increases in the latency of one or more BSER component with little change in wave amplitude (Stockard, Rossiter, and Wiederholt, et al., 1976; Robinson and Rudge, 1977; Stephens and Thornton, 1976). A decrease in conduction velocity due to axonal demyelination is considered the cause of this prolongation. A similar increase in BSER latency due to decreased conduction velocity was demonstrated with bilateral cryoprobes in the upper brain stem of the cat (Jones, Stockard, and Rossiter, et al., 1976; Stockard and Sharbrough, 1980). Cooling the pontine auditory pathway below the nuclei of the lateral lemnisci to 8-15°C produced progressive delays in the latencies of the BSER after wave III without reducing their amplitudes. This was interpreted as a slowing of conduction time in the ascending auditory tracts on both sides of the brain-stem.

An additional latency influence is indicated by other experiments in which latency was increased without accompanying amplitude effects by prolonging stimulus rise time (Hecox, Squires, and Galambos, 1976). These data indicate that, in addition to axonal conduction velocity, BSER latencies also reflect the rate at which threshold for synaptic activation is attained, i.e., as stimulus rise time is prolonged, synaptic threshold is more slowly attained, and latency for BSER generation is increased.

In contrast to the preceding effects that focused chiefly on latency, other studies have demonstrated significant effects on amplitude in the absence of any latency change. Patients with brain-stem tumors, for example, may show only a reduction in BSER amplitude (Stephens and Thornton, 1976). Administration of the muscarinic agonist oxytremorine or the mixed nicotinic-muscarinic agonist carbachol is reported to increase BSER amplitudes in the absence of latency changes; nicotine administration reduces amplitude without latency effects (Bhargava, Salamy, and McKean, 1978). These authors conclude that BSER amplitudes can be altered by changing the excitability of muscarinic or nicotinic receptors.

Other commonly used experimental procedures produce changes in both latency and amplitude. Examples are the increased latency and decreased amplitude which accompany an increase in stimulus rate (Pratt and Sohmer, 1976; Huang and Buchwald, 1978; Hyde, Stephens, and Thornton, 1976) or a decrease in intensity (Starr and Achor, 1975; Pratt and Sohmer, 1976; Huang and Buchwald, 1978). (Since the fastest click rate used, 200/sec, is much slower than axonal refractory periods, axonal transmission velocity would not be changed.) These latency increases suggest that the synaptic threshold is reached more slowly as a function of faster or less intense stimuli, while the concurrent amplitude decrements suggest that postsynaptic activation is attained in a diminished population of neurons.

From the foregoing data it is apparent that BSER latencies and amplitudes reflect different physiologic processes which can independently vary or which may concurrently change. These conclusions support the hypothesis that the BSER positive peaks reflect PSPs, insofar as PSP field potentials could predictably show latency changes as a function of altered input conduction velocity (e.g., as by axonal demyelination or cooling) without necessarily showing concurrent amplitude effects. PSP field potentials could also show amplitude (but not necessarily latency) changes as a function of altered excitability (e.g., as by drug actions) in cell membrane receptors. Alternative physiologic candidates, such as "axonal projections of the [brain-stem] nuclei rather than the nuclei themselves" (Stockard, Stockard, and Sharbrough, 1978), would appear incapable of causing the differential latency or amplitude changes summarized above.

BSER waves reflect functionally separable substrate systems. Selective changes restricted to a particular BSER wave as a function of some experimental variable suggests a generator substrate for that wave which is not shared with other BSER waves but, rather, is functionally separable.

This concept is supported by data such as the differential BSER sensitivity to binaural interactions. In numerous species it has been shown that when an equal number of BSER responses elicited by monaural stimulation of each ear are summed and compared with the same number of binaural responses, the amplitudes of waves I, II, and III are identical under the two conditions (cat, Jewett, 1970; Huang and Buchwald, 1978, Fullerton and Hosford, 1979; guinea pig, Dobie and Berlin, 1979b; Gardi and Berlin, 1979; Huang, 1980; rat, Huang, 1980). The same studies report that wave IV is larger by 25 to 50 percent with summed monaural than with binaural stimulation. This finding clearly indicates that a functional effect involving significant binaural interaction in the generator substrate of wave IV is not found in the generator systems of waves I to III.

One of the most common BSER procedures, the presentation of acoustic stimuli over a range of intensities, results in a uniform increase in BSER latencies as stimulus intensity is progressively decreased. This latency effect is due primarily to an increase in the latency of wave I with little or no latency increment added by the subsequent waves (cat, Huang and Buchwald, 1978; Mair, Elverland, and Laukli, 1978; human, Pratt and Sohmer, 1976; Starr and Achor, 1975; Stockard, Stockard, and Sharbrough, 1978). The differential sensitivity of wave I to intensity shows that its generator system reflects a functional characteristic clearly not shared by the generators of subsequent BSER waves.

Developmental studies also emphasize the concept of different generator systems for the different BSER waves, insofar as the course of their maturation proceeds differentially. During the third week of development in the kitten, a marked enhancement of wave III amplitude is produced by fast click rates in contrast to concurrent decremental effects on other BSER amplitudes (Shipley, Buchwald, and Norman, et al., 1980). Wave V in the kitten first appears significantly later than do waves I-IV (Jewett and Romano, 1972;

Shipley, Buchwald, and Norman, et al., 1980) and its latency-amplitude response to rapid click rates is slowest to attain adult values (Shipley, Buchwald, and Norman, et al., 1980). BSER interpeak intervals are incremently prolonged across waves I to V early in development; as a function of maturation, the interpeak intervals shorten differentially and become generally similar in the adult (cat, Shipley, Buchwald, and Norman et al., 1980; Jewett and Romano, 1972; rat, Jewett and Romano, 1972).

Taken together, the preceding parametric and developmental data suggest that individual BSER waves may reflect substrate systems which are functionally separable.

Summary of General Hypotheses

In this section, working hypotheses relating to the physiologic characteristics of the BSER generators based on data from a variety of experimental studies have been developed. Briefly restated, these hypotheses propose that: (1) BSERs reflect graded PSPs rather than APs discharged at cell somas or transmitted along the axonal projections; (2) BSER latency and amplitude measures reflect different physiologic processes which may interact, and (3) BSER waves reflect functionally separable substrate systems. The emergent composite portrays each BSER wave as a reflection of a generator system which can be differentially distinguished along parametric, developmental, or other dimensions. Within such separable substrate systems, latency is postulated as a function of fiber transmission time plus time to synaptic threshold of a target cell population, while peak amplitude is postulated as a function of graded PSP summation. In the subsequent section, hypotheses relevant to the generator system of individual BSER components, based on specific physiologic as well as anatomic characteristics, will be discussed.

HYPOTHESES OF BSER GENERATION

Wave I

Based on data from several species, there is general agreement that the first (I) vertex positive potential in the BSER sequence is produced by acoustic nerve activity (cat, Jewett, 1970; Lev and Sohmer, 1972; Buchwald and Huang, 1975; Achor and Starr, 1980a; rat, Jewett and Romano, 1972; mouse, Henry and Chole, 1978; Henry, 1979a, 1979b; monkey, Allen and Starr, 1978; human, Sohmer, Feinmesser, and Szabo, 1974; Jewett and Williston, 1971; Picton, Hillyard, and Krauz, et al., 1974; Streletz, Katz, and Hohenberger, et al., 1977; Starr and Achor, 1975; Stockard and Rossiter, 1977; Hashimoto, Ishiyama, and Mizutani, 1980; Hashimoto, Ishiyami, and Yoshimoto, 1981).

Wave I appears as a relatively small positivity when a vertex electrode is referenced to the pinna, mastoid, or tongue, or to a noncephalic reference on the sternum, neck, or tail (cat, Jewett, 1970; Lev and Sohmer, 1972; Plantz, Williston, and Jewett, 1974; Achor and Starr, 1980a; rat, Jewett and Romano, 1972; Plantz, Williston, and Jewett, 1974; mouse, Henry and Chole, 1979; monkey, Allen and Starr, 1978; human, Lev and Sohmer, 1972; Martin and Coats, 1973; Streletz, Katz, and Hohenberger, et al., 1977; Stockard, Stockard, and Sharborough, 1978). Wave I inverts to become a negative potential when an ipsilateral mastoid, pinna, or tongue electrode is recorded against a noncephalic reference (cat, Plantz, Williston, and Jewett, 1974; human, Streletz, Katz, and Hohenberger et al., 1977; Stockard, Stockard, and Sharbrough, 1978), as well as when the mastoid is referenced to tongue or nose (cat, Lev and Sohmer, 1972; rat, Jewett and Romano, 1972). Polarity inversion of wave I around the mastoid process is consistent with its postulated origin from acoustic nerve activity.

Lesion studies, in which the acoustic nerve was centrally sectioned at its exit from the internal acoustic meatus, have shown that wave I persists while all subsequent BSER waves are abolished (Fig. 7-3) (Buchwald and Huang, 1975; Henry and Chole, 1978b, Henry, 1979). Under some conditions, cochlear microphonic (CM) components may also appear in the wave I latency range. For example, after crushing the acoustic nerve (locus and extent not specified) in one cat, attenuation of 90 percent or more was reported for all BSER waves of neural origin; there was no effect on the CM, which was found to extend into the time domain of the first BSER wave (Achor and Starr, 1980b). These authors suggest that the CM can make a major contribution to wave I. However, when precautions are taken to define and minimize CM contributions by alternating stimulus polarity, shortening stimulus duration, or reducing stimulus intensity, wave I can be distinguished from the CM (Schwent and Jewett, 1976; Sohmer and Pratt, 1976; Ornitz and Walter, 1975; Henry and Lepkowski, 1978; Mair, Elverland, and Laukli, 1978). Under these conditions, acoustic nerve section still leaves a large, well defined BSER wave I of neural, not CM, origin (Henry and Chole, 1978b). These data are consistent with intracochlear recordings taken after potassium chloride (KCl) inactivation of the central end of the acoustic nerve which show the acoustic nerve neural response to clicks to remain clearly distinguishable from the CM (Legouix and Pierson, 1974).

The most common basis for relating the first BSER wave to the acoustic nerve, however, is its temporal correspondence with the acoustic nerve NI potential. It has been repeatedly noted in numerous recording configurations and across species that the peak latencies of the first BSER wave and the NI potential recorded from the round window or mastoid process are simultaneous (cat, Jewett, 1970; Lev and Sohmer, 1972; Achor and Starr 1980b; rat, Jewett and Romano, 1972; mouse, Henry and Chole, 1978b; Henry, 1979;

INTACT

PRE-COLLICULAR
DECEREBRATION

INFERIOR COLLICULUS
ASPIRATION

COCHLEAR NUCLEUS
ISOLATION

ACOUSTIC NERVE
ISOLATION

POST MORTEM

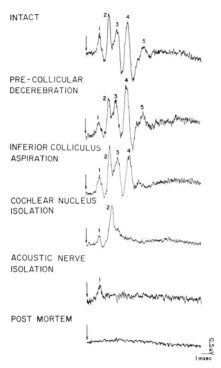

Figure 7-3. Auditory brain-stem responses after various lesions. The potential sequence recorded from the intact cat in response to binaural click presentations was unaltered following precollicular decerebration. Subsequent bilateral aspiration of the inferior colliculi largely eliminated BSER V. Following surgical isolation of the cochlear nuclei from the brain stem, waves III and IV disappeared. Isolation of acoustic nerve from the cochlear nucleus resulted in the loss of wave II. No potential remained in the post mortem recording (bottom trace). Positivity is above the baseline. (Reprinted with permission from Buchwald, J. S., and Huang, C. M. Far-field acoustic response: Origins in the Cat. *Science*, 1975, *189*:382-384. Copyright 1975 by the American Association for the Advancement of Science.)

human, Sohmer and Feinmesser, 1967; Terkildsen, Osterhammel, and Huis in't Veld, 1974a; Stockard, Stockard, and Sharbrough, 1978).

The two cochlear potential components originally described by Wever and Bray (1930) have commonly been identified as (1) *aurals*, or CM and (2) *neurals*, or acoustic nerve action potentials. It has been established in a variety of experiments that neurals are more sensitive than aurals to temperature changes, blood supply, anoxia, and death. These two kinds of potentials can be separated from each other in a number of ways. For example, with round-window recordings, the CM reverses polarity when stimulus polarity changes and the neural response does not; at low intensity, only the neural response appears; with increasing intensity only the neural response decreases in latency; and only the neural response is masked by noise and reduced by a preceding click (summarized by Rosenblith and Rosenzweig, 1951).

The Nl response has been identified as the neural component of round-window recordings and is commonly interpreted as a reflection of the acoustic nerve compound action potential (cat, Teas, Eldridge, and Davis, 1962; Antoli-Candela and Kiang, 1978; guinea pig, Legouix and Pierson, 1974; Nagel, 1974). From different locations within the middle-ear cavity and ear canal, as well as from extrabulbar recording locations on the mastoid process ipsilateral to the stimulus, potentials of the same polarity, latency, and duration as the round-window Nl response have been recorded (Fig. 7-4) (cat, Rosenblith and Rosenzweig, 1951; Montandon, Megell, and Kahn, et al., 1975). These results correspond with those cited above, which show that the BSER wave I recorded from the mastoid process as well as from the vertex has a latency which is identical with Nl, and a polarity inversion from negative to positive simply as a function of electrode configuration. Thus, evoked responses recorded from the scalp, the mastoid bulla, or within the middle-ear cavity have the same latency at the round window Nl response.

In contrast, when the compound action potential of the acoustic nerve is recorded from the central end of the nerve, it shows a peak latency which is 0.2 msec longer than that of the round-window Nl potential (Fig 7-5) (cat, Antoli-Candela and Kiang, 1978). An even longer latency of 0.4-0.5 msec has been noted for transmission from the spiral lamina in the first cochlear turn to the central end of the guinea pig's acoustic nerve (Nagel, 1974). These data introduce a curious paradox with regard to the generator substrate of BSER wave I. If wave I occurs simultaneously with the Nl round-window potential, it cannot be reflecting the longer latency compound action potential at the central end of the acoustic nerve. This makes it difficult to postulate an acoustic nerve dipole as the generator model for wave I. In the guinea pig, such a model would require a wave I latency increase up to 0.5 msec after the

Figure 7-4. Effects of electrode location on the waveform of potentials from an anesthetized cat. Preliminary measurements established that recordings were stable over long periods of time. The serial order in which recordings were made was location 5, 7, 4, 6, 3, 2, 1, 8, 9, 10. On the left is a drawing showing electrode placements. On the right are shown waveforms averaged over 500 responses to clicks (locations 3-7 on an expanded vertical scale shown in the dashed traces). Negativity at the recording electrode (referred to the headholder) is represented as downward deflections. (Reprinted with permission from Montandon, P. B., Megell, N. D., and Kahn, A. B., et al. Recording auditory-nerve potentials as an office procedure. *Annals of Otology, Rhinology and Laryngology*, 1975, *84*:2-100.)

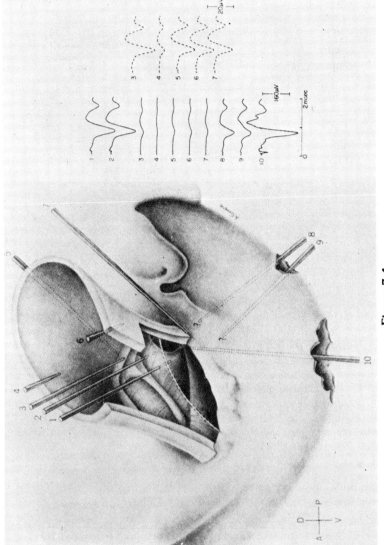

Figure 7-4.

169

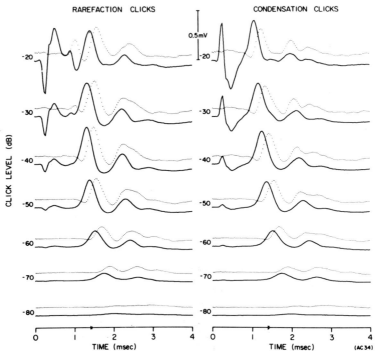

Figure 7-5. Gross potentials recorded simultaneously from the bone near the round window (solid traces) and the internal auditory meatus (dotted traces). Each trace is an average of between 16 and 512 responses to clicks. In most of the round window (RW) recordings, the early deflections represent the cochlear microphonic components which are negligible in the meatus recordings. In all traces, the N1 in RW recordings occurs approximately 0.2 msec earlier than N1 in meatus recordings. This probably represents the time needed for conduction of spikes from the site of spike origin in the cochlea to the recording electrode site in the internal auditory meatus (see Chapter 4). (Reprinted with permission from Antoli-Candela, F., and Kiang, N. Y.-S. Unit activity underlying the N_1 potential. In R. F. Naunton and C. Fernandez (Eds.), *Evoked electrical activity in the auditory neurvous system.* New York: Academic Press, 1978.)

Nl round window response and in the cat, a shift of at least 0.2 msec. As noted, however, the first BSER wave and the Nl response have simultaneous peak latencies. Thus, while acoustic nerve activity has been related to BSER wave I generation, acoustic nerve transmission of action potentials from cochlea to brain stem occupies a time course which is incompatible with wave I latency.

In the preceding section the significant role of graded PSPs in the generation of evoked field potentials was discussed. The relatively large current fields and long time constants of PSPs, in contrast to those of APs, have been causally related to evoked field potentials in a variety of experiments. The VIIIth nerve generator potentials, the graded activity in the terminal portion of the dendrites, have been observed with intracellular recordings in both goldfish (Furukawa and Ishii, 1967) and carp (Flock, Jorgensen, and Russell, 1973) (Fig. 7-6). In the mammalian cochlea, generator potentials are also assumed to occur in the unmyelinated terminals of the acoustic nerve which have been estimated to range from 700 μ to 1 or 2 mm in length (Dallos, 1978). Graded activity in other unmyelinated fibers (e.g., the motor cortex pyramidal cell apical dendrites) has been directly related to evoked field potentials recorded 0.4 mm distant (Humphrey, 1968). Such data suggest the possibility of a similar relation between generator potentials in the acoustic nerve dendritic terminals and the Nl potential recorded at the round window, i.e., that Nl reflects summated generator potential activity in the cochlea rather than a compound action potential transmitted along the course of the acoustic nerve. Such an hypothesis would be consistent with the previously noted parametric and physiological characteristics of Nl, insofar as generator potentials would necessarily display these characteristics at lower thresholds than their resultant APs.

Regarding BSERs, the results of lesion studies and the latency characteristics of wave I, i.e., its coincidence with Nl, suggest that wave I and Nl share a common acoustic nerve generator. Based on the preceding discussion we hypothesize that graded generator potentials in the dendritic terminals and *not* action potentials transmitted along the course of the acoustic nerve may be the physiologic and anatomic substrates most relevant to wave I. While CM activity can extend into the wave I time domain, a clearly defined wave of acoustic nerve origin persists in the absence of any CM contribution.

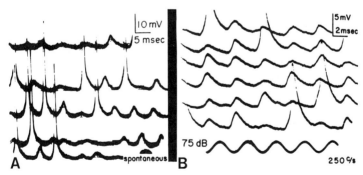

Figure 7-6. Generator potentials observed in VIIIth nerve fibers (small saccular fibers) in the hearing organ of the goldfish. A. Spontaneous activity. B. Responses to moderate intensity of sound, obtained from a different fiber. Subthreshold responses were graded to the sound intensity. (Reprinted with permission from Furukawa, T. and Ishii, Y., Neurophysiological studies on hearing in goldfish. *Journal of Neurophysiology*, 1967, *30*:1377-1403.)

Wave II

Across species, BSER wave II appears as a small-to-moderately-large positivity when a vertex electrode is referenced to the pinna, mastoid, or tongue, or to a noncephalic reference on the sternum, neck, or tail (cat, Plantz, Williston, and Jewett, 1974; Achor and Starr, 1980a; Jewett, 1970; Lev and Sohmer, 1972; rat, Plantz, Williston, and Jewett, 1974; Jewett and Romano, 1972; mouse, Henry and Chole, 1979; monkey, Allen and Starr, 1978; human, Streletz, Katz, and Hohenberger, et al., 1977; Martin and Coats, 1973; Lev and Sohmer, 1972; Stockard, Stockard, and Sharbrough, 1978). Wave II differs from wave I in that it does not become negative when a mastoid or pinna electrode is recorded against a noncephalic reference (cat, rat, Plantz, Williston, and Jewett, 1974; monkey, Allen and Starr, 1978; human, Streletz, Katz, and Hohenberger et al., 1977). Thus, as a function of electrode position, the polarities of waves I and II can be differentiated. Polarity inversion around the mastoid process for wave I is consistent with its postulated origin from acoustic nerve activity, while the absence of such inversion for wave II is consistent with its generation from a different far-field locus.

Wave II can be observed as two distinct peaks, termed IIA and IIB in this discussion, in the cat (Plantz, Williston, and Jewett, 1974; Stockard, Stockard, and Sharbrough, 1978; Shipley, Buchwald, and Norman, et al., 1980; Achor and Starr, 1980a) and in the monkey (Allen and Starr, 1978), when the vertex electrode is recorded against a noncephalic rather than a cephalic (e.g., pinna or tongue) reference. In the monkey, ipsilateral pinna-sternum recordings are reported to show a wave at the latency of IIA while vertex-ipsilateral pinna shows a wave at the latency of IIB (Allen and Starr, 1978). In the cat, the appearance of these two components is particularly pronounced early in development, when IIA amplitude may equal or exceed that of IIB (Fig. 7-7). As the waves shorten to adult latency and recovery cycle values, IIB becomes relatively more prominent. In the adult cat, wave IIB shows a latency which is comparable to that of wave II in vertex–cephalic reference recordings, whereas IIA occurs approximately 0.5 msec earlier (Shipley, Buchwald, and Norman, et al., 1980; Achor and Starr, 1980a) and has almost no definition when a cephalic reference (versus a noncephalic neck or sternum reference) is used (Jewett, 1970; Lev and Sohmer, 1972).

On the basis of similar latencies between wave IIA and a maximum voltage field in the cochlear nucleus (CN) area of acoustic nerve termination, the unmyelinated central terminals of the acoustic nerve have been suggested as the generator of wave IIA (Achor and Starr, 1980a). Consistent with these data is the finding that extensive lesions in the CN, sufficient to cause marked reduction or loss of the later waves, had no effect on wave IIA (Achor and Starr, 1980b).

A number of correlative surface BSER-depth evoked potential (EP) map-

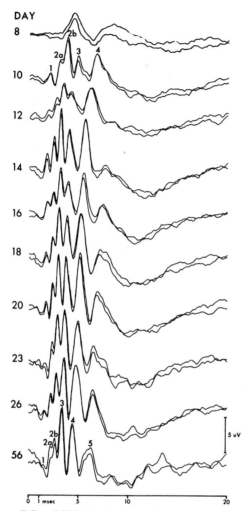

Figure 7-7. BSER developmental sequence from one kitten across the first two months of life. The stimulus (46 dB HL, 10/sec clicks) occurs at trace onset. (Reprinted with permission from Shipley, C., Buchwald, J. S., and Norman, R., et al. Brain-stem auditory evoked response development in the kitten. *Brain Research*, 1980, *182*:313-326.)

ping studies have been carried out in which wave II (or IIB) has been shown to occur at the same latency as that of the primary CN evoked potential (cat, Jewett, 1970; Lev and Sohmer, 1972, Achor and Starr, 1980a; mouse, Henry, 1979b), with both wave II and CN latency values comparable to those established in earlier studies of locally evoked CN potentials (Rose, Galambos, and Hughes, 1959; Moushegan, Rupert, and Galambos, 1962). A large positive voltage field in the trapezoid body as well as in the CN was reported to show the same latency as peak IIB in one study (Achor and Starr, 1980b). During the first 2 months of life, wave IIB shows an exponential decrease in latency with a developmental change in latency values (Shipley, Buchwald, and Norman, et al., 1980) that is similar to those of depth EPs recorded from the ventral CN of kittens during the same period (Pujol, 1972; Romand and Marty, 1975).

In a series of correlative recordings between surface BSER wave components and single units in the brain-stem auditory nuclei, a subpopulation of CN units has been described that shows a highly synchronized "onset" response to multiple stimulus presentations (less than 0.1 msec standard deviation in response latency). The mean response latency of these CN units (2.6 ± 0.4 msec) corresponded most closely with wave II (2.3 ± 0.4 msec) of the concurrently recorded BSERs (Huang and Buchwald, 1977).

The preceding electrophysiologic data indicate a consistent correlation between the latency of responses originating in the CN and BSER wave II. These findings have been supported by the results from various lesion studies. Marked reduction to complete loss of wave II has been reported following transection of the central end of the acoustic nerve (Buchwald and Huang, 1975) or partial to complete destruction of the ipsilateral CN (cat, Goldenberg and Derbyshire, 1975; Gardi, Merzenich, and McKean, 1979; Achor and Starr, 1980b; mouse, Henry, 1979b). After bilateral surgical isolation of the CN from the adjacent brain stem, waves I and II remained unchanged, whereas waves III, IV, and V disappeared (Fig. 7-3) (Buchwald & Huang, 1975). Similarly, following selective lesions or complete transection of the dorsal, intermediate, and ventral acoustic stria, waves I and II were unaffected, although all subsequent BSERs were markedly reduced (Buchwald and Huang, 1975; Fullerton and Hosford, 1979; Achor and Starr, 1980b; Gardi, Merzenich, and McKean, 1979). Moreover, extensive lesions of the superior olivary complex, which involved the adjacent trapezoid body fibers, had no effect on the BSERs prior to wave III (Achor and Starr, 1980b).

Insofar as interruption of the CN output produces no change in wave II, APs transmitted out of the CN through dorsal, intermediate, and ventral acoustic stria cannot play a role in wave II generation. Within the CN per se, both PSPs and APs are possible generator candidates. However, as discussed, given the greater length and time constants of the PSPs, their extracellular current fields are larger, more prolonged, and can be recorded as field potentials over a much greater distance than those of the somatic APs. Thus, the PSPs of CN neurons, particularly those which exhibit the highly synchronized "onset" responses which are necessary for a constant latency, short-duration EP, are suggested as the physiological substrate of wave II.

In summary, no tract or nucleus central to the CN has been convincingly implicated in the generation of wave II (or IIB), whereas data from a variety of different experiments consistently indicate that the CN contributes to and is essential for BSER wave II. PSPs generated by CN neurons are hypothesized as the significant anatomic and physiologic substrate of wave IIB.

Wave III

Wave III is recorded as a small-to-relatively-large positivity with either vertex-noncephalic electrode placements or with vertex referenced to the ipsilateral mastoid, pinna, or tongue during monaural stimulation (cat, Plantz, Williston, and Jewett, 1974; Shipley, Buchwald, and Norman, et al., 1980; Achor and Starr, 1980a; rat, Jewett and Romano, 1972; Plantz, Williston, and Jewett, 1974; mouse, Henry, 1979b; monkey, Allen and Starr, 1978; human, Stockard, Stockard, and Sharbrough, 1978; Streletz, Katz, and Hohenberger, et al., 1977).

Correlative recordings of surface BSERs and depth EPs in the same subject have shown that a potential of maximum amplitude in the superior olivary complex (SOC) of the ipsilateral and/or contralateral brain stem has a latency which coincides with that of wave III (cat, Jewett, 1970; Lev and Sohmer, 1972; Achor and Starr, 1980a; mouse, Henry, 1979b). In none of these mapping studies were similarly large EPs (latencies corresponding to wave III) recorded outside the SOC, e.g., in the CN, lateral lemniscus, or inferior colliculus, although a lower amplitude positivity at this latency was also reported in the trapezoid body (Achor and Starr, 1980a). While such data implicate SOC activity in the generation of wave III, the resolution of these depth EP recordings has been insufficient to differentiate nuclei of particular relevance.

Additional support for the importance of SOC contributions to wave III generation is provided by lesion studies. Extensive rostral brain-stem lesions which involved the inferior colliculus and lateral lemniscus, but spared the entire SOC or involved only the lateral superior olive (LSO) produced no change in wave III (cat, Lev and Sohmer, 1972; Goldenberg and Derbyshire, 1975; Buchwald and Huang, 1975; Gardi, Merzenich, and McKean, 1979; Achor and Starr, 1980b; guinea pig, Gardi and Berlin, 1979; mouse, Henry, 1979b). Lesions confined to the dorsal and intermediate acoustic stria likewise produced no change in wave III or in any other BSER (Gardi, Merzenich, and McKean, 1979; Achor and Starr, 1980b). However, a midsaggital section through the entire dorsoventral extent of the trapezoid body was shown to eliminate or markedly reduce the amplitude of wave III (Fig. 7-8) (Buchwald & Huang, 1975; Gardi, Merzenich, and McKean, 1979; Fullerton and Hosford, 1979), which suggests the importance of a contralateral generator. Following an extensive unilateral SOC lesion which destroyed most of the medial superior olive (MSO) and the decussating fibers of the trapezoid body, wave III was eliminated in response to ipsilateral stimulation while contralateral

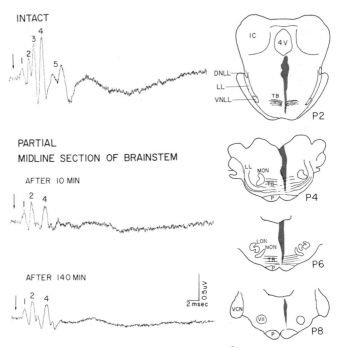

Figure 7-8. Changes in the BSER sequence rescorded from a decerebrate cat following midsaggital section of the brain stem. In this split-brain-stem preparation, a small amount of the ventral trapezoid body remained intact at the P4 level, as indicated in the lesion reconstruction diagrams on the right. Potential III showed a small residual positivity 140 minutes after the lesion. Potentials IV and V showed marked reductions, whereas potentials I and II remained at control levels. Key: inferior colliculus (IC); fourth ventricle (4V); dorsal nucleus of lateral lemniscus (DNLL); lateral lemniscus (LL); ventral nucleus of lateral lemniscus (VNLL); medial olivary nucleus (MON); pyramid (P); trapezoid body (TB); lateral olivary nucleus (LON); ventral cochlear nucleus (VCN); facial nucleus (VII). (Reprinted with permission from Buchwald, J. S., and Huang, C. M. Far-field acoustic response: Origins in the cat. *Science*, 1975, *189*:382–384. Copyright 1975 by the American Association for the Advancement of Science.)

stimulation produced a small residual positivity (Achor and Starr, 1980b). With smaller unilateral lesions of the SOC and adjacent trapezoid body, wave III was attenuated but not eliminated to either ipsilateral or contralateral stimuli (Achor and Starr, 1980b). Taken together, these depth-recording and lesion studies portray wave III as a compound potential which derives from both uncrossed input to the ipsilateral SOC and crossed input to the contralateral SOC. Insofar as wave III usually presents a single peak, such ipsilateral and contralateral contributions must have identical latencies so as to superimpose.

The suggestion that wave III consists of temporally overlapping components is supported by developmental observations of the kitten BSERs. With a vertex-noncephalic recording configuration, wave III consistently showed a double peak during the second week of life (Fig. 7-9) (Shipley, Buchwald, and Norman, et al., 1980). Thereafter, the two components, waves IIIA and IIIB, became less distinct and merged into a single wave III by the middle of the third week (Fig. 7-7). While a bimodal wave III was not observed in the adult cat, waves IIIA and IIIB were reported in the adult monkey with vertex-noncephalic electrodes (Allen and Starr, 1978). In this study, only a single-peaked wave III appeared when a vertex-ipsilateral pinna electrode configuration was used. In the adult human, two positive peaks within the latency range of wave III, waves IIIA and IIIB, have been reported as a normal variant with vertex-ipsilateral earlobe as well as vertex-contra- lateral earlobe recordings (Stockard, Stockard and Sharbrough, 1978; Chiappa, Gladstone, and Young, 1979; Edwards, Buchwald, and Tanguay, et al., 1982).

Particularly relevant to the role of the SOC in wave III generation is the comparative anatomy of this region. When the major olivary nuclei, i.e., the medial superior olivary nucleus (MSO), the lateral superior olivary nucleus (LSO) and the medial nucleus of the trapezoid body (MNTB), are compared across species in terms of number and size of cells/nuclei (Irving and Harri- son, 1967; Moore and Moore, 1971), three classes of SOC configurations are recognized: (1) MSO small, LSO relatively large, MNTB relatively large, as shown by the rat, mouse, and hamster; (2) MSO large, LSO large, MNTB large, as shown by the cat, guinea pig, dog, and chinchilla; (3) MSO large, LSO relatively small, MNTB relatively small, as shown by the human, ape,

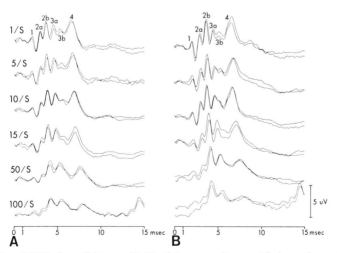

Figure 7-9.   BSERs from 2 kittens (A,B) of the same litter at 13 days of age. Note bimodality of wave III, which is transiently present only at this stage of development. (Shipley, C., and Buchwald, J., unpublished observations, 1980.)

178   Jennifer S. Buchwald

and monkey (Irving and Harrison, 1967). Indeed, in the human, the MNTB is too vestigial to be reliably identified and the LSO contains only 20 percent of the number of cells in the larger MSO (Moore and Moore, 1971).

The MNTB is innervated via large fibers of the trapezoid body from the ventral CN of the opposite side (Harrison and Irving, 1966). This entirely contralateral input has been confirmed by physiologic studies showing that MNTB cells respond only to stimulation of the contralateral ear (Goldberg, Adrian, and Smith, 1964). The LSO is ipsilaterally innervated via small fibers of the trapezoid body from the ipsilateral ventral CN; it receives contralateral input only indirectly through a projection from MNTB (Stotler, 1953; Harrison and Irving, 1966). The MSO, in contrast, receives direct projections from the ventral CN of both sides (Stotler, 1953), with fibers from the ipsilateral CN ending on the lateral dendrites and fibers from the contralateral CN ending on the medial dendrites of the same MSO cells (Fig. 7-10) (Stotler, 1953; Harrison and Irving, 1966). The MSO is the only SOC nucleus which receives direct projections from the CN of both sides. Moreover, in the human, it is not only the largest SOC nucleus but also the only known target for contralateral stimuli, since the MNTB, which can indirectly relay contralateral stimuli to the LSO, is vestigial.

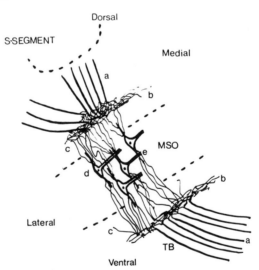

Figure 7-10. Diagram of the orientation and connections of cells in the MSO. Key: lateral olivary nucleus (S-Segment); medial olivary nucleus (MSO); trapezoid body (TB); contralateral and ipsilateral afferents (a); neuropil (b); preterminal afferents (c); cell bodies in the MSO (d); axons of cell bodies in the MSO (e). (Reprinted with permission from Clark, G. M., and Dunlop, C. W. Field potentials in the cat medial superior olivary nucleus. *Experimental Neurology*, 1968, *20*:31-42.)

The unique anatomical feature of direct inputs to the lateral and medial dendrites of the MSO from the ipsilateral and contralateral CN is paralleled by the distinctive electrophysiologic characteristics of the MSO. It has been postulated that depolarization of the CN afferent fibers to the MSO produces EPSPs which have a long time constant and which result in a current sink on the side of the cell membrane, i.e., on the dendrites adjacent, to the stimulated afferent fiber terminals (Clark and Dunlop, 1968). Summation of these EPSPs would then produce a negative field potential on the side of the MSO stimulated and a positive field potential on the opposite side. This interpretation is supported by both single-unit and field potential data. PSPs in the lateral dendrites have been shown to produce a large negative field potential at the lateral periphery of the MSO (Fig. 7-11) (cat, Tsuchitani and Boudreau, 1964; Clark and Dunlop, 1968). This negative EP characteristically inverted to a large positivity at the medial border of the MSO (Tsuchitani and Boudreau, 1964; Worden, Marsh, and Bremner, 1966; Clark and Dunlop, 1968; Guinan, Norris, and Guinan, 1972). With contralateral stimulation, PSPs in the medial dendrites were shown to produce a large negative field potential at the medial edge of the MSO; this potential typically inverted to a positivity at the lateral edge of the MSO (Fig. 7-11) (Tsuchitani and Boudreau, 1964; Clark and Dunlop, 1968). From the center of the MSO, a large amplitude positivity was recorded, with either ipsilateral or contralateral stimuli, which showed the same peak latency regardless of side of stimulation (Tsuchitani and Boudreau, 1964). These field potential data have been extended by other studies which indicate that binaurally excitable units are the most common type within the MSO, but not within the LSO or periolivary nuclei (cat, Goldberg and Brown, 1968; Guinan, Norris, and Guinan,

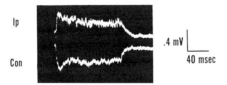

Ip

.4 mV

Con

40 msec

Figure 7-11. Reponses recorded at the dorsolateral border of the medial olivary nucleus (MSO) to ipsilateral and contralateral noise stimuli of long duration. The term "border" refers to the area immediately adjacent to the cell layer in which are located the long dendrites projecting from the MSO cells. When the electrode was in the cell layer, the potentials evoked by ipsilateral and contralateral stimulation were positive, of large amplitude, and equal latency. (Reprinted with permission from Tsuchitani, C., and Boudreau, J. C. Wave activity in the superior olivary complex of the cat. *Journal of Neurophysiology*, 1964, 27:814-827.)

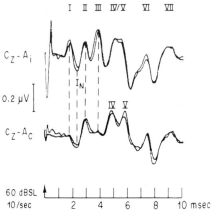

Figure 7-12. Effects of recording C_z − A_i (vertex to ipsilateral ear lobe) and C_z − A_c (vertex to contralateral ear lobe) on
BSER amplitudes in a normal subject. Waves I and III are selectively attenuated in C_z − A_c. (Reprinted with permission from
Stockard, J. J., Stockard, J. E., and Sharbrough, F. W. Nonpathologic factors influencing brain-stem auditory evoked potentials. *American Journal of EEG Technology*, 1978, *18*:
177-209.)

1972), and that such binaural MSO units have the same "best" frequency
with either ipsi- or contralateral stimulation (Guinan, Norris, and Guinan,
1972).

If BSER wave III reflected MSO field potentials, different electrode configurations might be anticipated to affect its amplitude. With ipsilateral stimulation, a vertex electrode referenced to a site which reflected the negative field
generated at the lateral edge of the ipsilateral MSO would predictably show a
larger net positivity than if it were referenced to a site which reflected the
positive field generated at the lateral edge of the contralateral MSO. The ipsilateral negativity, differentially inverted, would enhance the amplitude of a
vertex positivity, whereas the contralateral positivity, differentially inverted,
would subtract from the vertex potential. This predicted relation is indeed
supported by a number of observations. With the vertex electrode referenced
to the ipsilateral mastoid, wave III was reported to be consistently larger than
with vertex-contralateral mastoid recordings (Fig. 7-12) (mouse, Henry,
1979b; human, Stockard, Stockard, and Sharbrough, 1978). With the ipsilateral pinna or mastoid referenced to a noncephalic electrode on the neck,
sternum, or ankle, wave III appeared as a weak positivity (cat, Plantz, Williston, and Jewett, 1974; monkey, Allen and Starr, 1978; human, Stockard,
Stockard, and Sharbrough, 1978), or as a negativity (rat, Plantz, Williston,
and Jewett, 1974; human, Terkildsen, Osterhammer, and Huis in't Veld,
1974a; Streletz, Katz, and Hohenberger, et al., 1977). In contrast, a clear
wave III positivity appeared with the contralateral mastoid referenced non-

cephalically (Terkildsen, Osterhammer, and Huis in't Veld, 1974a). Taken together, these data suggest that the ipsilateral mastoid, like the region lateral to the ipsilateral MSO, is in a current field which is negative for wave III relative to the vertex or to the contralateral mastoid.

In summary, a variety of data links the MSO and its field potentials with wave III. Brain-stem levels rostral to the MSO are not important for the integrity of wave III, while the MSO and its crossed and uncrossed trapezoid body input are essential. The MSO is the only SOC nucleus which receives both ipsilateral and contralateral direct projections from the CN and displays evoked responses which occur at the same latency to either ipsilateral or contralateral stimuli, thus satisfying the wave III requirement for potential contributions from ipsilateral and contralateral generators which temporally superimpose. MSO field potentials produced by monaural stimulation are mirror-image dipoles with a negative field lateral to the ipsilateral MSO, and a positive field lateral to contralateral MSO, which is consistent with a wave III negative current field in the region of the ipsilateral mastoid. Finally, the PSPs of the lateral and medial MSO dendrites have a time constant and latency which are causally related to the large-amplitude MSO field potentials; these have, in turn, been correlated with the latency of wave III. In view of the direct and indirect links between MSO field potentials and wave III, the principal substrate for wave III generation is hypothesized as dendritic PSPs of the MSO.

Wave IV

A large single-peaked positivity has been recorded in a number of species as the fourth BSER wave when the vertex is referenced noncephalically (cat, Plantz, Williston, and Jewett, 1974; Shipley, Buchwald, and Norman, et al., 1980; rat, Plantz, Williston, and Jewett, 1974; mouse, Henry, 1979b; monkey, Allen and Starr, 1978), or when it is referenced to cephalic placements on tongue, nuchal ridge, ipsilateral or contralateral pinna (cat, Plantz, Williston, and Jewett, 1974; Shipley, Buchwald, and Norman, et al., 1980; Achor and Starr, 1980a; rat, Jewett and Romano, 1972; Plantz, Williston, and Jewett, 1974; mouse, Henry, 1979b; guinea pig, Dobie and Berlin, 1979b; monkey, Allen and Starr, 1978). The amplitude of wave IV is larger with vertex-to-noncephalic than with vertex-to-mastoid recordings (mouse, Henry, 1979b; monkey, Allen and Starr, 1978).

In the human, a IV-V wave complex can be recorded from the vertex. Several authors have suggested that this may be comparable to wave IV in the cat (Lev and Sohmer, 1972; Starr and Achor, 1978; Stockard, Stockard, and Sharbrough, 1978; Stockard and Sharbrough, 1980). As in the animal recordings of wave IV, the IV-V complex is also larger when the vertex electrode is noncephalically referenced than to the mastoid, presumably due to in-phase rejection of similar vertex and mastoid activity (Streletz, Katz, and Hohenberger, et al., 1977; Stockard, Stockard, and Sharbrough, 1978;

Chiappa, Gladstone, and Young, 1979). Separation of the IV-V components is reported to be maximized with vertex-contralateral mastoid and minimized with vertex-ipsilateral mastoid recordings (Stockard, Stockard, and Sharbrough, 1978). However, with vertex-ipsilateral mastoid recordings, a variety of IV-V configurations has been noted in normal subjects, e.g., a single peak in the latency range of wave V, a single peak V with IV as a leading shoulder, a single peak IV with V as a trailing shoulder, two distinct waves with peak IV lower, higher, or equal to peak V (Chiappa, Gladstone, and Young, 1979; Edwards, Buchwald, and Tanguay, et al., 1982).

In a correlative study of wave IV and depth EPs in the cat, Jewett (1970) reported that a large positive wave in the inferior colliculus (IC) and IC brachium shortened in latency and began to invert to a negativity as the electrode moved toward the lateral lemniscus (LL). This pericollicular potential showed a latency which was similar to that of wave IV, whereas the latency of a large negative wave recorded within the IC was intermediate between BSER waves IV and V (Lev and Sohmer, 1972). Achor and Starr (1980a) concluded that the IC does not substantially contribute to wave IV, insofar as the IC showed little evoked activity, while EPs with the latency of wave IV were found bilaterally in the region of the LL and SOC. Similarly, in a correlative BSER single-unit study, LL units showed a latency range corresponding to that of wave IV, whereas the latencies of units in the IC were more prolonged (Huang and Buchwald, 1977).

The independence of wave IV from the IC is further suggested by lesion studies. Following bilateral aspiration of the IC (cat, Buchwald and Huang, 1975; Gardi, Merzenich, and McKean, 1979; guinea pig, Gardi and Berlin, 1979), as well as after extensive IC lesioning (cat, Goldenberg and Derbyshire, 1975; Achor and Starr, 1980b; mouse, Henry, 1979b), no significant change was noted in the latency or amplitude of wave IV. Similarly, no change in the IV-V complex occurred after compression of the colliculi, severe enough to block the fourth ventricle and produce hydrocephalis, by a brain-stem tumor at the lower edge of the tentorium (human, Jerger, Neeley, and Jerger, 1980).

Other lesion studies have shown that, although selective destruction of the dorsal and intermediate acoustic stria had no effect on wave IV (cat, Gardi, Merzenich, and McKean, 1979; Achor and Starr, 1980b), lesions which included the ventral acoustic stria (trapezoid body) reduced wave IV amplitude by approximately 50 percent (Fig. 7-8) (cat, Buchwald and Huang, 1975; Gardi, Merzenich, and McKean, 1979; Fullerton and Hosford, 1979; Achor and Starr, 1980b). A large SOC lesion which also interrupted most of the decussating trapezoid body was shown to attenuate both waves III and IV, whereas an SOC lesion which did not include the trapezoid body still reduced wave III but had little or no effect on wave IV (Fig. 7-13) (Achor and Starr, 1980b). Taken together, these data suggest that wave IV consists of

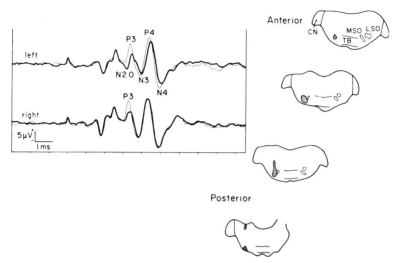

Figure 7-13. Reconstruction of superior olivary complex lesion in a cat and corresponding effects on the BSER. The unilateral lesion involved the lateral and medial superior olivary nuclei and the fibers of the trapezoid body. The BSER to contralateral stimulation ("right" in figure) had only one lesion effect, a 36 percent decrease in the amplitude of component P3. To ipsilateral stimulation ("left" in figure), component N2 shifted in a negative direction, and components P3, P4, and N4 decreased in amplitude by 45, 12, and 17 percent, respectively; all showed a slight increase in latency. (Reprinted with permission from Achor, L. J., and Starr, A. Auditory brain-stem responses in the cat. II. Effects of lesions. *Electroencephalography and Clinical Neurophysiology*, 1980b, *48*:174-190.)

one component, which depends upon fibers crossing the midline in the trapezoid body, and of another component, which is not dependent upon crossed projections. The data further suggest that the IC, the LSO, and the MSO are not essential for wave IV generation insofar as lesions of these nuclei (without extensive involvement of adjacent fiber tracts) produce no change in wave IV.

In other lesion studies, it was shown that unilateral or bilateral destruction of the dorsal portion of the LL and the dorsal nucleus of the LL (DNLL) had little or no effect on wave IV (cat, Buchwald and Huang, 1975; Achor and Starr, 1980b). In contrast, relatively small unilateral lesions in the ventral lemniscus produced transient changes in wave IV amplitude to contralateral stimulation and a sustained effect on the negativities preceding the following wave IV (Achor and Starr, 1980b). Larger unilateral lesions of the ventral leniscus, which included the VNLL and periolivary region, abolished the uncrossed component of wave IV, which remained after trapezoid body transection (Buchwald and Huang, 1975). Consistent with these effects, focal cooling with cryoprobes stereotaxically placed caudal to the LL nuclei was found to prolong wave IV latency without affecting BSER waves I and III (cat, Jones,

Stockard, and Rossiter, et al., 1976; Stockard and Sharbrough, 1980). These results suggest that the ventral region of the LL may be particularly important for the generation of wave IV.

Prominent binaural interaction effects displayed by wave IV suggest a similar conclusion. It has been shown that wave IV (but not waves I to III), is smaller by as much as 50 percent when a given number of stimuli are binaurally presented than when the same number of stimuli are monaurally presented to each ear and the responses summed (Fig. 7-14) (cat, Jewett, 1979; Huang and Buchwald, 1978; Fullerton and Hosford, 1979; guinea pig, Dobie and Berlin, 1979b; Gardi and Berlin, 1981; rat, Huang, 1980; dog, Huang, 1980). This difference between binaural and the summed monaural responses is reportedly abolished when crossing fibers in the trapezoid body are transected (Fullerton and Hosford, 1979). Binaural interaction data thus indicate that the generator of wave IV (1) responds to ipsilateral and contralateral stimuli with potentials of identical latency, and (2) responds to binaural stimuli with a potential which has the same latency but smaller amplitude than the sum of the potentials produced by ipsilateral and contralateral stimuli. Recordings from the LL indicate that EPs generated there share the foregoing latency and binaural interaction characteristics of wave IV. Electrodes in the ventral LL recorded field potentials with the same latency, threshold, and amplitude to ipsilateral and to contralateral stimulation (Fig. 7-15A) (cat, Kemp and Robinson, 1937; Rosenzweig and Sutton, 1958). Binaural stimulation produced EPs in each LL at the same latency as that observed for EPs produced by ipsilateral or contralateral stimulation (Kemp and Robinson, 1937). Thus, crossed and uncrossed projections to the LL result in EPs of identical latency. With regard to binaural effects, the sum of lemniscal EPs to ipsilateral and contralateral stimuli were shown to be greater than the EPs produced by the same binaurally presented stimuli (Fig. 7-15B) (Kemp and Robinson, 1937; Rosenzweig and Sutton, 1958). Single-unit recordings from the LL indicate that "onset" responses are common (Aitkin, Anderson, and Brugge, 1970; Guinan, Norris, and Guinan, 1972) and that the most synchronized, shortest-latency LL units respond with a mean latency which corresponds to that of BSER wave IV (Huang and Buchwald, 1978). LL cells typically are excited by ipsilateral as well as contralateral stimuli (Aitkin, Anderson, and Brugge, 1970; Guinan, Norris, and Guinan, 1972) and, as is true for the LL field potentials and BSER wave IV, the response of such LL units to binaural stimuli can be less than the sum of the unit-response to ipsilateral and contralateral stimuli (Aitkin, Anderson, and Brugge, 1970).

Relevant to the foregoing electrophysiologic and binaural interaction characteristics of the LL, generally similar to those of wave IV, are symmetrical input projections capable of mediating these effects. A possible candidate is the strong direct projection from the anterior ventral cochlear nucleus (AVCN), which crosses in the trapezoid body to provide major innervation of

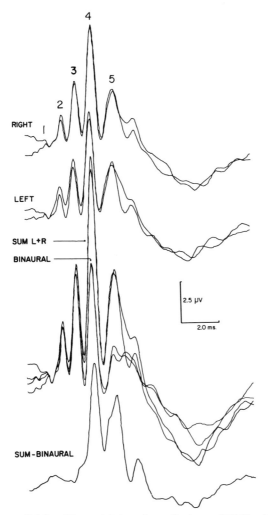

Figure 7-14. Binaural interaction effects on BSERs. From top to bottom, responses are shown to right and left monaural stimuli, to the sum of the right and left monaural responses, to the same number of binaural stimuli, and the summed monaural-binaural difference. Recordings are from an awake, restrained cat. Each trace represents an averaged response to 250 clicks. (Squires, N., and Buchwald, J., unpublished observations, 1980.)

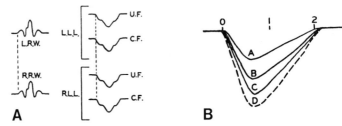

Figure 7-15. A. Semi-diagrammatic representation of responses from the lateral lemniscus to binaural click stimulation. Key: left and right round windows (LRW and RRW); left and right lateral lemniscus (LLL and RLL); uncrossed and crossed fibers of the tracts (UF and CF). All responses from both LLs appear at the same minimal latency, indicating perfect synchronization of ipsilateral with contralateral fibers. B. Tracings of LL click responses to stimulation of left ear alone (A), to stimulation of right ear alone (B), to simultaneous stimulation of both ears (C), and to the sum of the ordinates of the two monaural responses (D). The binaural response shows a smaller amplitude than the sum of the two monaural responses. All stimuli delivered at the same intensity. (Reprinted with permission from Kemp, E. H., and Robinson, E. H. Electric responses of the brain stem to bilateral auditory stimulation. *American Journal of Physiology*, 1937, *120*:316-322.)

Figure 7-16. Schematic diagram of the projection pathways from the posteroventral (PVCN) and anteroventral cochlear nuclei (AVCN). Solid lines indicate anatomically distinct fiber pathways. Branches of these pathways do not necessarily indicate collaterals of individual axons. Broken lines indicate that uncertainty exists concerning whether a given pathway is a source of a known input. Large solid arrowheads represent major inputs; empty arrowheads represent relatively minor inputs. Small arrowheads indicate direction of neural conduction. Key: anteroventral cochlear nucleus (AV); central nucleus of the inferior colliculus (CNIC); dorsal, cochlear nucleus (DC); dorsal nucleus of the lateral lemniscus (DLL); interstitial nucleus of Held's stria (IH); lateral superior olivary nucleus (LSO); lateral nucleus of the trapezoid body (LTB); medial superior olivary nucleus (MSO); medial nucleus of the trapezoid body (MTB); anterolateral periolivary cell group (PO_{al}); dorsolateral periolivary cell group (PO_{dl}); dorsomedial periolivary cell group (PO_{dm}); posterior periolivary cell group (PO_p); ventrolateral periolivary cell group (PO_{vl}); ventromedial periolivary cell group (PO_{vm}); posteroventral cochlear nucleus (PV); ventral nucleus of the lateral lemniscus (VLL); dorsomedial division of the ventral nucleus of the lateral lemniscus (VLL_{dm}); posteromedial division of the ventral nucleus of the lateral lemniscus (VLL_{pm}). (Reprinted with permission from Warr, W. B. Fiber degeneration following lesions in the posteroventral cochlear nucleus of the cat. *Experimental Neurology*, 1969, *23*:140-155.)

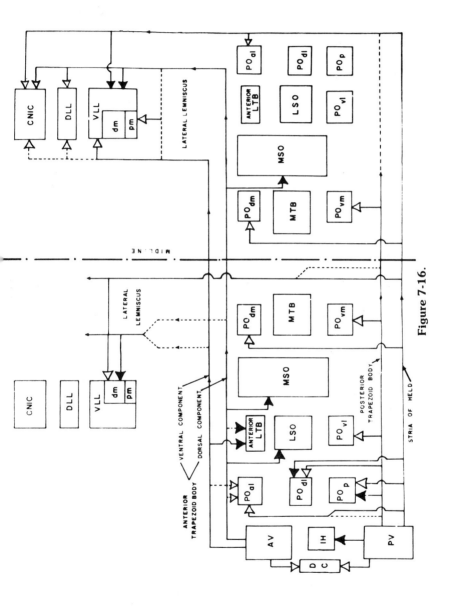

Figure 7-16.

187

the contralateral VNLL, with minor terminations in the DNLL (Fig. 7-16) (Warr, 1966, 1969). Ipsilaterally, the AVCN directly projects to the VNLL, but supplies no terminations to the DNLL (Warr, 1969, 1972). The ventral component of the trapezoid body, largely comprised of AVCN projections to the VNLL, has a mean fiber diameter of 1μ (excluding the myelin sheath), while the dorsal component, with AVCN projections to MSO, has a mean fiber diameter of 1.8μ (Fig. 7-16) (Warr, 1966, 1969). Transmission through the ventral component from AVCN to VNLL would be substantially slower than through the dorsal component from AVCN to MSO. The resultant AVCN activation of third-order VNLL neurons therefore should occur later than AVCN activation of third-order MSO cells. These predicted latency differences in MSO and LL activation are consistent with the latency differences of waves III and IV.

In summary, it is well substantiated that wave IV does not change following bilateral destruction of the IC, whereas it is markedly reduced in amplitude when the decussating trapezoid body is interrupted. SOC lesions sparing the trapezoid body have little effect on wave IV, whereas lesions or focal cooling of the ventral LL cause transient or permanent changes in wave IV without affecting the earlier BSER. A larger wave IV amplitude is produced when monaural stimuli are summed than when the same number of stimuli are delivered binaurally; this phenomenon has also been demonstrated in LL field potential recordings. Moreover, both LL EPs and single units show latencies similar to that of wave IV. The only crossed trapezoid body projection to the LL strongly innervates the VNLL fibers with approximately half the diameter of trapezoid body fibers innervating the MSO. These crossed projections originate from the AVCN, as do ipsilateral projections to the VNLL. Transmission through these crossed and uncrossed AVCN-VNLL projections is postulated as the major input, while the major substrate for wave IV generation is postulated as PSP activity within the VNLL cell population.

Wave V

Subsequent to wave IV, a lower amplitude, broader positivity, wave V, has been recorded with vertex referenced to noncephalic sites (cat, Achor and Starr, 1980a; Huang, 1980; Plantz, Williston, and Jewett, 1974; Shipley, Buchwald, and Norman, et al., 1980; rat, Huang, 1980; mouse, Henry, 1979a; guinea pig, dog, Huang, 1980; monkey, Allen and Starr, 1978), as well as to mastoid or pinna (cat, Achor and Starr, 1980a; Buchwald and Huang, 1975; Plantz, Williston, and Jewett, 1974; Lev and Sohmer, 1972; monkey, Allen and Starr, 1978), the tongue (cat, Jewett and Romano, 1972; Plantz, Williston, and Jewett, 1974; mouse, Henry, 1979a), or the nuchal ridge (guinea pig, Dobie and Berlin, 1979b). Wave V shows a similar amplitude with either noncephalic or mastoid references (cat, Plantz, Williston, and Jewett, 1974; mouse, Henry, 1979a; monkey, Allen and Starr, 1978).

In the studies cited above, wave V often was intermittently present and variable in wave form, in contrast to waves I to IV. Moreover, parametric studies of intensity effects indicate that the latency changes of wave V, although generally similar to those of waves I to IV, show a much larger standard deviation (cat, Huang and Buchwald, 1978; monkey, Allen and Starr, 1978). These differences are further emphasized during development, insofar as waves I to IV appear several days before the first appearance of wave V, and develop at a significantly faster rate (cat, Shipley, Buchwald, and Norman, et al., 1980).

While wave V appears to be qualitatively different from the earlier BSERs along dimensions of variability and maturation, binaural interactions affect the amplitude of wave V (Fig. 7-14) (cat, Fullerton and Hosford, 1979; Huang, 1980; Squires and Buchwald, 1980; guinea pig, rat, dog, Huang, 1980) and/or its preceding negative trough (guinea pig, Dobie and Berlin, 1979b), so that a smaller potential results from binaural stimulation than from the sum of an equal number of stimuli delivered monaurally to each ear. This effect is the same as that discussed in the preceding section for wave IV (cat, Jewett, 1970; Huang and Buchwald, 1978; Fullerton and Hosford, 1979; Huang, 1980; guinea pig, Dobie and Berlin, 1979; Huang, 1980; rat, dog, Huang, 1980). Following a midsaggital transection of the trapezoid body, both waves IV and V markedly decreased in amplitude (cat, Buchwald and Huang, 1975; Fullerton and Hosford, 1979) and lost this binaural-summed monaural difference (Fullerton and Hosford, 1979).

Thus, these data indicate that wave V (1) is less regularly present, shows more variability, and develops more slowly than waves I to IV, but (2) reflects the same binaural interaction effects shown by wave IV and loses these effects (concurrent with wave IV) following trapezoid body transection.

In the human, a relatively low-amplitude positivity subsequent to the IV-V complex, wave VI, is recorded with vertex referenced noncephalically (Stockard, Stockard, and Sharbrough, 1978; Streletz, Katz, and Hohenberger, et al., 1977; Terkildsen, Osterhammel, and Huis in't Veld, 1974a; Chiappa, Gladstone, and Young, 1979). Wave VI is similar or only slightly larger in amplitude with a noncephalic reference than with vertex-to-mastoid recordings (Chiappa, Gladstone, and Young, 1979; Streletz, Katz, and Hohenberger, et al., 1977; Stockard, Stockard, and Sharbrough, 1978). This is in contrast to the IV-V complex, which shows a 20 percent increase with a noncephalic reference (Chiappa, Gladstone, and Young, 1979). Wave VI was consistently ranked hardest to recognize of the BSERs in a "normal" population (Chiappa, Gladstone, and Young, 1979); in contrast to the earlier BSERs, wave VI was so irregularly present and variable in waveform that its clinical usefulness has been questioned (Chiappa, Gladstone, and Young, 1979; Stockard, Stockard, and Sharbrough, 1978). Insofar as the human IV-V complex has been related to the cat wave IV (Lev and Sohmer, 1972; Starr and Achor, 1978; Stockard, Stockard, and Sharbrough, 1978), wave VI might be compared to the cat wave V. Certainly, both waves share a broad, low-amplitude waveform, an irregularity of occurrence, and a variability which sharply contrasts to the earlier BSERs.

Correlative studies of BSERs and depth EPs indicate a correspondence in latency between wave V and EPs recorded in ipsilateral (cat, Jewett, 1970) and contralateral inferior colliculus (IC) (cat, Lev and Sohmer, 1972; mouse, Henry, 1979b). These potentials were largest in amplitude at the lateral edge of the IC (mouse, Henry, 1979b), and inverted from positivity to negativity as the electrode moved ventrally from the inferior margin of the colliculus (cat, Jewett, 1979). Although EPs with the latency of wave V were occasionally recorded rostral to the IC (Jewett, 1970), no correspondence was found between wave V and EPs recorded from the medial geniculate body (cat, Lev and Sohmer, 1972).

Similarly, in lesion experiments, complete transection of the brain stem rostral to the IC did not produce any appreciable change in wave V (Fig. 7-3) (cat, Buchwald and Huang, 1975; mouse, Henry, 1979b). Bilateral local cooling medial to the lateral lemniscus produced an increase in the latency of wave IV, which was directly reflected by the same latency increase in wave V (cat, Jones, Stockard, and Rossiter, et al., 1976; Stockard and Sharbrough, 1980). Following "deep" collicular lesions (cat, Gardi, Merzenich, and McKean, 1979) or restricted lesions in the dorsal LL (cat, Achor and Starr, 1980b), the negativity prior to wave V was reduced. After bilateral lesions which partially destroyed the central nucleus of the IC, i.e., the dorsal and medial regions (cat, Achor and Starr, 1980b; mouse, Henry, 1979a, 1979b) or produced an unspecified amount of collicular damage (cat, Goldenberg and Derbyshire, 1975; guinea pig, Gardi and Berlin, 1981), wave V showed little or no change. In one unilateral IC lesion of unknown extent, however, a 50 percent reduction of wave V was produced without effect on the preceding BSERs (Achor and Starr, 1980b). In contrast, more extensive bilateral IC lesions, which encompassed the lateral and ventral extent of the nucleus, resulted in marked reduction or loss of wave V (cat, Buchwald and Huang, 1975; mouse, Henry, 1979a, 1979b), an effect noted in chronic as well as in acute postoperative recordings (Fig. 7-3, 7-17). Similarly, loss of wave V followed lesions which interrupted lemniscal input just caudal and ventral to the IC (cat, Lev and Sohmer, 1972; Huang, 1980; mouse, Henry, 1979a, 1979b; guinea pig, rat, dog, Huang, 1980).

Taken together, the preceding correlative BSER and EP data and the results of lesion studies suggest that the deep ventrolateral portion of the IC is particularly important for wave V generation. On the basis of cell size and innervation, the large central nucleus of the inferior colliculus (ICC) has been divided into a large ventrolateral division and a smaller dorsomedial division (Rockel, 1971; Rockel and Jones, 1973a). The ventrolateral portion of the ICC has been further divided into a major region of medium and small cells,

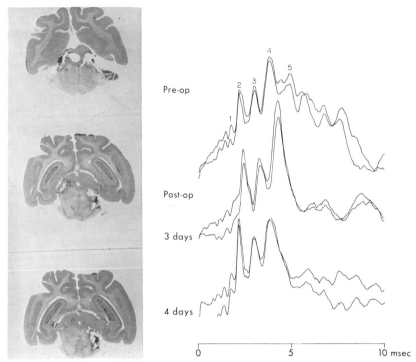

Pre-op

Post-op

3 days

4 days

0   5   10 msec

Figure 7-17. Effect of inferior colliculus (IC) aspiration on BSERs. Brain sections indicate extent of IC damage in cat from which BSER recordings are illustrated. No IC tissue remained in sections caudal to those shown. Post-operative recordings, which extended over a 1-week period, showed no distinguishable potentials after BSER wave IV. (Buchwald, J., and Hinman, C., unpublished observations, 1980.)

and an extreme ventrolateral anterior area of large cells (Rockel and Jones, 1973a). The ICC in turn is covered by a dorsal-posterior cap, the pericentral nucleus (ICP) (Rockel and Jones, 1973b), and by a lateral-posterior rind, the external nucleus (ICX). Lesions which included the ICP had no effect on wave V, and, although the ICX receives heavy innervation from auditory cortex and from the ICC, it receives few or no terminals from the LL (Goldberg and Moore, 1967; Rockel and Jones, 1973a). In contrast, the ventrolateral division of the ICC receives fibers only from the LL (Rockel and Jones, 1973a). Thus, on anatomic grounds, the ventrolateral ICC again appears to be the best candidate subdivision for wave V generation. This suggestion is supported by physiologic data which indicate marked habituation of ICP and ICX unit responses to stimulus rates of 1/sec, a characteristic shared neither by ICC units (Aitkin, Webster, and Veale, et al., 1975) nor by wave V. Since only those lesions which encompassed the ventrolateral margin of the IC resulted in clear alterations of wave V (Nagao, Roccaforte, and Moody, 1979), the extreme ventrolateral ICC region of large cells may be particularly relevant (Rockel and Jones, 1973a). A consistent physiological correlate is the finding that most cells in the deep ICC show only onset (or offset) responses to tone pulses, in contrast to the continuous responses of more dorsally situated cells (Merzenich and Reid, 1974).

One of the heaviest inputs to the ventral IC is provided by the ipsilateral VNLL, with cells of origin scattered throughout the entire dorsoventral extent of the nucleus (Adams, 1979). As discussed in the previous section, binaural interaction effects identical to those displayed by waves IV and V characterize evoked potentials recorded from the ventral lemniscus (Kemp and Robinson, 1937; Rosenzweig and Sutton, 1958). Given these and other data, the VNLL has been hypothesized as the principal generator of wave IV. The VNLL is also suggested as an essential relay in the production of wave V, since no other input to the ventral IC reflects a similarly symmetrical pattern of binaural innervation (Adams, 1979; Osen, 1972; Warr, 1966), a pattern which appears to be necessary for the binaural interactive effects which characterize both waves IV and V. In support of this additional synaptic relay for wave V, not postulated in the generator systems of waves III and IV, are the physiologic differences between wave V and the earlier BSERs in terms of its greater variability and slower maturation.

In summary, wave V differs significantly from waves I to IV along parameters of variability and rate of development. However, wave V reflects binaural interaction effects which appear to be the same as those of wave IV. These data suggest that the generator system of wave V incorporates the postulated VNLL generator of wave IV. The results of correlative BSER-depth EP recordings and of lesion studies, as well as supportive anatomic and physiologic data, lead to the hypothesis that wave V is generated in the extreme ventrolateral region of the ICC, a region cytologically characterized by large cells.

DISCUSSION

It is obvious that the acoustic nerve is necessary for the generation of all BSER waves but the auditory periphery in isolation produces only wave I; multiple responses from the lower brain-stem nuclei may contribute to the later BSER waves, but differential functional characteristics indicate that no two BSER generator systems are identical. The conceptual framework of this review has been that a finite generator system with a "knowable" anatomy and physiology underlies each BSER wave. Such an orientation neither implies a "simple" generator nor a number of interlocking "in-series" generators. In fact, the picture which emerges is a complex one of both parallel and serial projections to target pools of neurons with highly synchronized "onset" responses.

In the preceding sections, a number of working hypotheses relevant to BSER generation have been developed from electrophysiologic and anatomic data relevant to the brain-stem auditory pathway as well as from parametric, developmental, and correlative studies of the BSERs per se. An emphasis has been placed upon the functional differentiation of each BSER component, and upon the anatomy and physiology which appear to be singularly important for any particular wave. It is hoped that the resultant hypotheses will facilitate further experimentation and clarification of the origins of each BSER component.

Generator potentials in the unmyelinated terminal dendrites of the acoustic nerve are hypothesized as the substrate of wave I while PSPs in the CN are postulated as the generators of wave II. AVCN projections to the MSO of both sides which produce dendritic PSPs and resultant bilateral field potentials of equal latency and mirror-image polarity comprise the generator substrate hypothesized for wave III. Parallel to these projections, the AVCN output to the ventral LL of both sides produces longer bilaterally equal-latency field potentials which comprise the generator substrate hypothesized for wave IV. As the generator of wave V, bilateral PSP field potentials in the deep ventrolateral ICC are hypothesized, with input from the ventral LL region which shows binaural interactions identical to those of wave V. Thus, the hypothesized generator of wave V receives in series input directly from wave IV generator, whereas the generators of waves III and IV receive parallel but different input from the CN.

In general, the BSER positive peaks are hypothesized as originating from graded PSPs rather than from axonal or somatic APs on the basis of both theoretical and empirical data. Large PSP current fields result from large PSP space and time constants, and these current fields can be recorded over significant extracellular distances. In contrast, AP current fields that result from small AP space and time constants are small and cannot be recorded over similar distances. BSER amplitudes are presumed to reflect the size of the PSP current field, therefore, which is regulated by the strength of excitation and the number of neurons excited.

BSER peak latencies are hypothesized as reflecting axonal transmission time plus time to reach synaptic threshold in the target neuronal pool. According to this view, the interpeak interval between waves I and II reflects transmission time and synaptic delay from the acoustic nerve to the CN; the interpeak interval between waves II and III reflects transmission time and synaptic delay from AVCN to ipsi- and contralateral MSO; the interval between waves II and IV reflects transmission time and synaptic delay from AVCN to ipsi- and contralateral ventral LL; and the interval between waves IV and V reflects transmission time and synaptic delay from the ventral LL to the ventrolateral ICC. Other interpeak intervals, such as that between waves III and IV, have no particular significance, as these peaks reflect parallel, relatively independent generator systems.

While it is hoped that these hypotheses will be widely tested, a persistent problem in the interpretation of BSER data is the pervasive use of two active recording electrodes. Each of the most common reference placements (mastoid, pinna, ear canal, tongue, nasopharynx) has been shown to record BSER potentials when referenced to a second noncephalic electrode (neck or wrist). In contrast, a neck electrode referenced noncephalically to the tail or wrist provides a flat baseline essentially free of click-related potentials (cat, Plantz, Williston, and Jewett, 1974; Shipley, Buchwald, and Norman, et al., 1980; Achor and Starr, 1980a; rat, Plantz, Williston, and Jewett, 1974; human, Streletz, Katz, and Hohenberger, et al., 1977; Stockard, Stockard, and Sharbrough, 1978). To be sure, this recording is not totally devoid of auditory responses, which are theoretically volume-conducted over the entire body. However, under conditions appropriate for BSER recording, noncephalic references show no evoked potentials, whereas auditory responses of considerable amplitude may be present at cephalic reference placements. The interactive effects of two active recording loci may be used to advantage, e.g., the enhancement of wave I with vertex-mastoid as compared with vertex-noncephalic recordings. However, electrode interactions can become problematic whenever experimental or clinical variables are introduced.

A similar difficulty is posed by spatio-temporal mapping studies of the BSERs, in which a fixed electrode on the pinna or neck has been used as reference for a roving scalp electrode moved incrementally along midsaggital, parasaggital, and coronal planes (cat, Plantz, Williston, and Jewett, 1974; Jewett, 1970; rat, Plantz, Williston, and Jewett, 1974; Jewett and Romano, 1972; monkey, Allen and Starr, 1978; human, Streletz, Katz, and Hohenberger, et al., 1977; Martin and Moore, 1978; Stockard, Stockard, and Sharbrough, 1978). In all studies, the BSER waveform changed differentially as the electrode moved over the head. Because of these waveform changes, it was often difficult to identify a particular peak in one recording configuration as the same peak, partially inverted or distorted in latency, recorded with another electrode configuration. These data become particularly difficult to interpret when accompanied by the confounding effects of electrode interaction. However, for identifiable BSER waves, the peaks generally appeared within a narrow latency range regardless of recording locus. Such latency data suggest fixed generator substrates, which is in accord with the hypothesized PSP generation of BSER peaks.

In the summary of a 1979 international seminar on BSERs, it was concluded that "the anatomy and the physiology of the compact structures of the brain stem are so complex that the problem of generators is insoluble in the present state of the art. . . . The BSER can be used empirically but cannot at present be understood" (Davis, 1979). The hypotheses developed during the course of this review should, therefore, be considered with caution. However, the remarkable stability of the BSER latencies and waveforms across repeated recording sessions and varying arousal levels indicates that an extremely secure, highly synchronized, and constant generator system underlies each wave. It is hoped that the foregoing hypotheses may provide some insight into these systems.

SUMMARY

A number of hypotheses of BSER generation have been developed on the basis of current electrophysiologic and anatomic data relevant to the brain-stem auditory pathway and parametric, developmental, and correlative studies of the BSERs per se. General hypotheses proposed that (1) BSERs reflect graded PSPs rather than APs discharged at the cell soma or transmitted along the axons; (2) BSER latencies and amplitudes reflect interactive but different physiologic processes; and (3) BSER waves reflect functionally separable substrate systems. Hypotheses specific to the generation of each BSER wave were subsequently developed, and proposed that (1) generator potentials in the unmyelinated terminal dendrites of the acoustic nerve comprise the generator substrate of wave I; (2) PSPs in the CN comprise the generator substrate of wave II; (3) AVCN projections to the MSO of both sides produce dendritic PSPs, with resultant bilateral field potentials of equal latency and mirror-image polarity, and comprise the generator substrate of wave III; (4) AVCN output to the ventral LL of both sides produces bilateral field potentials of equal latency and binaural interaction which comprise the generator substrate for wave IV; (5) bilateral field potentials in the ventrolateral ICC, with input from the ventral LL region of binaural interaction, comprise the generator substrate of wave V.

Alfred C. Coats

8   Instrumentation

A choice had to be made in writing this chapter. Does one choose an approach built around his or her own laboratory? Certainly that would be biased, and would make for an unbalanced presentation. Does one focus on a particular commercially available system? This would not be instructive to beginning students, since they have not had the opportunity to work with different systems in order to determine which one is best-suited to answer their particular needs. Or, does one simply provide the bases for understanding various instrumentation systems, whether they be component parts, customized systems, or commercially available instruments. I chose the latter approach—for despite the fact that there are many excellent commercially available systems, the student of this area cannot avoid the necessity of understanding basic principles of AER recording.

PRINCIPLES OF AVERAGING

Averaging, to enhance a stimulus-time-locked response relative to non-time-locked background "noise," is the basic technological development upon which recording of evoked potentials is based (Dawson, 1954b). Averaging is especially necessary for recording very low amplitude evoked potentials from auditory periphery and brain stem, because these responses are buried

The preparation of this chapter was supported in part by grants P01 NS 10940 and R01 NS 12910 from the National Institute of Neurological and Communicative Disorders and Stroke, and by a grant from the Pauline Sterne Wolff Foundation.

in background noise up to 10 times their amplitude; they would be undetectable without averaging.

Figure 8-1 illustrates the principle of averaging. Background noise is random; hence, with repetition, its amplitude at any given instant will tend to average to zero. However, the time-locked response waveform will not "average out" in this way.

Averaging requires some method of data storage. Early averagers stored voltages by charging a series of capacitors on a rotating disk (Dawson, 1954b). These "analog" averagers have since been supplanted by digital instruments which store the voltages as numbers.

A complete description of an averaged response includes the number of individual responses included in the average (N), the total time period of the averaged waveform (the *epoch*), and the time relationship between the start of the average and delivery of the stimulus. Table 8-1 and Figure 8-1 summarize the terminology used to describe an averaged waveform.

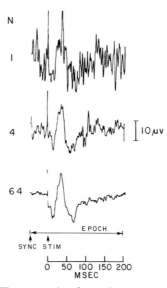

Figure 8-1. The principle of signal averaging to enhance a stimulus time-locked signal relative to random background "noise." The signal is an electroretinographic light flash response recorded from the eyelid. N = number of responses averaged. Arrow labeled SYNC denotes the pulse which starts the A-D converter. Arrow labeled STIM denotes the pulse which triggers the light flash. The interval between the SYNC and STIM pulses is the prestimulus delay; the trace recorded during the prestimulus delay is often used to establish a baseline for amplitude measurement.

Table 8-1

Basic Terminology of Evoked Potential Averaging

N—Number of individual responses included in the average

Epoch—Total period of time encompassed by the averaged waveform. May include a prestimulus baseline period

Signal-to-noise ratio—Ratio of amplitudes of the signal of interest (in our case the evoked potential) and background activity ("noise") upon which the signal of interest is superimposed.

Sync, or Timing Pulse—Pulse that initiates both average onset and stimulus delivery. A delay may be inserted between the sync pulse and either average onset or stimulus delivery.

Stimulus Pulse—Pulse that triggers the stimulus.

Relationship between number of responses averaged and background noise reduction. Reduction in noise amplitude is proportional to the square root of N. The example shown in Table 8-2 (which assumes a 1:1 signal/noise ratio in the unaveraged epoch) illustrates the significance of this principle to the clinical test situation—i.e., that as N is increased, there will be diminishing benefits in terms of increased signal/noise ratio. As this example shows, the first increment of 100 increases signal/noise ratio by a factor of 1000 percent. In contrast, signal/noise ratio increases only about 12 percent when the same increment of 100 is added to an N of 400.

Effects of non-random background noise. If the stimulus rate is an even multiple of the frequency of the non-random noise (e.g., 10/sec in the presence of 60 Hz hum), the background noise will "average out" at a slower rate than indicated by Table 8-2. If non-random noise is known to be present, one can therefore most effectively eliminate it by selecting a stimulus rate that is not an even multiple of the noise's frequency (e.g., 8/sec or 9.2/sec, rather than 10/sec, to eliminate 60 Hz hum).

Table 8-2

Change in Signal-Noise Ratio with Increases in N

N	Signal/Noise Ratio	% Increase in Signal/Noise Ratio
1	1/1 = 1.0	
100	100/1 = 10.0	1,000%
200	200/1 = 14.1	
300	300/1 = 17.3	
400	400/1 = 20.0	
500	500/1 = 22.3	11.8%

Instrument Overview

Basically, an auditory evoked potential instrument must accomplish four things. It must (1) generate an acoustic stimulus, (2) amplify the very small electrical signal from the patient, (3) numerically process the signal from the patient to obtain the averaged waveform, and (4) display and/or plot the averaged waveform. It is convenient to organize a discussion of the evoked potential instrument into four functional subsystems, each of which accomplishes one of these objectives. Figure 8-2 is a block diagram illustrating the functional interaction of an evoked potential instrument's four subsystems or sections. In early evoked potential systems, the subsystems were actually separate instruments, usually obtained from different manufacturers. In recent years, evoked potential systems which combine all four functions into a single instrument have become available.

In addition to the electronic instrumentation itself, electrodes will be discussed, because aspects of electrode design are at least as important as the instrumentation itself in determining the quality of results obtained—particularly in electrocochleography (ECochG).

STIMULUS SECTION

Principle of Operation

The stimulus section generates impulsive acoustical stimuli (clicks) which are synchronized with the epoch's onset. It may also generate continuous sounds (usually pure tones or broad-band noise) for contralateral or ipsilateral masking. The sound stimulus is generated by driving an acoustical transducer

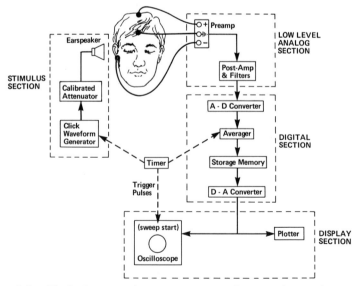

Figure 8-2. Block diagram of averaging system for recording auditory evoked potentials. A–D = analog to digital; D–A = digital to analog.

(often a standard audiometric earspeaker) with the output of a waveform generator. Sound intensity is controlled by routing the electrical signal through an attenuator which is calibrated is decibel steps. Thus, assuming that the earspeaker's acoustical output remains directly proportional to the voltage input (a reasonably safe assumption with audiometric earspeakers, but not as safe with commercial "high-fidelity" earspeakers), the intensity at all attenuator settings can be determined by calibrating at a single setting and referring all other settings to this initial calibrated setting. Besides intensity, the click's acoustical waveform and frequency spectrums must be specified. Further discussion of the control and calibration of acoustical stimuli may be found in Chapter 2.

Artifact Reduction

Stimulus artifact presents a special problem in designing a stimulating system for auditory evoked potential work. The earspeaker is a very effective generator of radiated electrostatic and electromagnetic energy. Since the earspeaker is located relatively close to the recording site, the energy it radiates is readily coupled to the recording electrodes to create an electrical artifact (Vurkek, White, and Fong, et al., 1981). The artifact's waveform will approximate that of the earspeaker's electrical input (Fig. 8-3).

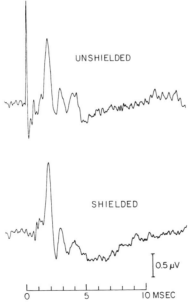

Figure 8-3. Radiated rectangular pulse artifact generated by an unshielded earspeaker, and its elimination by shielding the earspeaker. Click intensity was 115 dB pe SPL. Each waveform is an average of 1,000 responses.

Auditory evoked potential systems take three approaches to stimulus artifact reduction: (1) adding responses generated by opposite polarity stimuli (Aran, 1971; Spoor, 1974) or, with tone-burst stimuli, randomizing the phase relation between tone and burst onset (Yoshie, 1971); (2) separating the acoustical transducer from the subject, either by stimulating in free field (Aran, 1971) or by connecting the earspeaker to the patient by a flexible tube (Marsh, Brown and Smith, 1975; Montandon, 1976; Sohmer and Pratt, 1976); and (3) shielding the earspeaker (Coats, Martin, and Kidder, 1979; Elberling and Salomon, 1973; Moore, 1971; Terkildsen, Osterhammel, and Huis in't Veld, 1975a).

Adding responses to opposite-polarity clicks and randomizing burst-phase relationship selectively eliminate the stimulus artifact while preserving the neural response, because reversing click polarity reverses artifact polarity, but (at least under usual conditions of high-frequency or broad-band click stimulation) does not reduce the neural response's polarity. These methods are convenient and inexpensive. However, they preclude examination of polarity-reversing responses (e.g., the cochlear microphonics and the frequency-following response), and can generate distorted neural response waveforms, particularly when stimulating with low-frequency clicks (Coats, 1976) or when recording from a patient with a high-frequency hearing loss (Coats and Martin, 1977).

Reducing artifact by separating the transducer from the patient is cumbersome. With free-field separation, a sound-isolating room is required if threshold testing is to be done. Also, because free-field acoustical transmission selectively attenuates low frequencies, difficulties will be encountered when attempting to investigate low-frequency responses. Also, with free-field stimulation, movement of the subject's head and reverberation from test-room walls may introduce variability. However, when doing electrococh-leography with a needle electrode which protrudes from the external ear canal, free-field stimulation may be the only feasible method of applying the sound stimulus.

Figure 8-3 illustrates reduction of stimulus artifact by earspeaker shielding. Of the possible ways of reducing earspeaker artifact, this method is the most difficult to technically accomplish. It also increases headset weight, which compromises comfort. However, it does provide the best acoustical control of the stimulus and results in the most compact, convenient, and universally applicable means of applying acoustical stimulation for auditory evoked potential testing. Shielded earspeakers are now commercially available.

Low-Level Analog Section

The low-level analog section accepts the signal from the patient and amplifies it to the voltage level that is required by the digital processing section. The first amplification stage is contained in the preamplifier, which is often located near the patient and remote from the main instrument. The preamplifier's output is usually further amplified by one or more "post-amplification" stages, located in the main body of the averager. The low-level analog section also filters the analog signal to maximally reject interfering signals ("noise") while minimally distorting the desired signal (the evoked potential).

Following are principles of operation and instrument specifications of the preamplifier and filtering stages of the low-level analog section.

Preamplifier

Principle of operation.   As with almost all bioelectric recording instruments, the evoked-potential instrument employs a differential input preamplifier. Differential input preamplifiers record only voltage differences between input leads (differential signals); voltages that are the same (common mode signals) tend to cancel. In this way, the differential preamplifier selectively attenuates radiated electrical "noise" (e.g., from building power lines) which tends to be of equal amplitude at the two preamplifier inputs. Figure 8-4 illustrates this principle of operation.

Instrument Specifications and Characteristics

Gain.   The gain of an amplifier is specified as the amplitude of the *signal out* divided by the amplitude of the *signal in*. Thus, a 1 μV evoked potential at the input of an amplifier with a gain of 100,000 would have an amplitude of 100,000 μV, or 0.1 V, at the amplifier's output. Evoked potential instruments' low-level analog sections generally have gains in the range of 10,000 to 1 million. There is no best low-level analog gain for evoked potential systems. Gains are set according to the requirements of "downstream" sections (the filters and the digital analysis section), and these differ from instrument to instrument.

Common-mode rejection ratio.   The common-mode rejection ratio (CMMR) is a measure of the preamplifier's ability to selectively reject a common-mode signal while passing a differential signal. The higher the CMMR the better. CMMR may be measured by applying the same signal both differentially and in common-mode at the input leads. The ratio of the outputs yields the CMMR. Common-mode rejection ratios usually are expressed either as a proportion or in decibels. The frequency of the test signal should be included in the specification. Usually, the test signal is a 60 Hz sine wave, because power line hum is the most consistently troublesome radiated interfering signal. Preamplifiers for evoked potential systems generally have CMMRs of about 10,000:1, or 80 dB at 60 Hz.

Input impedance.   Input impedance is the electrical impedance (in Ohms) across the preamplifier inputs. Generally, the higher the input impedance the better, because high-input impedance reduces noise susceptibil-

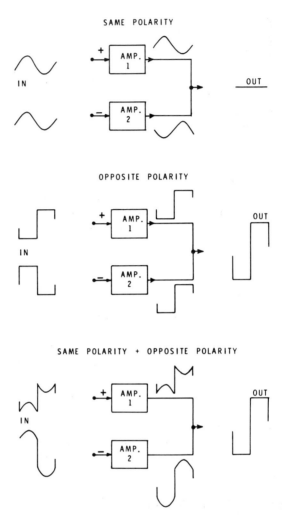

Figure 8-4. Principle of operation of a differential amplifier. The differential amplifier subtracts voltages applied at its two inputs. Thus, voltages that are the same at the two inputs ("common mode" signals, illustrated at top of the figure as a sine wave) are canceled. In contrast, voltages that are different at the two imputs ("differential" signals, illustrated in the center of the figure) are passed through and amplified. The diagram at the bottom of the figure illustrates how the common mode signal is removed from a mixed common mode and differential signal.

ity when high electrode impedance is unavoidable (as in extratympanic ECochG). High-input impedance also promotes patient safety by reducing the ability of electric current to flow between the electrodes. However, internal preamplifier noise tends to be higher in high input-impedance devices (good design can partly circumvent this problem).

Internal noise. Internal noise is defined as the electrical noise recorded when the input leads are shorted, or connected together through some standard resistance. Internal noise has a uniform (white) frequency distribution. It is generated by several types of component noise sources, including resistors which generate thermal noise and semiconductors which generate "shot noise" (Ott, 1976). Figure 8-5 shows the typical waveform of an evoked-potential system's internal noise.

The internal noise specification of an evoked potential instrument sets the lowest limit to which system noise can be reduced. This specification is particularly important when recording evoked potentials in the sub-microvolt range, as in ECochG and brain-stem audiometry.

The amplitude distribution of internal preamplifier noise is Gaussian in theory; it would be possible, by waiting long enough, to find a segment of noise of virtually any amplitude. Thus, in measuring peak-to-peak noise, only amplitude peaks occurring at least a specified percentage of the time (e.g., at least 0.01 percent) are considered. In specifying internal preamplifier noise, both the resistance of the input-shunting resistor and the amplifier's bandwidth must be included. A typical evoked potential system noise specification would be 6 μV peak-to-peak with a bandwidth of 20 Hz–10 kHz and a 10 kΩ shorting resistor.

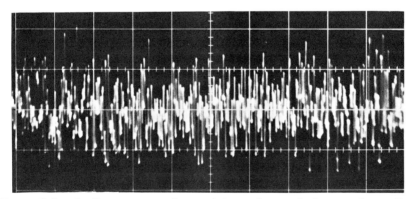

Figure 8-5. Oscilloscope trace of internal noise of an evoked potential recording system. System band pass was 20 Hz–10 kHz (rolloff of 12 dB/octave). Preamplifier inputs were shorted by a 10 kilo-ohm (kΩ) resistor. Amplitude scale is 2 μV/large division; time scale is 2 msec/division.

Patient isolation. In order to minimize electrical hazard to the patient, there must be very high electrical resistance between the patient and all sources of electrical power within the instrument. To achieve this, both the preamplifier power supply and patient leads must be isolated. Preamplifier power supply may be isolated either by powering it with batteries, or by special isolators, called DC-to-DC converters. To isolate the patient leads, many medical preamplifiers utilize optical couplers (Vurek, et al., 1981). Patient isolation is measured by connecting the input leads to ground and measuring the current flow across the connection. A typical specification is "current flow less than 20 mA."

Frequency Response

Principles and definitions. The "frequency response" of a system refers to its ability to pass signals of different frequency. Frequency response is usually measured by applying sine waves of varying frequency and constant amplitude and measuring relative outputs. The plot of relative amplitude out vs frequency is the frequency response curve of the system. Figure 8-6 illustrates the procedure for obtaining a frequency response curve.

Three characteristics of a recorder's frequency response curve are important: (1) its linearity, (2) its roll-off rate, and (3) its high and low cutoff points. Frequency response curves of recording devices typically have a relatively flat portion bounded on the high- and (except for DC amplifiers) low-frequency sides by declines to zero. The linearity of the curve in its flat portion is impor-

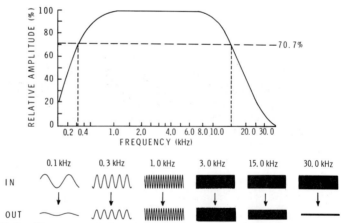

Figure 8-6. Illustration of the measurement of a recording system's frequency response. A sinusoidal signal of varying frequency but the same amplitude is applied at the input (signals labeled IN). Relative amplitudes at the output (waveforms labeled OUT) are measured, and the relative OUT amplitudes plotted against frequency (plot at top). The vertical dashed lines illustrate standard low and high 3 dB-down, or 70.7 percent, cutoff points, which are 0.32 kHz and 15.0 kHz.

tant, as significant peaks and valleys could create complex and unpredictable distortion in the recorded waveform (see Chapter 6). However, creating a very linear amplifier presents no design difficulties; hence, linearity per se is rarely included in published specifications.

Roll-off rate is the rate of decline of the frequency-response curve at its high and low ends. Biological amplifiers generally have equal roll-off rates at both ends. Roll-off rate may be expressed in dB/decade or dB/octave. Typical specifications, deriving from inherent characteristics of the Butterworth filter (the most commonly used type of electronic filter), are 6 dB/octave (first order Butterworth), 12 dB/octave (second order Butterworth), and 18 dB/octave (third order Butterworth).

High and low cutoff points are the high and low frequencies at which the output declines by 3 dB, or to approximately 71 percent of the maximum output amplitude. The band-pass of the recording system is the frequency range between the high and low cutoff points. Thus, for example, the band-pass of the system giving the frequency response curve (shown in Fig. 8-6) would be 320-15 kHz. The roll-off rate, as well as the high and low cutoff frequencies, must be included in the frequency-response specification.

Selecting the optimal frequency-response is critical in determining the performance of a biological recorder. The following discussion addresses this selection problem as it specifically pertains to an auditory evoked potential recording system.

Considerations in selecting frequency response for recording auditory evoked potentials. As with all bioelectric signals, evoked potentials are immersed in a milieu of competing electrical events. The quality of the averaged evoked potential record will be vastly improved if the recording system's frequency response is set to maximally reject the interfering signal. However, the system's frequency response must not be so restricted that the evoked potential is distorted. Tables 8-3 and 8-4 list frequency ranges of the most common interfering signals and of the various auditory evoked potentials, respectively. Recording-system frequency-response appropriate for the signal of interest can be selected with values from these tables. Those interfering signals which cannot be eliminated by filtering (e.g., muscle potentials and stimulus artifact) can be identified as well. Tradeoffs between signal distortion and noise elimination can be clarified. For example, by raising the low cutoff filter from 20 to 300 Hz the BSER is distorted (Fig. 8-7), but movement artifact is also greatly attenuated.

Digital Section

In essence, the digital section of the evoked potential instrument converts analog signals (from the patient) into numerical series (the analog-to-digital converter), and averages the digitized signals. Following are the principles of operation and important characteristics of these two subsections.

Table 8-3
Approximate Frequency Ranges of Interfering Signals

Signal	Cutoff Points (Hz) with 6 dB/Octave Roll-Off Low	High
Electrodermal response	0.01	5
Electrode junction potentials	0 (DC)	5
EEG	0.05	30
Movement potentials	0.05	50
60 Hz power line hum	60	60
Muscle potentials (EMG)	10	5k
Stimulus artifact (square wave)	10	20k
Radiated electromagnetic signals (e.g., FM station) after demodulation	10	20k
Internal amplifier noise	0 (DC)	∞

Analog-to-Digital (A-D) Converter

Principle of operation. Figure 8-8 illustrates the principle of operation. The A-D converter samples the signal from the low-level analog section at equal intervals. Sampling begins when initiated by a timing pulse that is time-locked to the click stimulus, and continues for a preset period of time (the epoch). At each sample point, the A-D converter converts the signal voltage into a number. Decimal numbers are shown in Figure 8-8 for illustrative purposes. The output of the A-D converter actually consists of binary numbers—numbers composed of strings of 1s and 0s, or *bits*. Figure 8-10 lists the binary numbers that correspond to decimal numbers from 0 to 31. The converted numbers are stored in memory as a series of words.

Table 8-4
Frequency Ranges (Cutoff Points Allowing Recording with Fidelity) of Auditory Evoked Potentials

Signal	Cutoff Points (Hz) with 6 dB/Octave Roll-Off Low	High
Cochlear microphonic	100	20k*
Summating potential (SP)	5†	3k
Auditory nerve action potential	20	3k
Auditory brain-stem response	20‡	3k
Middle potential	10	1k
Late (vertex) potential	2	100

*Cutoffs higher than 10k are rarely used in practice.
†Transient response SP. Steady-state SP would require a DC system.
‡Low cutoffs of 100-300 Hz are often clinically used. These cutoffs distort the BSER but make it easier to record.

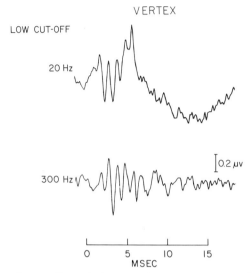

Figure 8-7. Effect of changing the recording system's low-cutoff frequency on the BSER waveform. The 300-Hz low cutoff is used by many clinical laboratories, in spite of the signal distortion that it creates, because this low cutoff frequency greatly attenuates movement artifacts.

Specifications and Characteristics

Time resolution. The time resolution of the A-D converter may be defined as the rate at which the converter is able to take digital samples of the waveform. The faster the sampling rate, the better the time resolution. Figure 8-9 illustrates the effect of sampling rate on fidelity of waveform reproduction.

Amplitude resolution. The amplitude resolution of the digitized waveform is defined as the number of discrete amplitude steps (or number of different numbers) available to represent signal voltage. As Figure 8-10 illustrates, amplitude resolution is determined by word length, that is, the number of bits contained in the digital word of the A-D converter. Thus, for example, a one-bit word would provide only two steps—0 and 1, whereas a two-bit word would provide four steps—00, 01, 10, 11. In specifying amplitude resolution requirements for BSER recording systems, one must consider the fact that background noise amplitude is typically 10 times that of the BSER; hence, only about 10 percent of A-D amplitude resolution is available to resolve the BSER waveform. In the context of practical clinical testing, the effect of increased A-D amplitude resolution is that it widens the voltage range through which data can be accepted and thus reduces the incidence of off-

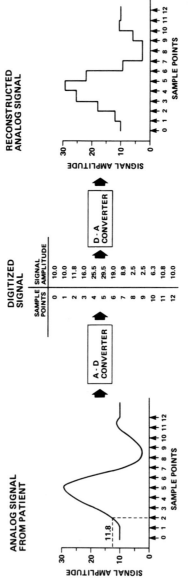

Figure 8-8. Diagrammatic illustration of the principle of operation of an analog-to-digital (A–D) converter. The A–D converter samples the input signal at a fixed rate. At each "sample point" it generates a number determined by the analog signal's voltage at that point. Thus, in this example, the converter obtains the number 11.8 at sample point 2. At right is shown the stepwise waveform which is obtained when the digitized signal is reconverted to analog form by a digital-to-analog (D–A) converter. In this figure, the amplitude numbers from the A–D converter are shown in decimal form for didactic purposes. Actually, the numbers would be in binary form, as illustrated in Fig. 8-10.

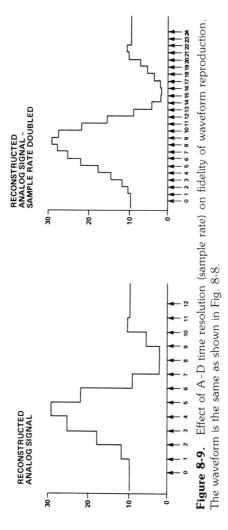

Figure 8-9. Effect of A–D time resolution (sample rate) on fidelity of waveform reproduction. The waveform is the same as shown in Fig. 8-8.

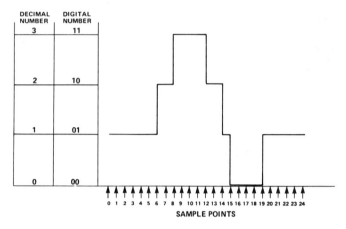

2 BIT RESOLUTION

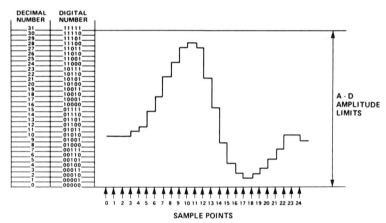

5 BIT RESOLUTION

Figure 8-10. Effect of A-D amplitude resolution on fidelity of waveform reproduction. The waveform is the same as shown in Fig. 8-8. The records are outputs of hypothetical D-A converters. An A-D converter with only a 2-bit word·length, allowing it to resolve amplitude into only 4 steps (2^2, or 2 x 2 = 4), is diagrammed at the top. A 5-bit A-D converter, capable of resolving amplitude into 32 steps, is diagrammed at the bottom. The amplitude limits of the A-D converter are also shown in the bottom diagram.

scale voltages encountered during average acquisition (see amplitude limits section, below). Amplitude reduction of A-D converters used in evoked potential systems generally ranges from 8 to 12 bits.

Amplitude limits. Input voltages corresponding to the highest and lowest numbers that the A-D converter is capable of outputting define the A-D converter's amplitude limits. All voltages below the converter's low limit or above its high limit are registered as a single minimum or maximum number (e.g., for a four-bit converter, 0000 or 1111). Signals that exceed the A-D converter's amplitude limits thus become "clipped" or "blocked" (Fig. 8-11). When signals are superimposed on high-amplitude noise, and the noise voltage exceeds the A-D converter's amplitude limits, the signal information is completely lost. Including such "blocked" epochs in an averaged waveform reduces its overall amplitude and also tends to blunt the sharpness of its peaks.

Signal amplitude at the A-D converter input must be kept within the converter's amplitude limits. However, to maximize amplitude resolution, signal amplitude should be also set as large as possible within these limits. Signal amplitude at the A-D converter's input is set by adjusting the low-level analog section's gain. To facilitate this adjustment, the evoked potential instrument should allow the operator to view the analog signal at the A-D converter's input on an oscilloscope screen. Such direct visual access to the analog signal is also helpful in minimizing noise interference.

Averager

Principle of operation. The averager repeatedly adds converted epochs (the sum) and also maintains a count of the number of epochs (N). On command (either entered by operator or internally generated), the averager divides the sum by N to obtain the average, then stores the result. When commanded to display the average, the averager reconverts the stored digital average into an analog signal by means of a digital-to-analog (D-A) converter. The reconverted analog signal is routed to the selected display device by appropriate switching.

Specifications and Characteristics

Sum-memory word length. With inadequate sum-memory word length, the magnitude of the summed responses may exceed the highest value which can be stored. This will appear in the averaged waveform either as wraparound (peaks going off the top of the display and reappearing at the bottom) or as blocking (Fig. 8-11). Sum-memory word lengths generally vary between 18 and 24 bits.

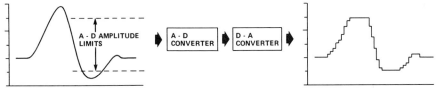

Figure 8-11. Effect of an input signal which exceeds A-D amplitude limits. The analog signal with A-D amplitude limits superimposed is shown at left. The same signal at the output of the system (after digitization then reconversion to analog form) is shown at right.

Number of data points/average.   The number of data points included in the average epoch determines the time resolution of the averaged waveform. Averagers normally hold this number constant and vary epoch duration by changing conversion time/point. Data points/average are generally powers of 2, and vary between 128 and 1024.

Artifact reject.   An averager with artifact reject capability selectively rejects epochs that contain points exceeding the A-D converter's limits. Artifact reject can greatly facilitate obtaining good quality records from "noisy" patients, particularly when such patients become noisy at irregular intervals. Artifact-reject is also helpful in situations where very large bioelectric signals (e.g., the electro-oculogram or electrocardiogram) cause intermittent interference. Provision of a means to adjust the reject criterion (e.g., from 1 to 256 off-scale data points) is a useful refinement of the artifact-reject function.

Display Section

Principle of Operation
Most evoked-potential recording systems display the acquired average on an oscilloscope; they also have some means of making a permanent copy of the average waveform. Following are briefly discussed the more commonly used means of making permanent records.

Oscilloscope camera.   Oscilloscope cameras generally mount on a frame (Bezel) around the oscilloscope face, and either swing aside or have a viewing port, which allows the operator to observe the oscilloscope when the camera is not in use. As a copying method for evoked potential work, the oscilloscope camera has the following advantages: (1) it is a direct representation of the signal as viewed by the operator, (2) it is commonly available in many laboratories and may thus be the most inexpensive means of acquiring the capability of making permanent copies, and (3) any text or numerical data displayed on the oscilloscope along with the average waveform is automatically registered by the oscilloscope camera.

The oscilloscope camera also has some disadvantages. (1) It is time-consuming. The operator must pause after each average has been acquired to operate the camera and (if a Polaroid unit is used) must also wait for film development. In the clinical test situation, this time expenditure is especially significant because it consumes patient- as well as technician-time. (2) If Polaroid film is not used, immediate feedback on the quality of the image obtained is not available. (3) The cost of supplies is relatively high. (4) The copy medium (film) is inconvenient, since it is relatively difficult to write directly on the film and the records must be pasted or otherwise mounted on a report page. (5) The white-on-black photographic image does not reproduce well.

Strip chart recorder.   The strip chart recorder usually is a standard heat- or ink-writing recorder. It registers time along the X axis by moving the paper at a fixed speed, and registers signal amplitude on the Y axis by pen movement. The advantages of the strip chart recorder are: (1) it is very easy to use; (2) it is compact, and lends itself well to portability; (3) it is a general-purpose instrument which can be used to register other bioelectric events [e.g., electroencephalogram, (EEG) eye movements]; (4) supply cost is minimal; and (5) it is relatively inexpensive.

The major disadvantages of the strip chart recorder are that multiple traces cannot be superimposed, and records must be pasted or mounted on a report form.

X-Y plotter. In contrast to the strip chart recorder, the X-Y plotter utilizes pen movement to provide both X (time) and Y (voltage) axes; the paper remains fixed. The X-Y plotter has the following major advantages: (1) traces can be superimposed; (2) multiple-color traces can easily be made, simply by changing pens; (3) a clinical report form can very easily be incorporated into the same chart on which the readout is made; and (4) supply cost is low.

Major disadvantages of the X-Y plotter are that it is relatively large and heavy (and therefore does not lend itself easily to portability), it is more expensive than the strip-chart recorder, and its time (X) axis is limited, (hence, it does not easily record continuous events, such as EEG and eye movements).

Electrostatic plotter. Electrostatic plotters duplicate on paper the exact image that is displayed on the oscilloscope face. These units are generally incorporated into larger systems which employ a general-purpose digital computer and a standard computer terminal as the oscilloscope readout device. The major advantages of the electrostatic plotter are that it is a fast and convenient means of copying the waveform; it allows registration of both textual and numerical data on the same chart as the record; and multiple traces can be easily superimposed, provided a memory scope is used as the readout device.

Disadvantages of the electrostatic plotter are: (1) they are the most expensive of the available readout devices; (2) they are bulky and heavy, hence do not lend themselves well to portability; (3) they are relatively expensive to interface with the cathode ray tube (CRT) terminal; and (4) they have a limited X (time) axis.

ELECTRODES

General Considerations

Electrode Placement and Electrode Types

Recording an evoked potential requires placement of three electrodes— two connected to the preamplifier inputs and a third *system-reference* or *ground* (depending on the type of system) electrode. One of the two electrodes connected to the preamplifier inputs is usually referred to as the *active* electrode and the other is referred to as the *indifferent* (or *reference*) electrode. It should be recognized that this convention is only partially accurate, since the indifferent electrode almost always makes at least some active contribution to the recorded waveform. Some laboratories utilize paired indifferent electrodes (generally located either over the mastoid processes or on the earlobes), and hence use four (rather than three) electrodes. However, this is not good practice because differences in impedances between the two indifferent electrodes can significantly affect the recorded waveform.

For recording the BSER and the middle and late auditory evoked-potentials, the active electrode is placed either on the scalp or high up in the center of the forehead. For recording the auditory nerve action potential and cochlear potentials, a specialized electrode, designed to place the contact point as close to the cochlea as possible, must be used. The indifferent electrodes for both ECochG and late evoked-potential recording are usually placed either over the mastoids, on the earlobe, or on the bridge of the nose (see Chapters 10-14).

Following are general requirements for good electrode design. They should be easy to place, allow for secure attachment, involve only minimal patient discomfort; have an electrically stable electrode-subject interface; and have an electrical impedance at the electrode-subject interface that is easily minimized by cleaning or penetrating the skin.

Electrode locations for auditory evoked-potential recording can be divided into three types (each location presents unique design and placement problems): (1) relatively large, flat surfaces (scalp, forehead, and mastoids); (2) curved surfaces, (bridge of nose, and earlobes); and (3) ECochG placements (as close to the cochlea as possible). Following are discussed the various electrodes that different laboratories use to meet these requirements.

Flat-surface electrodes. For scalp, forehead, or mastoid placements, standard EEG disc electrodes are commonly used (Fig. 8-12). These are metallic discs (usually of silver or gold) about 1 cm in diameter containing a recess for electrode paste. Some have a hole in the center to allow needle insertion to abrade the skin beneath the electrode. The electrodes are attached with adhesive tape or adhesive discs. Scalp electrodes are usually attached with collodion or with adhesive electrode paste and a cotton ball. Collodion attachment is relatively time consuming, and removal causes some patient discomfort. However, collodion provides a very secure electrode attachment. The use of adhesive electrode paste attaches the electrode somewhat less securely (though, generally, adequately for routine clinical evoked potential recording), but the attachment procedure is quick, removal is easy, and does not cause patient discomfort.

Electrical instability caused by battery potentials generated across the electrode-skin interface can create interference, which usually manifests as

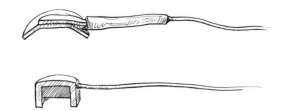

Figure 8-12. Surface electrodes used to record evoked potentials. Electrode at top is a standard EEG disc electrode, made either of silver or gold. The electrode at bottom is constructed of a silver chloride pellet contained inside a plastic cup. Both of these electrode types typically are about 6-10 mm in diameter.

increased movement artifact and occasional large baseline swings even when the patient is still. Polarization of silver-disc electrodes is minimized by electrolytically depositing a thin coat of silver chloride on the electrode surface (known colloquially as "chloriding" the electrode). Chloriding silver-disc EEG electrodes provides good (though far from perfect) protection against development of electrode junction potentials. However, this technique has the disadvantage that the silver chloride coat is relatively fragile; its benefits are lost if even a small area is scraped off. Thus, electrodes must be frequently rechlorided. A more effective way of utilizing a silver-chloride interface to reduce junction potentials is to recess a silver-chloride pellet into a plastic disc (Fig. 8-12). This not only protects the fragile silver-chloride material, but also holds the electrode's surface a constant distance from the skin to minimize movement potentials. The recessed electrode, however, is bulkier and more expensive than the simple disc electrode.

An alternative way of reducing electrode polarization is to make the electrode of a less-reactive metal (e.g. gold). This is less effective than chloriding, but the electrode is more durable. For routine evoked-potential work where the low-frequencies are filtered out, gold electrodes protect sufficiently against interference by electrode polarization.

Electrodes for curved surfaces. Although many laboratories use standard EEG electrodes for earlobe and bridge-of-nose placement, electrodes specifically designed to facilitate placement on these irregular surfaces are available. Figure 8-13 illustrates earlobe placement of one such electrode, which is constructed of a conductive cloth material, for earlobe placement. This electrode is obviously equally well suited for use on the bridge of the nose. In auditory evoked-potential recording, using the conductive cloth electrode on the earlobe (some labs use a plastic clip-on type carrier in which a flat-surface electrode is placed) minimizes the patient discomfort caused by earphones pressing against thicker standard EEG electrodes.

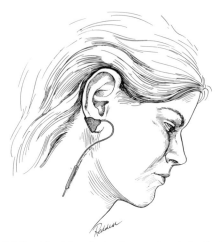

Figure 8-13. Flexible electrode constructed of electrically conductive cloth, specially suited for placement on irregularly shaped surfaces. The earlobe placement, often used as the reference location for auditory evoked-potential recording, is illustrated.

Electrodes for ECochG. The active ECochG electrode should be placed as close to the cochlea as possible, because (shown in Fig. 8-14), placement near the cochlea increases the size of all ECochG responses (action potentials, cochlear microphonics, summating potentials) (Coats, 1974; Simmons, 1976). The closer the electrode is to the cochlea, however, the more invasive and difficult is its placement. Electrodes for ECochG are usually placed either in the external auditory ear canal (extratympanic) or on the promontory (transtympanic or intratympanic).

Figure 8-15 illustrates placement of different types of ECochG electrodes. Two basic types of extratympanic ECochG electrodes have been used—needle electrodes that penetrate the canal skin (Coats and Dickey, 1970; Salomon and Elberling, 1971; Yoshie, 1968), and less-invasive electrodes that rest on the canal skin surface (Coats, 1974; Cullen, Ellis, and Berlin, et al., 1972; Montandon, 1976).

Needle electrodes were the first used for extratympanic ECochG (Yoshie, 1968). It was subsequently found that electrodes that did not penetrate the external ear canal skin recorded potentials just as large as those recorded by the needle electrode (Coats, 1974). Therefore, for extratympanic ECochG, the surface electrode has largely supplanted the more invasive needle electrode.

The promontory location records relatively large responses (Simmons, 1976; Yoshie and Ohashi, 1969). It is also a more invasive placement and, in pediatric patients, requires general anesthesia. However, because of higher response amplitude, many investigators—particularly outside the United

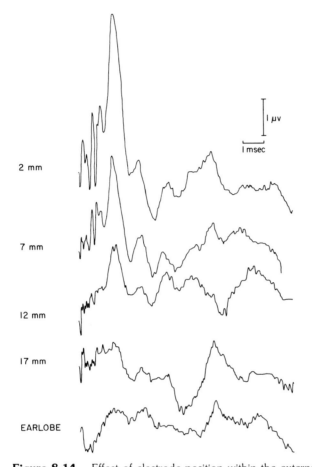

Figure 8-14. Effect of electrode position within the external ear canal on amplitude of recorded responses. A needle electrode (Figure 8-15B) placed at about 9 o'clock on the canal surface was used. Action potential and cochlear microphonic responses to a click generated by driving a PDR-10 earspeaker with an 0.01 msec squarewave pulse are shown. Click intensity was 107 dB peSPL (about 77 dB above normal threshold). (Reprinted with permission from Coats, A. C. On electrocochleographic electrode design. *Journal of the Acoustical Society of America.* 1954, 56:708-711.)

States—prefer promontory over the extratympanic placement (Aran, 1971; Spoor, 1974).

Earlobe electrodes have also been advocated for ECochG (Moore, 1971; Sohmer and Feinmesser, 1967). The earlobe provides a more convenient and less invasive ECochG placement, but responses recorded from this location are severely attenuated.

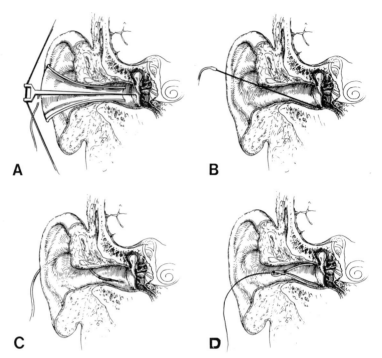

Figure 8-15. Four different types of electrodes used for electrocochleography. A illustrates the trans-tympanic needle, with point located on the promontory just above the round window (Aran, 1971). The needle is held in place by an elastic band, which is attached to a doughnut-shaped cushion (not shown) which surrounds the pinna. B, C, and D illustrate three extra-tympanic electrode types. B. A needle insulated except at its tip which is held in place by a droplet of glue on the pinna (Coats and Dickey, 1970; Yoshie, 1968). C. A needle which penetrates the external ear canal through a puncture wound placed posteriorly on the pinna and imbeds in the canal wall skin close to the tympanic annulus (Salomon and Elberling, 1971). D. A nonpenetrating electrode constructed of a flexible plastic leaf with a silver ball at the tip (Coats, 1974).

DISCUSSION

In this chapter, I have attempted to outline the basic principles for choosing, employing, and understanding auditory evoked-potential systems. No attempt has been made to advocate any particular system. Suffice it to say that the choice of equipment today is enormous, as are the number of different configurations that can be obtained. In order to choose a system, one must know precisely what the requirements are for the particular situation. It would also be instructive to visit different laboratories (or convention displays) so as to gain some "hands-on" experience with a system prior to final purchase. Many manufacturers will demonstrate their system on your premises; several will leave their system with you for a trial period of use and evaluation.

Ernest J. Moore

9   Effects of Stimulus Parameters

Previous chapters have explained that the auditory brain-stem evoked response (BSER) has emerged since 1967 as a distinct, although hybrid, indicant of peripheral and central electrophysiologic function. A unifying objective of investigative research in this area has been to clarify the electrophysiologic phenomena underlying the characteristic activity of the BSER. In several scientific reports, the basic tenet of the scientific method has been followed, i.e., gaining knowledge through the process of observation. The phenomena which have been subjected to observation have been the various waves that comprise the BSER. Given that we have already operationally defined our subject i.e., the BSER, it follows that we would soon become preoccupied with the stimuli that is used to evoke the phenomena, how the phenomena might vary according to changes in the stimuli, and how these phenomena are affected by yet other phenomena.

If one is allowed to formally define the BSER as a variable whose characteristics may differ according to a well defined classification scheme, continuing to reason along these lines indicates that the BSER can be classified according to its time of occurrence or latency, its magnitude or amplitude, and to its general structure and form. It can readily be seen that these characteristics create the dependent variable, i.e., that which is being measured. The independent variables which are under the researcher's direct control are the stimulus parameters. It follows that the independent variables can be manipu-

I wish to thank Ayalur Ananthanarayan, Barbara Brown, Marva Conley, Kris Douglas, Walter Grengg, Michael Piscotty, and Lynne Rowe for assistance in collection of portions of these data.

lated or controlled by the researcher, and can be predicted (within limits) to have an effect upon the dependent variables—the BSER waves.

With these properties in mind, this chapter will examine the effects of a series of independent variables (stimulus parameters) on the dependent variables (the BSER waves). This objective posits certain prerequisites common to the study of the auditory system using electrophysiologic methods: (1) isolation and identification of the components of interest, (2) analysis of the effects or interactions of the components upon each other, and (3) a description of the temporal and spatial relations of the components and their interactions with the activity of the intact organ under study. The underlying notion is the examination of the effects of the independent variables of frequency, intensity, and time. Another consideration are the effects of noise on the BSER waves.

INTERACTION OF STIMULUS PARAMETERS

According to Eisenberg (1965), several acoustic parameters are relevant to fundamental auditory neurophysiologic processes. In Figure 9-1, a schematic representation of several of these acoustic parameters are presented. The interaction of these acoustic or stimulus parameters is related to the auditory BSER. Note that there are only three primary stimulus parameters i.e., the acoustic stimulus is represented in a three-dimensional mode: frequency, intensity, and time. Bear in mind, however, that these parameters are in their physical or electrical state; their psychological counterparts are not the object of discussion.

In considering the neurophysiologic processes subserving these physical parameters, we see that *frequency* is related to the loci of stimulation along the basilar membrane and along the tonotopic configuration of the sensory and neural auditory pathways. *Intensity* is related to the spatial configuration of neural activity and the number of active neurons and fiber tracts. The variable of *time* can be further subdivided as to duration, rise–fall time, repetition rate or interstimulus interval, and phase-of-onset. The duration of the signal is related to the temporal configuration of activity in neural substrates. The rise–fall (or rise–decay) time is related to the intrinsic, temporal probability of the neural events at the onset of the auditory signal, and the tendency of the system to recover to prestimulus homostatic activity levels. Repetition rate, or its intrinsic counterpart, the interstimulus interval (ISI), is related to the integration of acoustic energy and the relative distribution of excitatory and inhibitory neural nets. Phase-of-onset determines the initial direction in which mechanical events in the cochlea occur, which in turn cause primary biochemical and neural aggregates to exhibit preferred times of occurrence.

The basic assumptions posited for the above notions owe a great deal to contemporary concepts of auditory electrophysiology. The assignation of

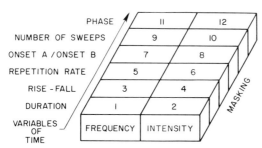

Figure 9-1. Interaction of stimulus parameters that are used in recording the auditory BSER. The three independent variables of frequency, intensity, and time (duration, rise-fall, repetition rate, onset A/onset B, number of sweeps, phase) are shown as variables that can be manipulated in the test situation. Masking adds another dimension to the complex nature of the test situation. (Modified from Berlin, C. I. Temporal and dichotic factors in central auditory testing. In J. Katz (Ed.), *Handbook of clinical audiology*. Baltimore: Williams & Wilkins, 1972.)

various changes in the BSER to the basic peripheral and central auditory neural substrates is related to a primary objective of presenting and manipulating the various stimulus-bound parameters so as to force the sensory neural system out of a position of equilibrium. With appropriate BSER recording techniques, one should be able to record the resultant dysequilibrium in the system's response. The transient changes (labelled as waves I, II, III, and so on) are far-field indicants of the electrophysiologic functioning of the auditory pathway, meaningful only when they are evoked by precisely specified and controlled stimulus variables. In other words, in order to understand the behavior of sensory, neural, and central substrates underlying the BSER, the acoustic signals must be precisely specified; they must bear upon the encoding capacities of the biological system under investigation (Eisenberg, 1965).

TYPE OF STIMULI

The ideal stimulus for evoking the BSER has long been the subject of considerable interest. From the very beginning of BSER research, (Suzuki, et al., 1966; Portman, et al., 1967; Sohmer and Feinmesser, 1967; Spreng and Keidel, 1967; Yoshie and Ohashi, 1967; Yoshie, et al., 1967; Jewett, et al., 1970; Moore, 1971), the search for the ideal stimulus was of major significance for these early investigators. What emerged from these studies was that each research group used some type of click. It can be argued, however, that each group of investigators had their own idea as to what constituted an "ideal" click stimulus, since all were defined according to the electrical input

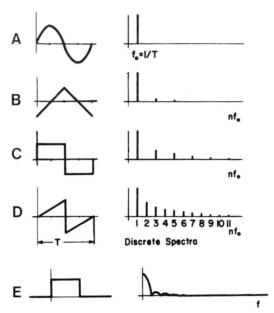

Figure 9-2. Representation of various spectra (relative amplitude vs frequency) to several basic waveforms (relative amplitude vs time). A–D. Examples of discrete spectra. E–G. examples of continuous spectra. H–J. examples of power spectral density functions. The discrete spectra are for periodic waveforms, the continuous spectra are for transient signals, and the power spectral densities exhibit the average contributions to total signal power as a function of frequency. The relative amplitudes and phase relationships are determined by the temporal structure of the signals and are mathematically described by a Fourier series. (Reprinted with permission from Pfeiffer, R. R., Consideration of the acoustic stimulus. In Keidel W. D., Neff W. D. (Eds.), *Auditory system, anatomy & physiology (ear), handbook of physiology*, vol. V/1. New York: Springer-Verlag, 1974, p. 13.)

(usually 0.1 msec; see Chapter 2) to the earphone. It is readily apparent, however, (Fig. 9-2) that the spectral shape of a signal is intrinsically related to the electrically generated signal. Additionally, Durrant (Chapter 2) has argued (and rightly so) that the final stimulus arriving at the cochlea will be influenced by the mode of delivery, (i.e., earphone vs speaker) and the acoustics of the auricle, ear canal, and the middle-ear space. We know that a "click" can be generated using a number of electrical equivalents, such as one or two cycles of a sine wave (Fig. 9-2A), the triangular wave (Fig. 9-2B), the square wave (Fig. 9-2C), the positive sawtooth wave (ramp) (Fig. 9-2D) or negative sawtooth wave (not shown), a positive (Fig. 9-2E) or negative- (not shown) going pulse, a short tone burst (Fig. 9-2F), the so-called haversine (Fig. 9-2G), and various forms of wide-band (Fig. 9-2H,I) and band-limited noise (Fig. 9-2J). Of paramount importance for each of these functions is their unique corresponding frequencies or spectral shapes (second panel of each signal shown in Fig. 9-2).

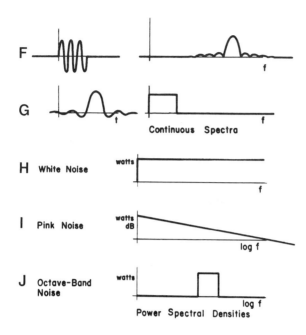

Continuous Spectra

H White Noise

I Pink Noise

J Octave-Band Noise

Power Spectral Densities

With these properties in mind, the audiologic and otologic objective has been to place stringent requirements on signal sources for greater frequency resolution and stability. For the most part, however, stimuli used for evoking the BSER have not been chosen based on the well known principles of spectra (frequency); rather, the wave forms had initially been chosen in the hopes of approaching or approximating an ideal spectrum or spectra. In the 1970s, the theoretical treatment of Gabor's (1947) elementary signal or "logon" theory (Davis, 1976) was revived in the literature. Here, the emphasis was on striking a compromise between an abrupt rectangular wave (see Fig. 9-2E) and a continuous, pure tone (see Fig. 9-2A). The logical sequel to these efforts is the desire to have a signal that is abrupt enough to synchronize primary auditory units, yet long enough to maintain frequency specificity. But one cannot have an abrupt signal in time and also have precision in frequency, and vice versa. Desire for compromise brought about the use of the tone pip (Davis, 1976), the ⅓ octave click (Naunton and Zerlin, 1976b), and the short tone burst (Bausch, Rose, and Harner, 1980; Brama and Sohmer, 1977; Davis and Hirsh, 1979; Funasaka and Abe, 1979; Klein and Teas, 1978; Kodera, Yamane, and Yamada, et al., 1977; Mitchell and Clemis, 1977; Moore, 1971; Parker and Thornton, 1978b; Picton, Quellette, and Hamel, et al., 1979; Stillman, Moushegian, and Rupert, 1976; Stockard, Stockard, and Westmoreland, et al., 1979; Suzuki, Hirai, and Horiuchi, 1977; Weber and Folson, 1977; Wood, Seitz, and Jacobson, 1979).

Other considerations of quantitative changes in signal spectra are changes in the temporal duration of the signal, the spectrum of a single pulse, and the spectra of different periodic representations of that pulse. These relations are depicted in Figure 9-3A and 9-3B. Each of the three single pulses in Figure 9-3A differ only in width (time duration). As the pulse becomes shorter in time, more of the overall signal content is at higher frequencies. This is an indication that there is an inverse relationship between temporal acuity and spectral bandwidth, or that stimulus systems with wider bandwidth capabilities will be able to generate narrower stimuli. In Figure 9-3B, both the envelope of the continuous spectrum of a single pulse and the discrete spectra of the periodic representations maintain the same shape. The envelope of the spectrum of the base signal is necessary to specify the necessary spectrum handling requirements of the stimulus system (Pfeiffer, 1974).

The discussion that follows will emphasize, for the most part, the use of

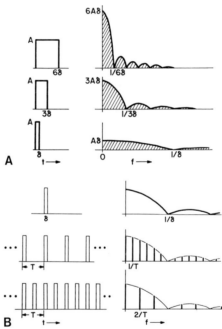

Figure 9-3. Representation of the relationship between time (t) and frequency (f). A. The quantitative changes in signal spectra with changes in time duration of the signal. B. The relationship between a continuous spectrum of a single pulse, and the spectra of two different periodic representations of the single pulse. (Reprinted with permission from Pfeiffer R. R., Consideration of the acoustic stimulus. In Keidel W. D., Neff W. D. (Eds.), Auditory system, anatomy & physiology (ear), handbook of physiology, Vol V/1. New York: Springer-Verlag, 1974, p. 15.)

he short tone burst in eliciting the BSER. At this juncture, however, it would ɔe instructive to consider those principles which assist in standardizing our ɑuantitative measurements.

CALIBRATION OF STIMULI

As specification of intensity is discussed in Chapters 2 and 8, a brief ·eminder will suffice. The best physical designations for the intensity of the ;hort duration signals employed in BSER testing is the peak-equivalent sound ɔressure level (PE dB SPL).

Two other stimulus parameters exist in addition to intensity: *frequency* ɑnd *time*. A precise calibration of these two dimensions should also be conducted prior to performing ECochG and BSER tests. In specifying physical ·requency, the ideal device is an electronic frequency counter, or universal ɔounter.

The analog oscilloscope, an indispensable, general-purpose, and basic aboratory or clinical tool, provides a method for calibrating all of the variables ɔf time (see Figure 9-1), including duration, rise–fall or rise–decay time, ·epetition rate, the occurrence of signal "A" as related to signal "B," phase of ɔnset, and the onset and offset of sweep (epoch) time or a "trigger" signal. Ɔne might also use an electronic counter. The oscilloscope can additionally ɔrovide amplitude measurements of numerous input signals, including clicks, ɔone bursts, continuous tones, ⅓ octave clicks, and bursts of noise, or longasting noise sources.

EFFECTS OF FREQUENCY

Figure 9-4 displays the BSER to various audiometric frequencies. The ɛlectrical equivalents of the signals used to evoke these responses were short ɔone bursts having a linear rise–fall time of 1.0 msec, a plateau of 3.0 msec, ɔr an overall duration of 5.0 msec. In other instances, rather than maintain ɑ constant duration, we have employed the Olsen and Carhart (1966) ·echnique using equivalent durations (Moore and Schlafman, in preparation). The BSER waveforms displayed in Figure 9-4 do not, on visual inspection, ɗiffer appreciably as a function of frequency. However, differences manifest ᴡhen one quantifies the peak latencies, e.g., for wave I, slight differences ɑcross frequencies are apparent (see Fig. 9-5). That is, latency values at the owest intensity level employed (– 40 dB of attenuation) do show a difference n time of occurrence. On the other hand, at the highest intensity (– 10 dB of ɑttenuation), for all practical purposes, a shift in latency as a function of freɑuency is not apparent. Interestingly, the effects of intensity at the low (1000 Ƕz) and high frequency (8000 Hz) are evident. In other words, the very

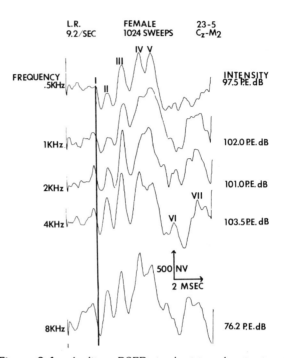

Figure 9-4. Auditory BSERs to short tone bursts at various frequencies: 0.5 KHz, 1 KHz, 2 KHz, 4 KHz, and 8 KHz. Each tone burst was shaped using a 1.0 msec linear rise-decay time and a 3.0 msec duration. Repetition rate was 9.2/sec; a total of 1024 responses were averaged. For this illustration, intensity was not equated across the various frequencies. Responses obtained from a normal-hearing 23-year-old female subject. Electrodes were attached to vertex-right mastoid.

highest intensity level (− 10 dB) revealed overlapping data for all frequencies employed (Bausch, Rose, and Harner, 1980). However, as intensity decreased, latency increased and a clear separation of the 1000 Hz data and the 8000 Hz data is readily apparent. Accordingly, it can be inferred that the results at the highest intensity level primarily originate from the most basal region of the cochlea, but as the stimuli are decreased, the components originate from a more apical region (Elberling, 1974).

The effects of frequency on wave V are depicted in Figure 9-6. A clear separation in latency between 1000 and 4000 Hz is apparent, regardless of the intensity levels employed. A decrease in intensity also shows a corresponding increase in latency, for both 1000 and 4000 Hz. The separation of wave V latency at 1000 and 4000 Hz was obtained by Picton and his colleagues (1981) while employing the technique of "derived responses" (Teas, Eldridge, and Davis, 1962). Several investigators have noted this frequency-dependent relation (Don and Eggermont, 1978; Don, Eggermont, and

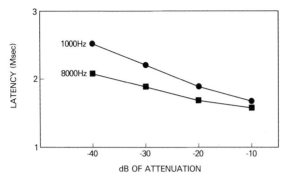

Figure 9-5. Input-output latency functions for wave I at 1000 and 8000 Hz. At the − 10 dB attenuation level (3.2 volts p-p), the latency of wave I for 1000 or 8000 Hz does not differ. As the intensity is decreased, the functions tend to separate from each other, until at − 40 dB attenuation, a clear separation is observed. A monotonic relation is assumed; extrapolating these curves to threshold should reveal a significant separation as a function of frequency. This would portend specific loci of stimulation along the cochlear partition and frequency specific stimuli.

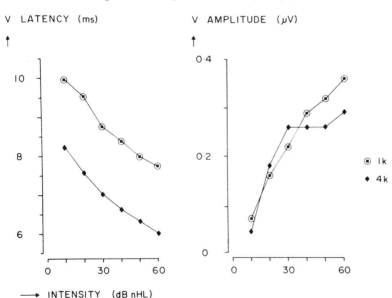

Figure 9-6. Input-output latency and amplitude functions for wave V at 1000 and 4000 Hz. Separation of the two functions at the highest (60 dB) and lowest (10 dB) sensation levels for latency are apparent. As intensity increased, the magnitude of both the 1K and 4K data increased, but note the saturation effect for the 4K response. These data are consistent with several published reports. (Reprinted with permission from Picton, T. W., Stapells, D. R., and Campbell, K. B. Auditory evoked potentials from the human cochlea and brainstem. *Journal of Otolaryngology*, 1981, *10*:1-41.)

Brackman, 1979; Eggermont and Don, 1980; Elberling, 1974; Parker and
Thornton, 1978a, 1978b, 1978c; Wood, Seitz, and Jacobson, 1979), and
have concluded that the wave V peak recorded from normal hearing subjects
is thought to mainly derive from the 2000-4000 Hz region of the cochlea
This notion is predicated on the findings that wave V progressively increases
as the center frequency of the derived response decreases, and the latency
change is similar to latency changes observed for the auditory nerve N
response (Eggermont and Don, 1980; Elberling, 1974).

Further evidence of the spatial representation of frequency along the
cochlear partition can be inferred from the psychophysical tuning curve (Durrant, Gabriel, and Walter, 1981) to short tone bursts presented at low sensation levels (see Chapter 2). While the sharpness of the tuning function seems
to be level-dependent, reasonably discrete stimulation using very brief tone
bursts is possible. It is noted, however, that the "tip" of the tuning curve is not
well-preserved for intensity levels far above normal hearing thresholds. A
psychophysical function using a Békésy tracking procedure shows similar
results when tracking short tone bursts at threshold (Fig. 9-7). The classical
input-output function characteristic of long tones is present, except that the
curves separate as a function of the power integration function (Moore and
Conley, in preparation). Of course, as the intensity of the stimuli is increased,

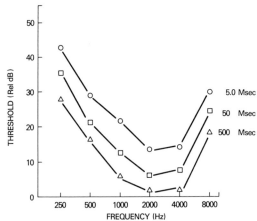

Figure 9-7. Thresholds for short tone bursts as a function of
frequency. The parameters are the duration of the stimuli for
5.0, 50, and 500 msec tone bursts. There is a clear separation
between each of the stimulus conditions, with a 10-15 dB difference between the 5.0 and 500 msec durations. Since the 5.0
msec curve parallels the 500 msec curve, and both are at threshold, the 5.0 msec thresholds are assumed to be frequency-
specific even at the lowest frequencies. It follows that loci of
stimulation along the basilar membrane should also be specific.
The tracking procedure of Békésy was used as the psychophysical method. Ten normal hearing subjects were tested.

equency splatter becomes problematic. To what extent frequency spread
an be tolerated is related to how precisely one wishes to chart the "pure
one" audiogram (see Chapter 2) and relate the loci of stimulation along the
ochlear partition. These fundamental observations and the boundaries be-
ween which audiologist and otologist can operate are detailed by several investigators (Naunton and Fernandez, 1978; Davis and Hirsh, 1979; and
Funasaka and Abe, 1979).

EFFECTS OF INTENSITY

We have already learned that stimulus intensity is related to the spatial
configuration of neural aggregates and the number of active neural elements
present. In other words, the intensity of a stimulus influences the frequency of
neural firing, and the number of neural elements capable of firing. These rela-

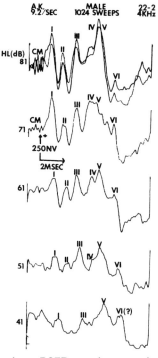

Figure 9-8. Auditory BSERs as a function of various intensity
levels. Each tone was shaped using a 1.0 msec linear rise-decay
time and a 3.0 msec duration. Repetition rate was 9.2/sec;
1024 responses were averaged. As intensity decreased, amplitude decreased and latency increased for all components. Responses shown were obtained from a normal-hearing 22-year-
old male subject with electrodes on vertex-right mastoid; right
ear stimulated.

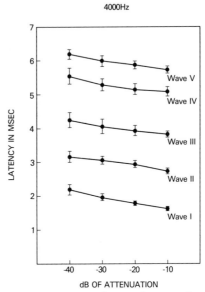

4000Hz

Figure 9-9. Input-output latency functions for auditory BSER at 4000 Hz. The parameters are the various waves of the BSER, I through V. Stimuli was shaped using a 1.0 msec linear rise-decay time and a 3.0 msec duration. All waves display a monotonic relation to intensity; there is a decrease in latency as intensity is increased. At − 10, 3.2 volts (p-p) generated 115 PE dB SPL.

tions can be represented in the BSER waveform as a function of different intensity levels (Fig. 9-8). A distinct series of waves is accordingly labeled (for 4000 Hz only) in the Figure. Each 10 db decrease in the intensity of the stimuli shows a corresponding increase in the latency of each wave. These relations are quantitatively depicted in Figure 9-9. Similar input-output functions were generated by other frequencies, and therefore, are not presented here (to do so would be redundant). The salient feature of this illustration is that all five waves decrease in latency as a function of increasing intensity, or conversely, that there is an increase in latency as the intensity of the stimuli is decreased. This is seen over the entire range of intensities investigated and suggests an approximately linear relation to the logarithm of the stimulus intensity. In certain definite regions, note also the increase in the variability measure (vertical bars) as intensity is decreased, and that the variability score also increases when comparing wave I to wave V. As expected, the BSER waves (Fig. 9-8) at the 41 dB level are losing much of their "peakness." Further intensity decreases will increase the amount of the variability score and make it extremely difficult to identify wave components from the variations in background noise. Interestingly, the robustness of wave V causes it to remain long after the other waves have receded.

EFFECTS OF TIME PARAMETERS

Several time parameters that influence the BSER will be considered. First, the overall *duration* of the input signal will be shown to be important. Second, we will point out that the effects of the *rise-decay* (or rise-fall) time of the signal will be reflected in the resultant BSER waves. Third, the *repetition rate* of the input signal will be shown to make the BSER waves less stable. Fourth, presenting to the auditory system one signal followed in time by another (*onset of A vs the onset of B*) will cause the BSER waves to reflect a kind of refractoriness. On the other hand, the *number of stimuli* of epochs tend not to appreciably influence the BSER. Finally, we will demonstrate (experimentally) that the *phase-of-onset* of the input signal produces perturbations in the time of occurrence of certain of the BSER components.

Duration and Interstimulus Interval

The association between BSER components and the duration and interstimulus interval (ISI) of the input signal are depicted in Figure 9-10. In recording these BSER waves, the frequency and intensity of the short tone burst were held constant at 4000 Hz and at 90 PE dB SPL, respectively. Consider also that the rise-fall time (1.0 msec), repetition rate (9.2/sec), number of sweeps or epochs (N = 1024), and phase-of-onset (rarefaction, $\varnothing$ = 0) all remained constant.

By simple visual inspection, it is to be noted that as duration is increased from 3.0 to 100 msec, the latency of all components increased (see also Harkins, McEvoy, and Scott, 1979). Note also that the amplitude of the various components decreased. Furthermore, the various components are observed to become less distinct, however, all waves can readily be identified at the longest duration, although the double-peaked wave IV-V complex has merged into one broad, identifiable peak. Note further that since we chose to hold the repetition rate constant, the ISI is decreasing while the duration is increasing, or, conversely, as the ISI is decreased, the various BSER waves are less distinct and show an increase in latency but a decrease in amplitude.

For comparison, note the quantitative data for the duration-ISI relations in Figure 9-11. The input-output functions for waves I and V confirm our initial visual observations that an increase in duration (or a corresponding decrease in ISI) will result in a slight increase in the latency of waves I and V. For both waves, the shift in latency, for all practical purposes, is nearly identical. The numerical values are on the order of 250-300 μsec (0.25-0.30 msec). While these changes are minimal, they are extremely important when establishing clinical norms that generally range in microseconds (e.g., see Brackman, 1977; Brackman and Selters, 1976, 1978; Selters and Brackman, 1977, among others).

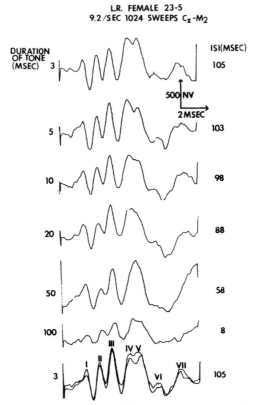

Figure 9-10. Auditory BSERs as a function of the duration of the tone burst and corresponding interstimulus interval (ISI). Stimuli was a 4000 Hz short tone burst shaped by a 1.0 msec linear rise-decay time and a 3.0 msec duration. Repetition rate was held constant at 9.2/sec; 1024 responses were averaged; intensity level 115 PE dB SPL (3.2 volts p-p). As duration increased, or ISI decreased, amplitude decreased and latency increased.

Rise–Decay Time

The BSER may equally be influenced by various rise-decay times of the input signal (Kimmelman, Marsh, and Yamane, et al., 1979; Kodera, Hink, and Yamada, et al., 1979; Suzuki and Horiuchi, 1981). In this case, a point is reached where response identification becomes extremely difficult as rise-decay time increases. The BSER response to various rise-decay times are illustrated in Figure 9-12, which illustrates that the neural impulses that make up the BSER are best excited by fast-rising stimuli. The latency of the various components are also seen to shift to a later time of occurrence for longer rise-decay times. To be true, we may also note a decided dimunition in the magnitude of the various components. Seen thus, a rise-decay time of

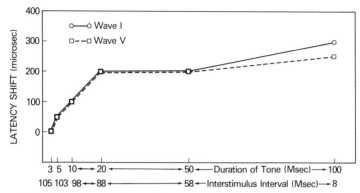

Figure 9-11. Input-output latency functions of auditory BSER for various durations and corresponding ISI. Three normal-hearing subjects were tested 5 times each for a total of 15 times. (See Fig. 9-10 for a complete description.) The shift in latency is parallel for waves I and V up to a duration of 50 msec; there is a slight separation of about 50 μsec at the 100 msec duration.

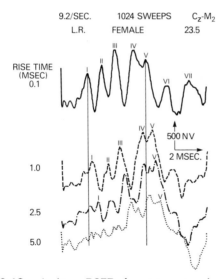

Figure 9-12. Auditory BSERs for various rise-decay times. Stimuli was a 4000 Hz short tone burst shaped by a 0.1, 1.0, 2.5, or 5.0 msec rise-decay time. A 3.0 msec duration was used in each case. Repetition rate was 9.2/sec; 1024 responses were averaged (see Fig. 9-10 for a complete description). As rise time increased, amplitude decreased, latency increased, and response identification became more difficult.

5.0 msec causes wave I to disappear into the ongoing background noise of
the response trace so that waves I and II are not readily perceptible. Continuing to reason along these lines reveals, on the other hand, that waves III, IV,
and V can still be detected, although waves VI and VII are out of the range of
visual detection. Once again, what is demonstrated is that distinct BSER
potentials depend upon a synchronous discharge of auditory nerve fibers.
Since we learned in Chapter 4 that it is primarily the fibers innervating the
basal turn of the cochlea that synchronously fire to a brief transient stimulus,
we suffer no illusions over the fact that the BSER components arising from the
100 μsec rise-time is disproportionately weighted toward the basal end of the
cochlea. That a longer rise-decay time can be interpreted as causing a delayed neural discharge is certainly not out of the question. These relations
have been quantified and are displayed in Figure 9-13. The successive components consistently increase in latency as a function of increasing rise time
(Fig. 9-13). That is, the points on the curve do not oscillate in relative value,
but each of the values is greater than the preceding value. In mathematical
terms, we would say that we have a monotonic relation, or an ordered set of
quantities.

Repetition Rate

Increasing the rate of stimulation also increases the latency, but decreases the magnitude of the BSER waves (Campbell, Picton, and Wolfe, et

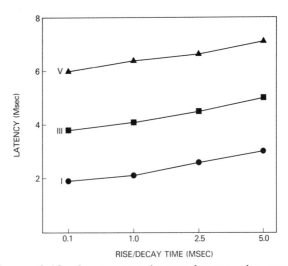

Figure 9-13. Input-output latency functions for various
rise-decay times. Three normal-hearing subjects were tested 5
times each for a total of 15 times. (See Figure 9-12 for a more
complete description.) Data plots are for waves I, III and V. A
monotonic relation emerges for increasing duration of the rise-
decay time. Waves II and IV were similar but are not plotted.

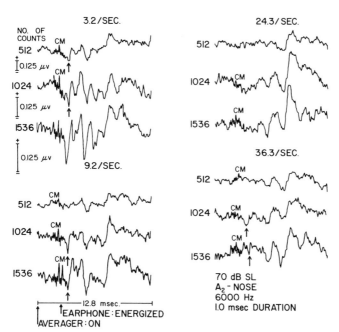

Figure 9-14. Cochlear microphonic (CM), action potentials (AP), and BSER for repetition rates of 3.0, 9.2, 24.3, and 36.3 stimuli/second. Electrodes on bony bridge of nose and ipsilateral earlobe. Responses were obtained at 70 dB SL at 6000 Hz. Rise-decay time was 0.1 msec, overall duration was 1.0 msec; 512, 1024, or 1536 responses were averaged. Three normal hearing subjects were tested. The averager was turned on 2.0 msec prior to click presentation. Responses decrease as a function of increasing repetition rate. Positivity of the nose electrode is plotted downward. (From Moore, E. Human Cochlear Microphonics and Auditory Nerve Action Potentials from Surface Electrodes. Unpublished Ph.D. dissertation, University of Wisconsin, Madison, Wisconsin, 1971.)

al., 1981; Chiappa, Gladstone, and Young, 1979; Don, Allen, and Starr, 1977; Harkins, McEvoy, and Scott, 1979; Moore, 1971; Picton, et al., 1981; Pratt, Ben-David, and Peled, et al., 1981; Rowe, 1978; van Olphen, Rudenburgh, and Vervey, 1979; Weber and Fujikawa, 1977; Yagi and Kaga, 1979). The effect is most pronounced for repetition rates greater than 10/sec, but the effect does not go unnoticed at rates below 10/sec. Figure 9-14 depicts analog data; Figure 9-15 summarizes the quantitative data as amplitude input-output functions for auditory nerve N_1 amplitude.

We have since quantified these associations for all BSER waves; the data are not significantly different from the N_1 data. The parameter (in this case) was the number of responses or epochs summed; sensation level and frequency were held constant. The relation of decrement in amplitude as repetition rate is increased can be recognized. An increase in latency has also been demonstrated (Antonelli, Cazzavillan, and Gaini, et al., 1981; Baschek and

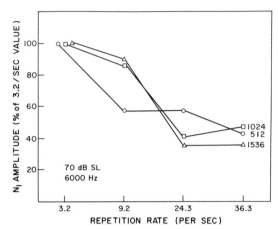

Figure 9-15. Input-output amplitude function for increasing repetition rate. (See Fig. 9-14 for a complete description.) Responses decrease in magnitude by about 15 percent at 9.2/ sec to about 60 percent at the 36.3/sec rate. Positivity of the nose electrodes is plotted downward. (From Moore, E. Human Cochlear Microphonics and Auditory Nerve Action Potentials from Surface Electrodes. Unpublished Ph.D. dissertation, University of Wisconsin, Madison, Wisconsin, 1971.)

Steinert, 1980; Mair, Elverland, and Laukli, 1979; Picton, et al., 1981). Note that the cochlear microphonic does not decrease as a function of repetition rate; this probably reflects its non-neural or mechanical origin.

Number of Responses (Epochs) Averaged

In certain clinical situations, there is a need to sum or average responses beyond the generally accepted number of about 1000, as when testing small children or other "uncooperative" subjects, when electrodes are not firmly held in place, etc. Such conditions require that we have some notion as to the effects on latency and amplitude to the number of responses (epochs) that exceed 1000. We investigated these factors for a minimum of 256 responses to a maximum of 57,344 (a little over 2 hours of recording time) responses, collected in multiples of 1024 (lk). In this publication, only those data from 1024 to 7168 responses are displayed (Fig. 9-16). We found no significant effects as a function of epochs averaged. There was, however, a tendency at around 8000 responses, to "smooth" the wave IV-V complex so that wave IV was no longer a distinct and separate peak. Whether this observation has any significance (as an electrophysiologic phenomenon) or whether it is an instrumentation problem is unknown. In theory, there is no apparent reason to suspect that the BSER would be electronically altered during a long averaging process, since most signal averagers use digital circuitry (only a few averagers

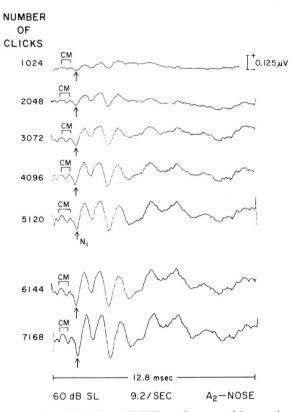

NUMBER
OF
CLICKS

1024   CM $\left[^+_-0.125\,\mu V\right.$

2048   CM

3072   CM

4096   CM

5120   CM N_1

6144   CM

7168   CM

|———————— 12.8 msec ————————|

60 dB SL   9.2/SEC A_2–NOSE

Figure 9-16. CM, AP, and BSER as a function of the number of responses averaged. Clicks (0.1 msec) were presented at 60 dB SL, 9.2/sec repetition rate. As few as 256 responses and as many as 57,344 (not shown above) were averaged in 1K (1024) steps. Electrodes on bony bridge of nose and ipsilateral earlobe. Only two subjects were tested due to the inordinate amount of time needed to complete this task. The X-Y plotter was adjusted for the 1024 condition so as to be able to write out the larger conditions on the same paper (not a true average, but rather, a summation). Positivity of the nose electrode is plotted downward. (From Moore, E. Human Cochlear Microphonics and Auditory Nerve Action Potentials from Surface Electrodes. Unpublished Ph.D. dissertation, University of Wisconsin, Madison, Wisconsin, 1971).

239

still in use utilize capacitative circuits). Practice, however, is less predictable than theory. For example, we have experienced several clinical test situations in which a sleeping patient will suddenly awaken, move abruptly, and "throw points" (data points or addresses of the computer memory) near the end of an average. As a result, certain BSER wave peaks will be shifted by an appreciable latency and/or amplitude factor.

Onset of A/Onset of B

Another time-dependent phenomenon that has been rather extensively used in psychoacoustic experimentation is the temporal masking paradigm (Durrant and Lovrinic, 1977). Temporal masking is a masking effect in which two sounds are not simultaneously presented. If a signal (e.g., signal A) occurs before, say, a masker (e.g., signal B), a backward masking paradigm is operative. On the other hand, if signal A is presented after signal B, a forward masking paradigm is operative. Simultaneous masking occurs if signal A and masker B are on at the same time. There are numerous examples in life in which two stimuli follow one another, for instance, in music where notes played on the same instrument usually appear sequentially in time, yet no masking effects are apparent. Since this phenomena has been extensively investigated by psychoacousticians, it follows that electrophysiologist would replicate certain of these experiments using the BSER (Ananthanarayan and Gerken, personal communication; Brinkmann and Scherg, 1979; Mogensen and Kristensen, 1979).

Ananthanarayan and Gerken (personal communication) recorded the BSER using a tone-on-tone forward-masking paradigm. A masking stimulus of 4000 Hz preceded the 4000 Hz probe stimulus by Δt in msec. All stimulus pairs were monaurally presented (rate: 2/sec) and at an intensity level 60 dB above the masker threshold. The Δt intervals (masker preceding the probe, offset to onset) were 5, 15, 45, and 135 msec. The BSER obtained from one subject are shown in Figure 9-17. Wave V is prolonged in latency when compared to the unmasked condition; this is similar for wave III. A larger wave V latency shift occurred for the simultaneous-masking condition and for the t = 5 and 15 msec forward-masking conditions. Wave V amplitude was greater at the t = 5, 15, and 45 msec conditions, while wave III amplitude was smaller for these values of Δt than in the unmasked condition. Latency shifts decreased monotonically with increasing Δt, and latency for both waves III and V did not return to the unmasked value, even at a Δt of 135 msec, suggesting a forward-masking effect at this longer interval.

Regarding amplitude, wave III exhibited a general reduction in amplitude for the simultaneous-masking condition, and a tendency toward recovery of amplitude values with increasing Δt. Wave V also exhibited a reduction in amplitude for the simultaneous-masking task, but exhibited an increment in amplitude in the forward-masking conditions; thus, wave enhancement was Δt dependent.

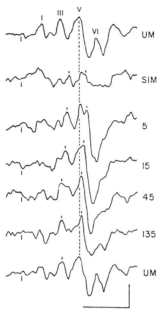

Figure 9-17. Auditory BSERs using a tone-on-tone forward-masking paradigm. A masking stimulus A of 4 KHz preceded the probe stimulus B of 4 KHz by Δt (5, 15, 45, 135 msec). Intensity level presented 60 dB above masker threshold. Waves III and V are prolonged in latency for various Δt. The calibration marker is 5 msec and 0.5 μv. (Reprinted with permission from Ananthanarayan, A. K. and Gerken, G. M. Masking and enhancement. A contrast of processes in the auditory brain-stem response, personal communication.)

A reduction in amplitude and an increase in latency appear to be related to varying durations of neural firing subserving the BSER of interest, and thus, a desynchronization of individual units. These effects are attributed to a peripheral masking effect (Ananthanarayan and Gerkin, personal communication). The enhancement effected noted for wave V, however, was not thought to be peripheral but rather some type of central effect, and, further, that wave V enhancement was not compatible with a forward-masking interpretation. The temporal sequence that resulted in wave V enhancement was compared to the manner in which rapid spectral change affects medial geniculate evoked responses. The investigators note that such an enhancement process could facilitate the analysis and discrimination of sound sequences that occur in speech perception (Ananthanarayan and Gerken, personal communication).

Morgensen and Kristensen (1979) investigated the effects of multiple clicks in MS patients. They presented single and pairs of click stimuli monaurally and binaurally. Waves I, III, V, and FFP7 were evaluated. Interpeak conduction times as well as peak latencies proved fruitful in disclosing abnormalities among the subjects tested. A high percentage (about 83 percent) of BSER abnormalities were revealed using this approach.

Phase of Onset

In the early 1970s, very little attention was paid to the phase-of-onset of the input signal, i.e., whether the stimuli was presented in a condensation or rarefaction phase, and the starting time from zero. In fact, the usual practice was to alternate the polarity of the stimuli so as to eliminate stimulus artifact. Today, with the widespread use of electrostatically/magnetically shielded earphones (first used over 10 years ago (Moore, 1971)), as well as artifact rejection circuitry there is no longer a need to alternate the polarity between condensation and rarefaction stages. This is important since audiogram shape and lesion location can influence the BSER waves when condensation and rarefaction responses are mixed (Coats and Martin, 1977; Ornitz and Walter, 1975; Ornitz, Mo, and Olson, et al., 1980). Figure 9-18 displays these salient features. We would do well to heed the warnings described in Chapters 2 and 10 about these relationships.

EFFECTS OF MASKING

In this section, we review the topic of masking, or the effects of noise on the BSER. We address the question of the possible mechanism(s) responsible for ipsilateral and contralateral masking effects. Latency and amplitude effects

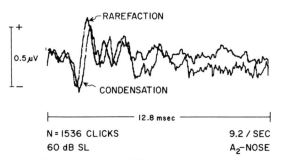

Figure 9-18. Auditory BSER obtained to rarefaction and condensation clicks with initial onset from zero degrees. A total of 1536 clicks (0.1 msec) were presented at 60 dB SL at a repetition rate of 9.2/sec. Electrodes on bony bridge of nose and ipsilateral earlobe. A slight latency shift can be seen for the earlier waves. Positivity of the nose electrode is plotted downward. (From Moore, E. Human Cochlear Microphonics and Auditory Nerve Action Potentials from Surface Electrodes. Doctoral thesis, University of Wisconsin, Madison, Wisconsin, 1971.)

are discussed. Recent data generated in our laboratory are qualitatively and quantitatively presented. But first, we begin with a brief discussion of some relevant psychoacoustic considerations about masking.

Masking is said to occur when one sound makes another sound difficult or impossible to hear, or when the threshold of the signal (the maskee) has been elevated by a second signal or noise (the masker). The phenomenon of masking is a convenient method of study in frequency analysis (Wegel and Lane, 1924); if a signal of known frequency is interfered with by the introduction of another signal, frequency analysis has been altered. With these properties in mind, a strategy was devised in which we investigated the representation of frequency in the BSER. Our experimental paradigm is displayed in Figure 9-19 (Moore and Ananthanarayan, 1978).

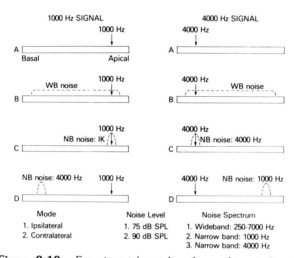

Figure 9-19. Experimental paradigm for masking studies. A. Probe tones of 1000 and 4000 Hz were used to elicit the BSER. Subsequently, the BSER was obtained to either the (B) 1000 or 4000 Hz probe tone in the prescence of a wide-band noise (250 Hz-7 KHz); (C) a narrow-band noise (1000 Hz or 4000 Hz) centered at the probe tone (1000 Hz tone, 1000 Hz noise or 4000 Hz tone, 4000 Hz noise); or (D) away from the probe tone (1000 Hz tone, 4000 Hz noise or 4000 Hz tone, 1000 Hz noise). Presentation of the noise was either ipsilateral or contralateral; intensity of the noise was 75 or 90 dB SPL. The probe tones had a rise-fall time 0.1 msec, an overall duration of 3.0 msec; repetition rate 9.2/sec. Electrodes were placed on the vertex-ipsilateral mastoid. (From Anathanarayan, A. K. Effects of Ipsilateral and Contralateral Noise on Auditory Nerve and Brain Stem Evoked Responses. Unpublished Master's thesis, Memphis State University, 1978.)

The BSER was elicited with probe frequencies of 1000 and 4000 Hz (Fig. 9-19A). Subsequent responses were obtained in the presence of wide-band noise (Fig. 9-19B), at the center frequency of two narrow bands of noise (Fig. 9-19C), or away from the narrow bands of noise (Fig. 9-19D). Note that the paradigm called for the masking noise to be simultaneously presented with the probe stimuli. The mode of presentation for the noise was either ipsilateral or contralateral, and sounds were presented at a SPL of 75 or 90 dB. The noise sources were a 250–8000 Hz wide-band noise (Fig. 9-19B), a 1000 Hz band-limited noise (Fig. 9-19C), or a 4000 Hz band-limited noise (Fig. 9-19D).

Figure 9-20 depicts the analog waveforms to the 1000 Hz probe tone using the ipsilateral mode. In the top panel, a clearly identifiable BSER is present. However, when the wide-band noise was introduced, responses tended to decrease in amplitude and latency was prolonged. At the 90 dB level, only the wave V component is discernable. There are no significant effects on the BSER in the presence of the 1000 Hz narrow band of noise. In contrast, the presence of the 4000 Hz narrow band of noise is seen to

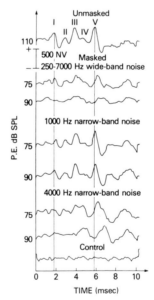

Figure 9-20. Ipsilateral masking condition for 1000 Hz probe tone. (See Fig. 9-19 for a more complete description.) The wide-band noise diminished the amplitude of the BSER and prolonged latency. A similar effect is noted for the 4000 Hz narrow-band noise. Note, however, that the 1000 Hz narrow-band noise exerts no masking effect. (From Anathanarayan, A. K. Effects of Ipsilateral and Contralateral Noise on Auditory Nerve and Brain-Stem Evoked Responses. Unpublished Master's thesis, Memphis State University, 1978.)

diminish BSER amplitude and latency is prolonged, particularly at the 90 dB level. We interpret these data to indicate that the 1000 Hz probe stimulus is mainly evoking activity from a more basal, or high frequency, part of the cochlea, rather than the apical, or low frequency, end. This is apparent from the quantitative data (Figs. 9-21, 9-22). Figure 9-21 shows the latency values; Figure 9-22 shows amplitude values. (We did not calculate values for wave IV since it was often too small and variable.) Note that certain of the Cartesian coordinates do not contain a full complement of data, e.g., wave II for the wide-band noise condition and the 4000 Hz narrow-band noise condition. This is because wave II was not distinguishable for certain of these masking conditions.

In order to understand the behavior of the 4000 Hz probe stimulus, we collected the analog data noted in Figure 9-23. Here again, we see the ubiquitous wave I–V complex (top panel). With the introduction of wide-band noise or the 4000 Hz narrow-band noise, response amplitude decreased, while latency increased. On the other hand, in the presence of the 1000 Hz narrow-band noise, minimal amplitude and latency effects are observed when compared to the wide-band, or 4000 Hz narrow-band, of noise. These observations can be viewed as input-output functions in Figures 9-24 (latency) and 9-25 (amplitude). Our interpretation of these data is that the 4000 Hz stim-

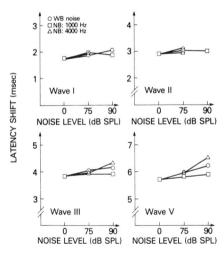

Figure 9-21. Input-output latency functions for the ipsilateral masking condition for the 1000 Hz probe tone. (See Fig. 9-19 for a more complete description.) Latency tends to remain constant for the 1000 Hz narrow-band noise, while the wide-band noise and 4000 Hz narrow-band noise cause shifts in latency. (From Anathanarayan, A. K. Effects of Ipsilateral and Contralateral Noise on Auditory Nerve and Brain-Stem Evoked Responses. Unpublished Master's thesis. Memphis State University, 1978.)

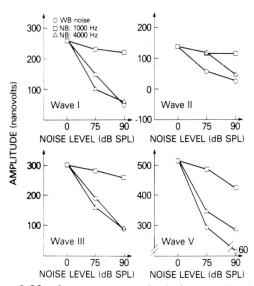

Figure 9-22. Input-output amplitude functions for the ipsilateral masking conditions for 1000 Hz probe tone. (See Fig. 9-19 for a more complete description.) BSER amplitude for the 1000 Hz narrow-band noise decreased, but there are greater effects for the 4000 Hz narrow-band noise and the wide-band noise. (From Anathanarayan, A. K. Effects of Ipsilateral and Contralateral Noise on Auditory Nerve and Brain Stem Evoked Responses. Unpublished Master's thesis, Memphis State University, 1978.)

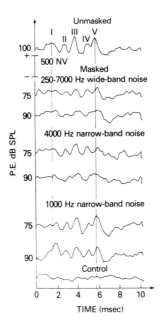

Figure 9-23. Ipsilateral masking condition for the 4000 Hz probe tone. (See Fig. 9-19 for a more complete description.) Latency increased and amplitude decreased for the wide-band noise and the 4000 Hz narrow-band noise. The 1000 Hz narrow-band noise exerts minimal effects. (From Anathanarayan, A. K. Effects of Ipsilateral and Contralateral Noise on Auditory Nerve and Brain Stem Evoked Responses. Unpublished Master's thesis, Memphis State University, 1978.)

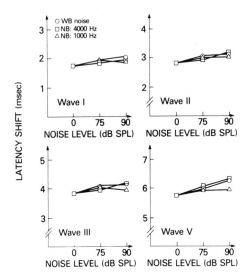

Figure 9-24. Input-output latency function for the ipsilateral masking condition for the 4000 Hz probe tone. (See Fig. 9-19 for a more complete description.) While a small shift in latency is seen for all conditions, the effect is less for the 1000 Hz narrowband noise condition. (From Anathanarayan, A. K. Effects of Ipsilateral and Contralateral Noise on Auditory Nerve and Brain Stem Evoked Responses. Unpublished Master's thesis, Memphis State University, 1978.)

ulus is evoking responses in a more basal direction. Whether the responses are frequency-specific or place-specific is up for argument; we tend to subscribe to the idea that a little bit of both are involved.

You will recall that the experimental paradigm called for placing the various noise sources in the contralateral ear. In viewing the data in Figures 9-26 (1000 Hz stimulus) and 9-27 (4000 Hz stimulus), the series of brainstem components are quite apparent for all masking conditions. We do note perhaps an earlier latency for wave V to the 1000 Hz stimulus, in the presence of the 1000 Hz and the 4000 Hz narrow-band noise. This, however, was not a consistent finding for all subjects. Whether there is some possibility of a potentiating effect (either peripherally or centrally) demands further observation. Ananthanarayan and Gerken (personal communication) subscribe to a central effect.

These masking studies can be summarized by considering possible physiologic mechanisms that might provide for the frequency selectivity, or lack of it, as seen in our masking data. It may be that there is some kind of mechanical tuning involving a filtering process (von Békésy, 1960). The notion that there is some tuning as measured in VIIIth nerve fibers cannot be dismissed (Kiang and Moxon, 1974). Another notion is the so-called lateral

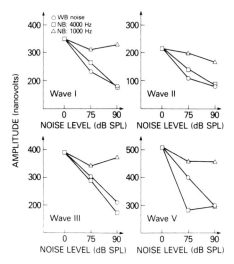

Figure 9-25. Input-output amplitude functions for the ipsi-lateral masking conditions for the 4000 Hz probe tone. (See Fig. 9-19 for a more complete description.) A slight decrease in amplitude is evident for the 1000 Hz narrow-band noise, but a much larger decrease in amplitude is seen for the wide-band noise and the 4000 Hz narrow-band noise. (From Anathanar-ayan, A. K. Effects of Ipsilateral and Contralateral Noise on Auditory Nerve and Brain Stem Evoked Responses. Unpub-lished Master's thesis, Memphis State University, 1978.)

inhibition phenomenon as first seen in the visual system, and with a possible analog in the auditory system (Houtgast, 1972). In a real sense, what seems to emerge is that our data at 500 and 1000 Hz at very high intensity levels are perhaps neither frequency- or place-specific. Data from 2000 Hz and above are probably both frequency- and place-specific. With reasonable assurance, we can infer that at or near threshold, our data is perhaps frequency- and place-specific. The psychophysical stimuli used to evoke the BSER is cor-roborated in the psychophysical tracking experiments (see Fig. 9-7).

Other investigators asking these same questions have used different ex-perimental paradigms. Most notable has been the derived response technique (Don, et al., 1979; Don and Eggermont, 1978; Eggermont and Don, 1980; Parker and Thornton, 1978a; Picton, et al., 1981; Teas, et al., 1962), and the band-reject technique (Picton, et al., 1981). Both techniques have ad-vantages and disadvantages, as does our own. What seems consistent among all three approaches is that similar conclusions have been obtained about fre-quency spread, or lack thereof (see Beagley and Butler, 1981; Fialkowska, Janczenski, and Sulkowski, et al., 1980; Lehnhardt and Battmer, 1979).

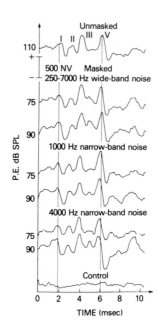

Figure 9-26. Contralateral masking condition for the 1000 Hz probe tone. (See Fig. 9-19 for a more complete description.) Noise conditions tend not to affect the BSER. A few subjects showed a decrease in the latency of wave V for the 4000 Hz narrow-band noise; the effect was not highly consistent. (From Anathanarayan, A. K. Effects of Ipsilateral and Contralateral Noise on Auditory Nerve and Brain Stem Evoked Responses. Unpublished Master's thesis, Memphis State University, 1978.)

DISCUSSION

The BSER is a dependent variable with certain measurable properties. These properties can be specified in precise terms only when the input to the system is well-known. The input, for the most part, is some type of acoustic stimulus generated by a sinusoid or some other periodic (and at times, non-periodic) function. Precision in the measurement of the dependent variable (the BSER) is influenced by a host of independent variables, e.g., intensity, frequency, and several time parameters. We have learned that it would be ideal to maintain a certain amount of precision, since we are concerned with abnormal auditory systems forced out of equilibrium by certain auditory disease processes. To minimize errors in specifying abnormality, the transfer function of the biological system under investigation must have a precisely controlled input, so as to make the most reliable inferences about the condition of the system, based on the output.

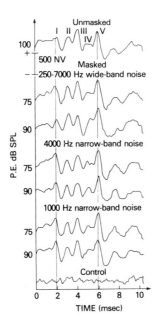

Figure 9-27. Contralateral masking condition for 4000 Hz probe tone. (See Fig. 9-19 for a more complete description.) Noise conditions tend not to affect the BSER. (From Anathanarayan, A. K. Effects of Ipsilateral and Contralateral Noise on Auditory Nerve and Brain Stem Evoked Responses. Unpublished Master's thesis, Memphis State University, 1978.)

These fundamental observations lead us to the consideration of BSERs in clinical practice. The general scheme is that in practical test situations, one will attempt to optimize the protocol by adhering to certain fundamental recording principles. The idea is then to proceed to the task at hand, knowing that these and other intervening variables will manifest themselves, depending on the nature of the test situation and the test material. It is recognized that complete knowledge of the interaction of stimulus parameters does not constitute a "closed book," and, therefore, this chapter is little more than a glimpse of a larger field of view. Mastering other aspects of the basic fundamental processes presented throughout this treatise should assist in widening one's view of the field—the auditory BSER.

III CLINICAL APPLICATIONS

Janet E. Stockard
James J. Stockard

10 Recording and Analyzing

Early studies of the human auditory brain-stem evoked response (BSER) placed little emphasis on recording technique or normal variability. The discussion centered on the predictability of response behavior with changing stimulus variables and on the relative invulnerability of BSER central (interpeak) latencies to stimulus, subject, or recording variables. The complexity of interactions of central and peripheral factors and of subject and recording variables is now apparent, and an understanding of these effects is a prerequisite to any clinical application of the test.

This chapter provides an analysis of these technical factors in "normal" controls and neurologic and otologic patients. Examples of central deficits influencing measures of peripheral auditory function are included, but more of the discussion will deal with the strong dependence of BSER central latencies on peripheral or subject factors and the implications for the neurologic application of the test.

In the adult patient population, neurologic and otologic applications of the BSER require different stimuli; tones or filtered clicks are preferred for the otologic application. To date, little has been published about the BSER using frequency-specific stimuli in infants. Consequently, at present, simultaneous neurologic and otologic screening is conventionally performed in newborns using the same broad-band stimulus. Risk factors for hearing and brain-stem deficits overlap considerably in infants, and the neonatal intensive care unit provides a concentrated population of high-risk patients. Since many laboratories will be called upon to assess both hearing and neurologic status in these patients, discussion of the neonatal BSER will cover both neurologic and otologic applications.

255

PROCEDURE

The analysis of normal BSER variability in this chapter draws from data acquired from 100 normal premature (N = 22) and full-term (N = 78) newborns (64 males and 36 females), and 64 neurologically and audiometrically "normal" adults (30 males and 34 females) aged 18 to 75 years (mean age 29; standard deviation (sd), 10 years).

Bipolar electroencephalogram (EEG) activity recorded between vertex and ear electrodes was amplified 100,000 times and filtered (100 Hz to 3000 Hz, 6 dB down) using Grass Model (Quincy, Massachusetts) P511 J amplifiers. It was analyzed for 10 to 15 msec following stimulus onset, using Grass Model 10 or Nicolet (Madison, Wisconsin) CA1000 signal averagers (10 to 30 µsec sampling interval). Trials (2000 to 8000 samples) were replicated at least once and written out on an X-Y plotter. Latencies were measured with a digital cursor to within 10 to 20 µsec.

Broad-band clicks with peak power at 2000–4000 kHz were generated by passing a 100 µsec square-wave pulse through shielded TDH-39 headphones (Fig. 10-1). Intensity was varied in 10 dB steps from 0 or 30 dB HL to 70 dB HL (re:average normal-hearing subjects' threshold in newborns), and from 0 or 30 dB SL to 70 dB SL (re:subject's click threshold to within one decibel in adults). Contralateral 40 dB HL broad-band masking was used with 70 dB click stimulation. Both rarefaction and condensation clicks (Fig. 10-2) were employed in separate recordings. Rate of click presentation was 10 or 80/sec.

Comparisons of vertex (C_z) to periaural electrodes ipsilateral (A_i) vs contralateral (A_c) to click stimulation and, in some cases, vertex to ipsilateral earlobe or ipsilateral mastoid were made. Ear-to-ear (A_i-A_c) waveforms could

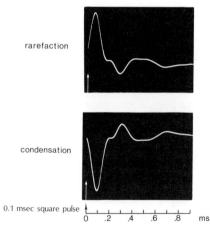

Figure 10-1. Response of TDH-39 earphone to 0.1 msec square wave pulse as displayed on oscilloscope.

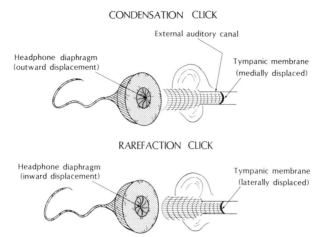

Figure 10-2. Schematic representation of physical properties of rarefaction and condensation clicks, differences in their generation, and effects on tympanic membrane.

be derived by digital subtraction of the averages recorded in the above derivations on the Grass Model 10 system.

STIMULUS VARIABLES

The first vertex positive peak (I) of the BSER, which is the surface reflection of the auditory nerve action potential, provides the necessary reference point from the peripheral auditory pathway for the calculation of central auditory conduction (brain-stem transmission time) time. Results of early BSER studies suggested that the subtraction of wave I latency from that of other components adequately corrected for most peripheral variables. Specifically, it was felt that the BSER behaved much like volume-conducted activity from a relay of generators linked in series, with intensity-related latency shifts in wave I being reflected precisely in later components (Terkildsen, Osterhammel, and Huis in't Veld, 1973; Hecox, and Galambos, 1974). This led to the conclusion that conductive hearing deficits would not influence central (interpeak) latencies; little effort was made to standardize the intensities employed between and within laboratories. Similarly, effects of the initial acoustic phase of the click were felt to be negligible (Terkildsen, Osterhammel, and Huis in't Veld, 1973). This factor often was uncontrolled in human BSER studies. It has since been shown that events at the periphery strongly influence central conduction times as measured by interpeak latencies (Coats, 1978; Rossi, Solero, and Cortesina, 1979; Stockard, Stockard, and Westmoreland, et al., 1979), and that separate interpeak latency (IPL) norms must be applied to each combination of stimulus parameters used.

INTENSITY

Latency Effects

When click intensity is reduced from 70 to 30 dB SL in adults, the magnitude of the latency shift is greatest in wave I and least in wave V. The largest shift usually appears between 50 and 40 dB SL where amplitude dominance is transferred from the first to the second major peak of the VIIIth nerve action potential (AP), causing a sudden jump in latency (Eggermont and Odenthal, 1974a). This jump is not paralleled by the shift in wave V. An abrupt decrease in the I-V IPL occurs at this point, as shown in Figure 10-3. Smaller but significant decreases are also seen in IPLs involving wave I between 70 and 60 dB SL (I-III, $p < 0.02$), 60 and 50 dB SL (I-III, $p < 0.02$; I-V, $p < 0.001$), and 40 and 30 dB SL (I-V, $p < 0.01$). Significant IPL alterations are also seen in newborns. Figure 10-4 illustrates the effect in a normal premature infant. These small, progressive decreases probably reflect, in part, the greater effects of traveling wave delay on wave I than on later components, which appear to have contributions from a more extensive length of the cochlear partition than wave I (Terkildsen, Osterhammel, and Huis in't Veld, 1975a, 1975b). Figure 10-5 summarizes the non-linear latency shifts for the major components in response to 10 decibel changes in stimulus intensity from 70 to 30 dB SL in adults.

Latency-intensity functions are covered in Chapters 11 and 12, but it is noteworthy that the 0.28 msec (sd 0.07) latency shift in wave V/10 dB intensity change found in adults in this study, although in agreement with Pratt and

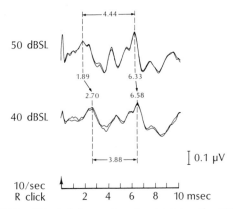

Figure 10-3.   Effect of decreasing stimulus intensity at "transitional" intensity zone (male, age 25). The jump in wave I latency caused by the transfer of amplitude dominance from the first to the second peak of the auditory nerve potential is not paralleled by the shift in wave V latency. The I-V IPL is altered by the differential effect of intensity on the two components.

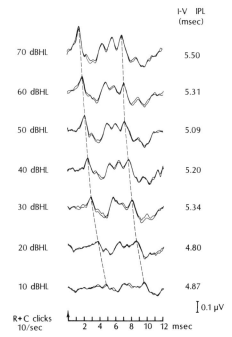

Figure 10-4. Intensity-related alteration of the I-V interpeak latency (IPL) in a normal premature newborn (male, 34 weeks gestation, age 15 days). IPL intensity effects are more variable in newborns than adults.

Sohmer (1976), is well below the 0.4 msec cited by Galambos and Hecox (1978). These authors state that a latency-intensity slope of less than 30 μsec/dB "virtually ensures" a high-frequency hearing deficit. Figure 10-6 demonstrates such a "shallow" wave V latency-intensity function in an audiometrically and neurologically normal subject. The discrepancy is probably mainly due to the lower intensity range (10 to 60 dB SL) used by these authors (Hecox and Galambos, 1974), as compared to our 30 to 70 dB SL range, since the largest shifts are seen near threshold. As can be seen in Figure 10-5, the degree of wave V shift varies greatly among intensity ranges but approaches 0.4 msec/dB only at the lower intensities. The conclusions to be drawn from this are that, when latency-intensity norms are applied, they must be specific for the intensity range tested and the portion of that range under consideration. Non-linearity of latency-intensity functions makes "slope" alone an unreliable measure.

It is of interest that the intensity-related shortening of interpeak latency (described earlier) cannot be duplicated by effective lowering of click intensity with the introduction of white noise masking, presented ipsilateral to click stimulation. When the masking noise and broad-band clicks are presented

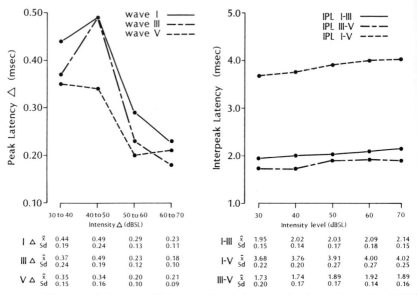

I △	$\bar{x}$	0.44	0.49	0.29	0.23	I-III	$\bar{x}$	1.95	2.02	2.03	2.09	2.14
	Sd	0.19	0.24	0.13	0.11		Sd	0.15	0.14	0.17	0.18	0.15
III △	$\bar{x}$	0.37	0.49	0.23	0.18	I-V	$\bar{x}$	3.68	3.76	3.91	4.00	4.02
	Sd	0.24	0.19	0.12	0.10		Sd	0.22	0.20	0.27	0.27	0.25
V △	$\bar{x}$	0.35	0.34	0.20	0.21	III-V	$\bar{x}$	1.73	1.74	1.89	1.92	1.89
	Sd	0.15	0.16	0.10	0.09		Sd	0.20	0.17	0.17	0.14	0.16

Figure 10-5. Left. Degree of latency shift/10 dB intensity change for major BSER components in different portions of the 30 to 70 dB SL intensity range in adults. Right. IPL intensity function. (Reprinted with permission from Stockard, J. E., Stockard, J. J., Westmoreland, B. F., et al. Brainstem auditory evoked responses. Archives of Neurology, 1979, 36:823-831.)

through the same TDH-39 earphone, wave I latency is unaltered; later components are prolonged, causing an *increase* in the IPLs involving wave I, as shown in Figure 10-7. The resistance of wave I latency to ipsilateral masking noise in this experiment is consistent with the findings of Kiang, Watanabe, and Thomas, et al., (1965) in single-fiber auditory nerve recordings. The differential effect of competing noise on the early and later BSER components was reported in Chapter 9. These dramatic alterations of IPL further demonstrate both the sensitivity of central latencies to peripheral factors and the importance of controlling ambient noise when feasible, since the latter can, like masking noise, differentially alter latencies of various BSER components.

Amplitude Effects

The amplitude of the IV-V complex[1] is also less affected by stimulus intensity than are earlier components (Terkildsen, Osterhammel, and Huis in't Veld, 1973; Pratt and Sohmer, 1976). The change in mean amplitude from 0.49 µV at 70 dB SL to 0.28 µV at 30 dB SL in adults represents an

---

[1]Measured from the most vertex-positive peak, whether wave IV or V, to the negative trough following wave V.

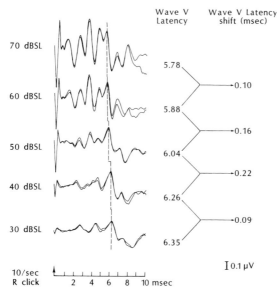

Figure 10-6. Intensity series in a normal adult subject (female, age 23). Over the 30 to 70 dB SL intensity range, wave V intensity-related latency shifts remain below 25 μsec/dB (mean shift = 14 μsec/dB) in this subject. Wave I shifts an average of 33 μsec/dB. The 40 dB change in stimulus intensity resulted in a 0.73 msec change in the I-V IPL in this subject. Note that wave I amplitude is greatly reduced at 50 dB SL as compared with all other intensities.

average 41 percent reduction in amplitude over the 40 dB range. Wave I amplitude over the same range is reduced by 81 percent. The most abrupt change in amplitude is seen between 60 and 70 dB, where wave I doubles in amplitude in both newborns and adults. In many individuals, wave I amplitude is lower at the "transitional" intensity (usually 45-55 dB SL) than at 30 dB SL (Fig. 10-6). Routinely employed intensities should be well above the "transitional" region in order to avoid the large shifts seen in both amplitude and latency.

It is clear that stimulus intensity requires careful control in clinical studies when either peak or interpeak latencies are compared to normative data. Use of sensation level (SL) rather than hearing level (HL) intensities will correct for relatively flat conductive losses when the subject's threshold can be determined. This is not possible in infants and, when larger interaural differences in wave I latency are encountered, asymmetries of interpeak latency may result (Fig. 10-8) or may be enhanced (Fig. 10-9). Interaural IPL differences cannot be attributed to central conduction delays when there is significant asymmetry of wave I latency, since the I-V IPL may vary by as much as 0.7 msec over a 40

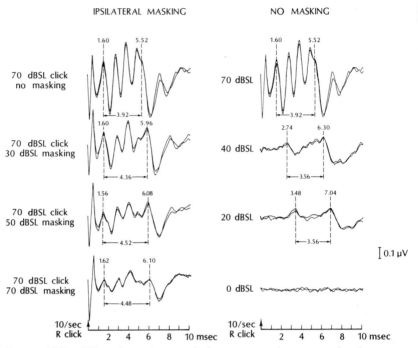

Figure 10-7. Effect of introduction of white-noise-masking to stimulated ear as compared with simple reduction of stimulus intensity (no masking) (female, age 24). The latter has a greater effect on wave I than on wave V, resulting in a decrease in the IPLs involving wave I. Simultaneous white-noise-masking at progressively higher intensity levels competing with the click, on the other hand, has a greater effect on later BSER components than on wave I, resulting in *increases* in IPLs involving wave I.

dB range of intensity. In certain adults, on the other hand, in whom integrity of the peripheral auditory apparatus can be established by conventional audiometry, the close inter-ear symmetry of IPLs (Fig. 10-10) can be used to increase the sensitivity of the test. In normal-hearing patients, for example, interaural asymmetries in I–V IPL of 0.5 msec or greater are abnormal, whether or not the IPLs considered separately from each ear are normal (Fig. 10-11).

REPETITION RATE

The effects of increasing stimulus rate on wave V latency and IPLs of the BSER is widely appreciated (Pratt and Sohmer, 1976; Zollner, Karnahl, and Stange, 1976; Don, Allen, and Starr, 1977; Rowe, 1978). These effects are enhanced by immaturity, as evidenced by the greater shifts seen in newborns as compared to adults (Stockard, Stockard, and Westmoreland, et al.,

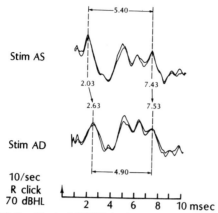

Figure 10-8. Typical BSER finding in small, premature infants of asymmetric wave I latency and I-V IPL asymmetry, probably both resulting from mild conductive hearing deficit AD (female, 29 weeks gestation, age 5 weeks). Contralateral 50 dB HL masking was used. Normal child on 8-month follow-up.

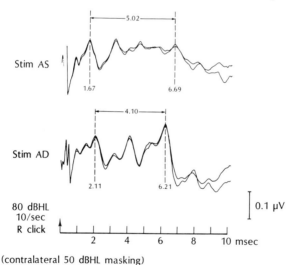

(contralateral 50 dBHL masking)

Figure 10-9. Prolonged wave I latency with stimulation AD in this patient prevents valid assessment of central conduction from that ear (male, age 18 months). I-V IPL with stimulation AS is prolonged. Since wave V latency with stimulation AD as compared with AS is *shorter*, while wave I AD as compared with AS latency is *longer*, the 0.92 msec I-V IPL asymmetry is attributable to both central and peripheral factors.

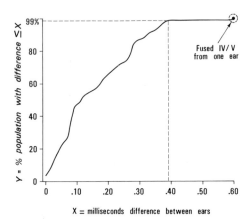

Figure 10-10. Cumulative frequency distribution of inter-aural I-V IPL differences in 100 neurologically and audio-metrically normal subjects. Note that 99 percent of normal subjects have interaural I-V IPL difference of less than 0.4 msec. The subject with a higher value had a fused IV-V complex in the BSER from one ear and discrete waves IV and V from the other ear, yielding a spuriously high inter-ear asymmetry (I-V IPL vs I-IV-V IPL); this emphasizes the importance of proper component identification in such assessments of interaural IPL symmetry.

1979). Rate effects have reportedly been enhanced by advanced age (Fugi-kawa and Weber, 1977).

There are striking inconsistencies in adult studies regarding the effect of rate on wave I latency (Yagi and Kaga, 1979; Pratt and Sohmer, 1976). The disagreement might be attributed to the different intensity levels and acoustic phases employed by investigators, since both variables interact with stimulus rate. In five normal adults we studied, rate effects on wave I latency were much greater when a 50 dB SL click (as compared to a 70 dB SL click) was used (Fig. 10-12). This probably reflects the fragility of the balance between action potential (AP) peak dominance in this intensity range, and the differential sensitivity of the two major AP peaks to stimulus rate (Eggermont and Odenthal, 1974a). Figure 10-13 demonstrates the instability of wave I latency at the "transitional" intensity. In this case, the I-V IPL actually decreased with 80/sec stimulation, because of the large jump in wave I latency with transfer of peak dominance. Note that wave V rate-related shifts are equivalent at the two intensities in Figure 10-12. Since wave I shifts, on the other hand, are highly dependent on intensity, rate-related IPL changes are difficult to predict.

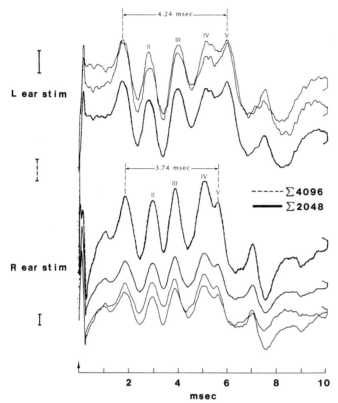

Figure 10-11. Abnormal interaural asymmetry of I-V IPL (0.5 msec) in audio-metrically normal subject despite normality of IPLs from each ear when considered separately (female, age 26, history of right visual blurring, no brain stem signs). Inter-ear asymmetry of IPLs, in addition to case history suggestive of optic neuritis, helped to established early diagnosis of multiple sclerosis in this patient, who was asymptomatic at the time of testing, but subsequently proved to have demyelinating disease.

ACOUSTIC POLARITY (PHASE)

It has been shown that the first firing of the auditory nerve coincides with movement of the basilar membrane toward the scala vestibuli, which corresponds to the rarefaction phase of the acoustic stimulus and lateral displacement (Fig. 10-1) of the tympanic membrane (Kiang, Watanabe, and Thomas, et al., 1965). This fact alone would predict a wave I latency delay of one-half the cycle of the stimulus to condensation (C), as compared to rarefaction (R), stimuli. It was initially suggested that, when brief click stimuli are employed, this factor is insignificant (Terkildsen, Osterhammel, and Huis in't Veld, 1973); however, more recent studies have demonstrated large C-R differ-

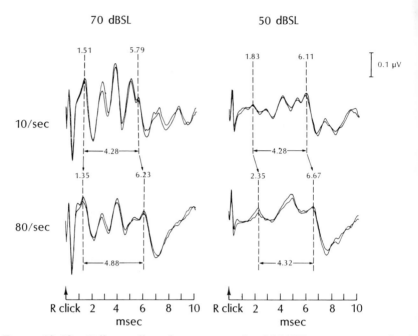

Figure 10-12. Differing effect of rate on wave I and I–V IPL at two intensity levels with R click stimulation (female, age 33). At 50 dB SL ("transitional" intensity zone), wave I latency increased with higher rate, while at 70 dB SL, wave I latency decreased with increased rate. In contrast, rate effect on wave V is approximately equal at the two intensities. The differential effect of rate and intensity on components I and V results in a change in the magnitude of the rate effect on the I–V IPL with stimulus intensity.

ences for both peak (Ornitz and Walter, 1975; Coats and Martin, 1977) and interpeak (Stockard, Stockard, and Westmoreland, et al., 1979) latencies.

Of the major BSER components, only wave I latency was affected by acoustic phase in our normal subjects. Since this latency is shorter in response to R clicks than to C clicks while waves III and V are usually unaffected, IPLs involving wave I are also influenced by phase. Table 10-1 summarizes the effects of phase on peak and interpeak latencies of the BSER. In some individuals, BSER vertex-positive peaks II–IV may also be altered by phase, in either direction. This is particularly true in infants (Stockard, Stockard, and Westmoreland, et al., 1979) and children (Ornitz and Walter, 1975), as illustrated in Figure 10-14. The magnitude of C-R wave I differences is also greater in newborns, resulting in rather large IPL C-R differences (Fig. 10-15).

At 70 dB SL in adults, preditable morphologic changes occur with inversion of stimulus phase. Wave V amplitude was increased in 73 percent of our normal controls by the use of condensation clicks. With rarefaction stimuli, the amplitude of waves I and IV were usually enhanced. In most cases, at 70 dB SL, the first six BSER waves can be clearly resolved when both R and C

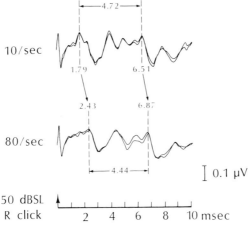

10/sec

80/sec

⊥ 0.1 µV

50 dBSL
R click   2   4   6   8   10 msec

Figure 10-13. Seven-year-old child with brain-stem tumor (female, age 7). At 50 dB SL (R click), increased rate caused a dramatic latency shift in the double-peaked wave I as dominance shifted from the first to the second peak. Since the rate effect is greater on wave I than on wave V at this intensity, the I-V IPL actually *decreased* with the higher rate. This was not the case at 70 dB SL (not shown), where wave I was relatively unaffected by the high rate.

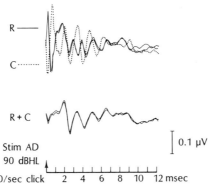

R ——

C ·······

R + C

Stim AD   ⊥ 0.1 µV
90 dBHL
10/sec click   2   4   6   8   10   12 msec

Figure 10-14. Five-year-old child with pontine glioma and bilateral otitis media (no sensori-neural deficit) (female, age 5). Rarefaction (solid line) vs condensation (dashed line) responses show the large out-of-phase component for all waves often seen in young children. It is rare, however, for wave V latency to show a significant phase difference.

267

Table 10-1

Effect of Acoustic Phase on BSER Peak and Interpeak Latencies

	I		II		III		IV		V		VI		V_N*		I-III		I-V		III-V	
	C	R	C	R	C	R	C	R	C	R	C	R	C	R	C	R	C	R	C	R
Adult x̄	1.69	1.62	2.78	2.80	3.77	3.75	4.92	4.89	5.64	5.62	7.26	7.14	6.35	6.26	2.08	2.13	3.95	4.02	1.92	1.94
sd	0.19	0.12	0.19	0.19	0.20	0.17	0.25	0.23	0.25	0.23	0.36	0.29	0.31	0.25	0.20	0.15	0.26	0.24	0.37	0.38
t	4.31		0.57		0.88		0.57		0.98		2.68		2.83		1.99		2.70		0.62	
df	46		27		46		24		37		30		30		41		35		35	
p	0.001		0.50		0.30		0.50		0.30		0.02		0.01		0.10		0.02		0.50	
Newborn x̄	1.94	1.81	3.15	3.11	4.66	4.62	5.78	5.73	6.71	6.72	8.31	8.20	7.61	7.60	2.72	2.80	4.79	4.92	2.08	2.13
sd	0.25	0.22	0.40	0.28	0.25	0.29	0.41	0.35	0.27	0.32	0.33	0.43	0.34	0.39	0.17	0.21	0.30	0.26	0.24	0.23
t	4.01		0.49		1.11		0.86		0.55		2.40		0.45		2.80		3.46		1.39	
df	54		32		52		18		49		31		52		53		50		48	
p	0.001		0.60		0.20		0.40		0.50		0.02		0.60		0.01		0.005		0.20	

*V_N is the vertex negative trough following wave V.

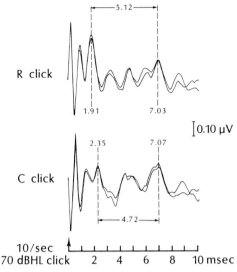

Figure 10-15. Rarefaction (R) and condensation (C) responses in this normal, premature infant show typically large out-of-phase component, particularly in wave I (male, 35 weeks gestation, age 9 days). I-V IPL in C response is reduced when compared with R response.

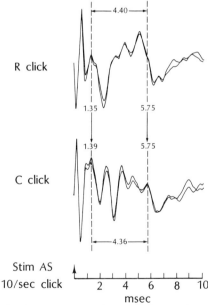

Figure 10-16. Exaggerated morphologic phase effect on waves IV and V in a normal subject (female, age 51). Wave V is enhanced by the use of condensation clicks.

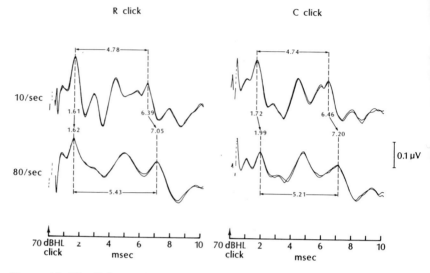

Figure 10-17. Differential effect of rate on R vs C wave I latency and resulting IPL interaction of rate with phase in a normal newborn subject; this interaction is also seen in adult subjects (full-term female, age 1 day).

clicks are used in separate recordings. Figure 10-16 shows an exaggerated morphologic phase effect in a normal-hearing subject.

As mentioned above, stimulus phase also influences the magnitude of the rate effect on wave I latency (and on IPLs involving that component). At 70 dB SL, wave I latency is either unaltered or decreased by high rates of R click presentation. In contrast, 80/sec C clicks always produce a longer wave I latency, in comparison to 10/sec C click stimulation (Fig. 10-17). The result is a significantly ($p < 0.001$) greater I-III and I-V IPL rate-related change for R clicks than for C clicks. Since phase differences are large in children and at high rates of stimulus presentation, summation of R and C responses should be avoided when possible in these cases. Cann and Knott (1979) have outlined reliable methods for determining the acoustic polarity of the click at the output of any earphone.

EFFECTS OF SUBJECT VARIABLES

Age

Maturational changes in central conduction time have repeatedly been demonstrated (Hecox, 1975; Salamy, McKean, and Buda, 1975; Starr, Amlie, and Martin, 1977; Stockard, Stockard, and Westmoreland, et al., 1979). In our subjects, the major change occurred in the I-III IPL, which averaged 2.77 msec (sd 0.23) in the newborn, as compared to 2.13 msec (sd

Table 10-2

Infant Normative Data Peak and Interpeak Latencies

Author	Age	Intensity	Rate	Phase		I	V	I-III	I-V	III-V
Stockard, Stockard, and Westmoreland, et al., 1979	Newborn	70 dB HL	10/sec	R	x̄	1.81	6.72	2.77	4.90	2.15
					sd	0.22	0.32	0.23	0.28	0.23
					N	54	49	63	60	59
Salamy, McKean, and Pettett, et al., 1978	Newborn	55 dB HL	10/sec	R+C	x̄	2.12	7.11		4.99	
					sd	0.36	0.28		0.31	
					N	15	15		15	
	6 weeks	55 dB HL	10/sec	R+C	x̄	1.63	6.55		4.92	
					sd	0.18	0.21		0.28	
					N	20	20		20	
	3 months	55 dB HL	10/sec	R+C	x̄	1.71	6.44		4.73	
					sd	0.38	0.33		0.12	
					N	12	12		12	
	6 months	55 dB HL	10/sec	R+C	x̄	1.69	6.24		4.55	
					sd	0.20	0.25		0.15	
					N	10	10		10	
	3 years	55 dB HL	10/sec	R+C	x̄	1.68	5.99		4.18	
					sd	0.20	0.64		0.43	
					N	8	8		8	

0.15) in the adult. Interpeak latencies have been shown to attain adult values by 1 to 3 years of age (Salamy and McKean, 1976; Ochs and Markand, 1978). Maturational peak and interpeak latency changes as reported by Salamy, McKean, and Pettett, et al., (1978) are shown in Table 10-2 along with our norms for full-term newborns.

Jerger and Hall (1980) studied the effects of aging on wave V latency in gender-matched and audiometrically normal adults. They found a 0.2 msec increase from 25 to 55 years of age. Interpeak latencies were not analyzed in the above study. Although Rowe (1978) demonstrated an increase in IPLs with advanced age, groups were not matched for gender or hearing. Rosenhamer, Lindström, and Lundborg (1980) failed to detect any effect of advanced age interpeak latencies. This has also been our experience (p > 0.5, t test) for young vs old adults with respect to mean latency values. Unfortunately, while our older adults were audiometrically normal, we were unable to exactly match audiograms in the two groups—our older subjects showing 5-15 dB higher thresholds at 4000-8000 Hz. Thus, the effects of advancing age per se on BSER latency, if any, remain obscure; any age-related IPL increases could have been offset by slight audiogram-related (mild high-frequency hearing loss) decreases in IPL. Although the mean I-V IPL values for the two groups are similar, the larger standard deviation in the older group (0.28 msec) increases the upper limit of normal.

Gender

Peak latencies and I-V IPLs are significantly longer in males than in females (Stockard, Stockard, and Sharbrough, 1978; McClelland and Mc-Crea, 1979; Rosenhamer, Lindström, and Lundborg, 1980). Possible gender differences were ignored in almost all early BSER studies; normal control populations generally tended to be dominated by young females. The shorter mean values and smaller standard deviations in this population resulted in spuriously low upper limits of normal in some clinical studies. Differences in sex ratio may account for the large differences in upper limit of normal values from lab to lab. Sex differences in interpeak latency were not seen in our newborn group (p > 0.3).

Audiogram

While flat conductive hearing losses are easily corrected for in adults by the routine use of sensation level rather than hearing level or sound pressure level, the effects of sensorineural deficits on BSER amplitude, peak, and interpeak latencies cannot be controlled when broad-band clicks are applied (as is convenient to do in the neurologic application of the test). Shortening of the I-V IPL in this population at a given intensity level (because of the greater effect of the deficit on wave I than on later components) has been reported

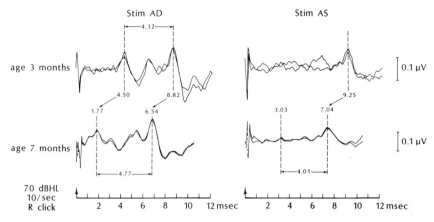

Figure 10-18. Premature infant with birth asphyxia, chronic otitis media AD and high-frequency hearing loss AS (male, 28 weeks gestation). Left. At age 3 months, wave I grossly prolonged. Short I-V IPL probably due to confirmed otitis media (and reduced effective intensity of stimulus). Right. Age 3 months (41 weeks conceptional age), wave I absent AS and wave V prolonged. At 7 months, small, prolonged wave I present with less marked prolongation wave V latency. Short I-V IPL probably due to sensorineural hearing deficit. At age 7 months, the otitis media resolved and wave I latency normalized. I-V IPL was found within normal limits for conceptional age. Interaural asymmetry of I-V IPL at 7 months is artifact of reduced hearing AS. Contralateral 50 dB HL masking was used.

(Coats and Martin, 1977). An example is shown in Figure 10-18. Furthermore, the intensity-related decrements in IPLs involving wave I may be enhanced by the deficit (Coats, 1978).

Peak latency (and IPL) *phase* differences may also be enhanced in persons with sensory hearing deficits. Since high sound pressure levels must be used in these patients for clear wave I resolution, stimulus phase is often alternated during sampling to cancel stimulus artifact. This may result in cancellation of wave I and other components when the C-R out-of-phase component is large. In these cases, it may be necessary to conduct a single-phase click (using tubing) in order to introduce a delay between the stimulus artifact and wave I.

Temperature

In most patients, core temperature is of little concern; however, when large fluctuations are likely to occur, as in newborns and comatose adults, temperature should always be measured prior to testing. Central temperature reductions below 35°C, as commonly occur in obtunded or severely intoxicated patients, are likely to result in spurious hypothermia-related prolongations of IPL which mimic the BSER effects of structural brain-stem lesions (Stockard, Sharbrough, and Tinker, 1978).

EFFECTS OF RECORDING PARAMETERS

Recording Derivation

In a study by Hashimoto, Ishiyama, and Tozoka, et al., (1979), use of vertex-to-periaural electrodes contralateral to click stimulation was proposed to uncover abnormalities of interpeak latency which were not seen in the routine vertex-to-ipsilateral-ear derivation. These authors failed to consider, however, the normal increase in interpeak latency in this recording derivation as compared to the standard recordings referenced to the stimulated ear (Stockard, Stockard, and Westmoreland, et al., 1979). While wave I (and $I_N{}^2$) latencies are slightly altered between these derivations, wave V is significantly prolonged, resulting in a mean difference in the I_N-V IPL of 0.11 msec ($p < 0.01$).

Predictable morphologic changes related to these recording derivations are useful for proper identification of BSER components in clinical studies (Stockard, Stockard, and Sharbrough, 1978). While waves I and III are reduced in amplitude in contralateral recordings, waves I_N and II amplitudes are relatively unaffected. Waves II and III often merge into a single component, and the IV-V IPL is increased. In most studies, proper identification of all components is assured by simultaneous recordings in these two derivations.

In our comparison of vertex-to-mastoid and vertex-to-earlobe derivations, wave I amplitude was highest in the latter, indicating that the earlobe is the better "reference" site for purposes of resolving wave I.

High- and Low-Frequency Filter Settings

Although interpeak latencies are relatively unaffected by filter settings, absolute latencies and amplitudes, as well as relative amplitudes, highly depend on both high- and low-frequency filtering. Absolute latencies and amplitudes decrease with increases in low-frequency cut-off and with decreases in high-frequency cut-off. Relative amplitudes of BSER components are altered, since amplitude alterations (due to filtering) are dependent on the rise time and duration of the component; these vary among component (see Chapter 6).

HEARING SCREENING IN NEWBORN INFANTS

Hearing screening programs in newborn infants using various physiologic and behavioral observation techniques have met with little success in the past because of the subjective nature of response interpretation. The BSER offers the first objective means of assessing peripheral auditory function, which is unaffected by level of arousal or attention (Amadeo and Shagass,

---

[2]Vertex-negative trough following wave I.

1973). The technique has been assessed by several laboratories (Chisin, Perlman, and Sohmer, 1979; Finitzo-Hieber, Hecox, and Cone, 1979; Galambos and Hecox, 1978; Montadon, Cao, and Engel, et al., 1979), and has been proven to be useful. In our experience, the BSER is useful as a screening tool only when stimulation parameters are carefully controlled and serial studies are obtained in cases of abnormal response. Even under optimal technical conditions, BSER findings consistent with deafness or hearing loss can occasionally be seen in infants who prove, on conventional audiometric testing and clinical follow-up, to have normal hearing.

In our estimation, the validity of the various BSER criteria upon which otologic diagnoses are made has yet to be demonstrated in newborns. Demonstration of the prognostic value of BSERs in this age group inevitably requires relatively long-term follow-up of a large patient population, such capabilities as have only recently become available to prove the clinical utility of the test in adult neurology. The BSER measures upon which otoneurologic applications in newborns must tentatively be based are reviewed below.

Peak Latencies

Wave V is the most commonly used component in both newborns and adults in peak latency criteria for otologic diagnosis. Montandon, Cao, and Engel, et al. (1979) advocate the use of both AP and wave V latencies for hearing assessment in newborns. We have also found use of the surface-recorded AP (wave I) latency, together with wave V latency, a practical and effective approach to screening. Wave I latency (as compared to wave V latency) is a more precise and sensitive index of middle- (Mendelson, Salamy, and Lenoir, et al., 1979) and inner- (Coats and Martin, 1977) ear function; it is less affected by abnormalities of central auditory conduction which may not involve hearing acuity.

Of the 19 infants in our series with prolongations of wave V latency but normal wave I latency, none has shown any evidence of decreased hearing sensitivity on follow-up at 10 to 22 months of age. Maturational changes are also greater in wave V than wave I latency, leading to greater chance of error in interpretation when this component is measured alone.

The main advantage of using wave V latency is its ease of resolution at low intensities; however, we have found wave I quite easy to obtain at moderate intensities when 10/sec single polarity clicks are employed.

Latency–Intensity (L–I) Functions

Most laboratories measure wave V latency at more than one intensity so that the slope of latency change related to stimulus intensity can be plotted and compared to the normal curve. Our L–I function data, while similar to those of Schulman-Galambos and Galambos (1975), are at odds with Hecox (1975), who found a more shallow wave V slope in newborns (28 μsec/dB) than adults (44 μsec/dB). We found the opposite, with newborns showing an average shift over the 40 decibel range of 36 μsec/dB (sd 7) as compared to 28 μsec/dB (sd 7) in our adults. Only four of the newborn subjects showed a slope of less than 30 μsec. This discrepancy might be explained by the smaller range of intensities at which Hecox found a measurable wave V peak in newborns, since the largest shifts occur at the lowest intensities.

Figures 10-19 and 10-20 demonstrate the variability in the magnitude of intensity-related latency shifts in newborns at the levels tested. Because the degree of shift is not stable over the 40 decibel range, L-I functions plotted over small intensity ranges are of little clinical value. Unfortunately, in newborns with sensorineural deficits and in some with conductive deficits, wave V cannot be recorded over a wide intensity range (at safe levels). Of the eight infants in our series with sensorineural deficits (confirmed later), BSERs were absent in three and, in five, consisted of one or two small potentials with 70-85 dB HL stimulation only. Because of the paucity of information regarding the relative vulnerability of the newborn cochlea to noise exposure, use of higher intensities was not considered advisable.

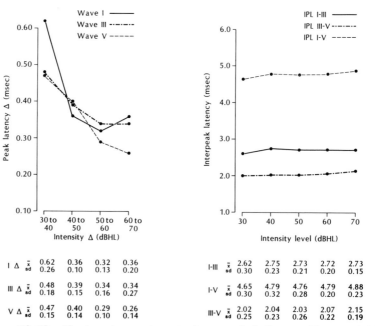

Figure 10-19. Newborn latency-intensity function. Left. Degree of latency shift/10 dB intensity change for major BSER components in different portions of the 30 to 70 dB SL intensity range in normal, full-term newborns. Right. IPL intensity function.

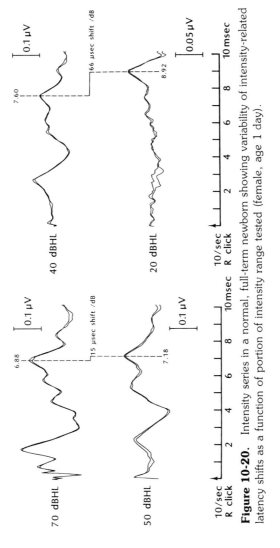

Figure 10-20. Intensity series in a normal, full-term newborn showing variability of intensity-related latency shifts as a function of portion of intensity range tested (female, age 1 day).

277

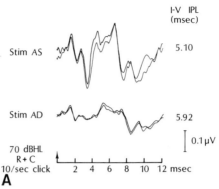

Figure 10-21. Asphyxia seizures (full-term female). A. Initial BSERs on asphyxiated newborn showed normal IPLs with stimulation AS but prolonged I-III and I-V IPL with AD stimulation (age 2 days). B. Intensity series were performed at ages 9 days, 9 months, and 21 months. Early studies revealed normal BSER latencies and threshold with AS stimulation but an elevated BSER threshold and a steep amplitude-latency (A-I) function with stimulation AD. At 21 months, AS response threshold normalized, but the A-I function was still steep when compared with AD responses. Audiometric examination (monaural visual reinforcement audiometry) at 21 months revealed normal behavioral thresholds. In the latter examination, pure tones were delivered through earphones; thresholds in either ear, at 500 Hz, 1000 Hz, 2000 Hz, 4000 Hz, and 6000 Hz, were below 30 dB HL. Test reliability was excellent. At 2 years, the child is microcephalic and has delayed motor development, but is developing speech and is alert and responsive. Contralateral 40 dB HL masking was used in BSER studies.

Amplitude

The most nebulous BSER abnormalities are those of amplitude reduction. Responses may be unrecordable at moderate intensities in normal infants before 28 to 31 weeks of conception (Starr, Amlie, and Martin, et al., 1977; Krumholz, Goldstein, and Felix, et al., 1978; Galambos and Hecox, 1978). Thereafter, response amplitudes approach adult values, but at a slower rate than response latencies. Relative amplitudes (amplitude ratios), which in adults provide a "hedge" against the high degree of normal amplitude variability, are of little clinical value in newborns since maturational changes in amplitude proceed at different rates for the various components and head size changes rapidly at this age, altering the distance between the periaural electrode and the auditory nerve.

We have seen markedly attenuated responses of normal latency (including wave I) in serial studies in a neurologically and audiometrically normal infant, but in 11 other cases, severely reduced amplitudes in repeated studies were associated with a poor neurologic or otologic outcome.

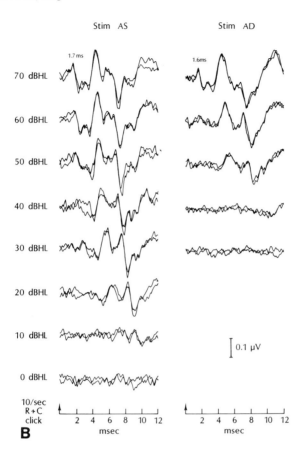

A–I Function and Threshold Measurement

A further refinement of the screening technique involves the plotting of BSER wave IV-V or I amplitude against stimulus intensity, either to establish the threshold of a recordable response or to detect the abnormally steep rises in amplitude associated with recruitment (Odenthal and Eggermont, 1974).

In newborns, wave I shows an average amplitude reduction of 66 percent when intensity is decreased from 70 to 30 dB HL, while wave IV-V is only reduced by 33 percent. We have seen elevated BSER threshold and very steep A-I functions, supposedly characteristic of recruitment, in an infant with normal hearing but with neurologic sequelae of birth asphyxia (Fig. 10-21).

Threshold determination in cases of conductive loss can provide crucial information, as demonstrated by the case illustrated in Figure 10-22. Presence of a response at 50 dB HL on stimulation of an ear with congenital atresia of the external meatus confirmed the presence of a functional inner ear. The normal response with stimulation of the other ear suggested normal hearing in that ear. Finitzo-Hieber, Hecox, and Cone (1979) also report excellent

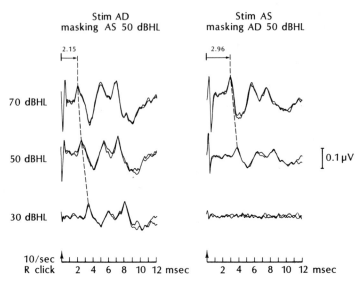

Figure 10-22. Goldenhar's syndrome. Intensity series in a newborn with atresia, left (full-term female, age 4 days). High amplitude wave I at 70 dB HL, normal latency-intensity function, and minimal threshold elevation with stimulation AS primarily suggest conductive deficit and presence of a functional inner ear.

results in the application of the BSER in this type of patient. Bone-conduction of acoustic stimuli has potentially important clinical neuro-otologic applications in cases where middle-ear function is either impaired or questionable (Moore and Harris, 1982).

Absence of Response

Although the total absence of BSERs (including wave I) would seem to be a certain indication of either severe functional or structural abnormality of the peripheral auditory apparatus or VIIIth nerve, there were some surprising clinical correlations with this BSER finding in our series. In 7 of our 10 patients with absent BSERs in the newborn period, clinical or pathologic evidence of either peripheral auditory impairment or irreversible brain-stem damage was present. Three of the infants had sensorineural deficits, confirmed later, and four either expired of birth injuries shortly after the BSERs were performed or developed a response in later recordings. However, in three patients in the group, hearing was found to be normal (to the extent that it could be assessed by conventional audiometry at their present age), despite the absence of BSERs.

These latter three infants (at this writing, ages 12, 21, and 24 months), showed low behavioral thresholds at all frequency ranges with excellent test reliability on serial standard audiometric examinations. Results of the audiometric evaluation of the 12-month-old child must be considered tentative because of the limitations of the examination in this age group. BSERs were performed on the three infants at least three times over the first 6 to 10 months of life. All three infants have neurologic sequelae of birth injuries with signs of brain-stem dysfunction, as in the cases illustrated in Figures 10-23 and 10-24. In two of the three infants, the initial study (performed in the newborn period) showed a small early neural component that disappeared in subsequent recordings. Although an VIIIth nerve AP might have been revealed in subsequent studies on these infants with a transtympanic electrode, conventional BSER technique failed to demonstrate the peripheral auditory function which must exist for the degree of function demonstrated by these infants. In the two older infants, the pediatrician and audiologist were convinced that amplification would be inappropriate, although they did not rule out the possibility of a more subtle otologic deficit which cannot be demonstrated in such young children. The findings in these three infants may represent those of clinically insignificant cochlear or VIIIth nerve changes and severe brain-stem injury, together accounting for the gross reduction in all BSER components. One can only conclude that amplification should not be initiated on the basis of absent BSERs alone.

Figure 10-24 illustrates how click artifact may resemble biologic potentials when high intensities are employed. Artifact may be large, of long duration, and can mimic or obscure wave I. Alternating rarefaction and condensation clicks should be used to cancel the artifact only in combination with

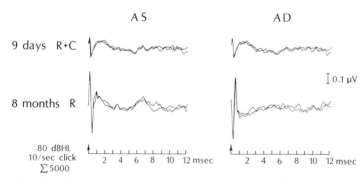

Figure 10-23. Premature male twin with neonatal seizures of uncertain etiology (35 weeks gestation). Initial BSER studies using both single and alternating polarity clicks, up to 85 dB HL, showed no response. At 8 months, with AS stimulation, one or two small potentials (3 to 7 msec), 80 dB HL could be produced. AD stimulation produced no response. Tympanometry was normal in the newborn period and at 8 months, but was relatively flat at 15 months when the child had a cold. At 8 months, standard audiometric evaluation revealed low behavioral thresholds at all frequency ranges, and at 15 months (when the tympanometry was abnormal) thresholds were obtained at moderate intensities. At 21 months, the child has a choreoathetotic diplegia and a VIth nerve palsy. Development is delayed in all areas. The EEG is normal. The child is alert, sociable, and responsive to low-level speech.

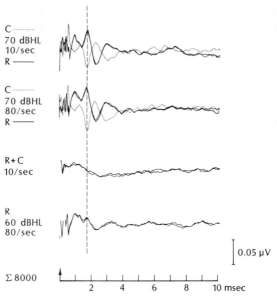

Figure 10-24. Full-term male whose neonatal course was complicated by a pulmonary hemorrhage, seizures, and hyperbilirubinemia (age 9 months). On audiometric examination, the child reliably localizes sounds of all frequency ranges at low intensities. He presents at 12 months with spastic choreoathetotic diplegia, impairment of vertical extraocular movements—severe limitation upward and mild limitation downward, no horizontal limitation. Child displays delayed development but is alert and responsive to low-level speech. BSERs at 2 weeks, 3 months, and 6 months were identical to those shown here. Note that the peak at 1.75 msec is 180° out-of-phase when R and C recordings are compared. High stimulus presentation rates produced no amplitude or morphologic change. Latency did not change with the intensity change. All of these factors indicate a nonneural source of the potential. Testing at 85 dB HL with R + C clicks revealed no neural response.

single-polarity recordings, since early components may also be cancelled. If the source of an early potential is still in doubt when both R and C responses have been plotted, altering stimulus rate and intensity can also help distinguish non-neural and neural components. High stimulus presentation rates should significantly reduce the amplitude of wave I, but not of a non-neural potential. Reduced stimulus intensity would not alter the latency of a nonneural potential. Although the appearance of the potential in Figure 10-24 would be typical for wave I in any single tracing, the complete polarity inversion with reversal of the click phase from C to R, and lack of rate effect on the amplitude of the potential indicates its artifactual origin. Some stimulating devices allow simultaneous presentation of masking noise and clicks to the test ear; when this is possible, a masking noise of greater intensity than the click should drastically alter any neural activity but would not affect a non-biologic potential (see Chapter 9). Such potentials can be distinguished from microphonics by acoustic coupling (tube-conduction) of the stimulus, which will prolong the latency of a cochlear microphonic but not of electromagnetic stimulus artifact. Mechanical click artifact is abolished by acoustic coupling.

Occasionally in newborns, BSERs may be present in earlobe-to-earlobe recording derivations but absent in the conventional vertex-to-earlobe derivation. For this reason, simultaneous recording of the two derivations (Okitsu, Kusakari, and Ito, et al., 1980) is advised when BSER amplitude is severely reduced.

As mentioned earlier, BSERs may normally be absent in early prematurity unless very high click intensities are employed. Figure 10-25 is an example of a premature infant who showed no response at 29 weeks of conceptional age but a normal response (except for a peripheral abnormality) at 35 weeks of conceptional age. This child was normal when examined at 6 months of age.

BSERs may be reversibly absent or severely depressed in amplitude in critically-ill newborns. Such a case is shown in Figure 10-26. BSERs were unrecordable in initial studies, but later appeared with prolonged latency and reduced amplitude when the child had clinically stabilized.

The conclusion to be drawn from the studies in this group of patients is that the absence of BSERs must be interpreted with caution. Infants should be

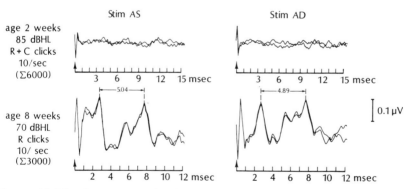

Figure 10-25. Premature male whose neonatal course was complicated by RDS (respiratory distress syndrome) and hyperbilirubinemia (27 weeks gestation). At 12 months, developmental, audiologic, and neurologic examinations were normal. Initial studies (at 29 weeks conceptional age) at 70 and 85 dB HL showed no response; both single- and alternating-polarity stimuli were used. At 35 weeks of conceptional age, response was normal, except for mild prolongation of wave I latency.

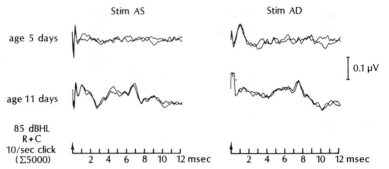

Figure 10-26. Full-term male with congenital myotonic dystrophy. Infant showed gradual improvement of hypersomnolence and poor responsivity over first 2 weeks of life. Initial BSERs at age 5 days showed no response to 85 dB HL clicks (both single- and alternating-polarity used). At 11 days, when the child had shown clinical improvement, a small, prolonged response was elicited. At 10 months, he is reported (by his private pediatrician) to localize low-intensity sounds; he has not had formal audiometric evaluation.

tested when mature, stable, and normothermic. Serial studies together with standard audiometric examination are prerequisites to decisions regarding management and rehabilitation.

Interpeak Latencies

Selective vulnerability of the brain-stem auditory nuclei to both asphyxia (Hall, 1964) and bilirubin toxicity (Gerrard, 1964; Dublin, 1951) has been pathologically demonstrated in newborns. These common complications of birth and the neonatal period have been strongly implicated in the develop-

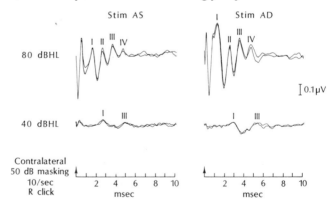

Figure 10-27. Twenty-five-year-old male with clinical and radiologic evidence of midbrain lesion following head trauma. At 80 dB HL, only waves I–IV are present with stimulation of either ear, despite the patient's inability to perceive the stimulus. Waves I–III are present with stimulation of either ear at 40 dB HL.

ment of hearing as well as neurologic disorders. Although end-organ or caudal pontine (cochlear nuclei and projections) structures are probably involved in most cases of neonatally acquired hearing loss, it is known that deafness can result from midbrain lesions (Howe and Miller, 1975) as in the case shown in Figure 10-27. Abnormalities of central conduction time may only rarely be accompanied by decreased hearing sensitivity; however, any effective screening program should include measurement of both peripheral and central auditory conduction. Either abnormality will have implications for the child's otoneurologic development; the two abnormalities indicate different therapeutic or rehabilitative approaches. For example, amplification was attempted and repeatedly revised (at great expense to the patient in Fig. 10-27) until BSERs indicated a central deficit. In four cases in our newborn series, combined peripheral and central BSER abnormalities were found (Fig. 10-28). In these cases, simple calculation of wave V latency might have led to the conclusion that the total delay was due to peripheral factors. If a hearing deficit were confirmed by conventional audiometry in such a case, the presence of a severe abnormality of central auditory conduction, combined with the peripheral abnormality, would assume considerable significance in decisions about the type and extent of therapy.

Masking

Although Finitzo-Hieber, Hecox, and Cone (1979) suggest that contralateral masking is not necessary in clinical BSER studies, Chiappa, Gladstone, and Young (1979) have demonstrated BSER responses with stimulation of a "dead" ear due to cross-hearing of the click stimulus. We have seen the same in a patient with a severed auditory nerve. Masking should be routinely used

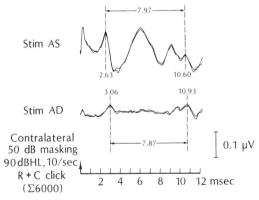

Figure 10-28. Trisomy-18 by chromosomal examination (full-term male, age 15 days). Responses to 90 dB HL clicks reveal prolongation of wave I latency but more pronounced delay to wave V; I-V IPLs are grossly prolonged.

in adult BSER studies and in infants with low amplitude, late responses, or with interaural asymmetries of latency or amplitude. A masking intensity at an effective level sufficient enough to eliminate significant cross-hearing should be routinely employed. In small infants for whom a single stimulating earphone is held to the ear, the masking earphone can be imbedded in a foam rubber mattress and the infant positioned on his or her stomach with the non-test ear facing that earphone.

DISCUSSION

Rigorous control of stimulus, subject, and recording variables, and a knowledge of normal BSER variability as a function of these factors are prerequisites to the accurate interpretation of the BSER for either neurologic or otologic diagnosis. The potential for false-positive and false-negative interpretations, particularly of central latencies, in the absence of proper controls, is enormous.

While technical advances in adult applications of the BSER have accelerated, the state of the art in the newborn and infant population demands considerable refinement. The standardization of recording with bone-conducted stimuli in all ages would do much to close the technical gap between the cooperative adult population and those patients in whom subjective stimulus thresholds cannot be determined. The very common problem of transient conductive impairment in newborns is a serious limitation in both the neurologic and otologic applications of the test.

The most glaring inadequacy at present is the paucity of normative data of responses to more frequency-specific stimuli. Tone-pip generators are currently available on many BSER test units and will probably come to be routinely applied in those neurologic patients with sensorineural hearing deficits. Such stimuli will be even more important in newborn hearing screening. When normal response variability to more suitable stimuli has been described in a large newborn control population, the very crude screening techniques outlined in this chapter should be considered obsolete. Because of the inherent technical disadvantages of both bone-conducted and frequency-limited stimuli (stimulus artifact and suboptimal synchronization properties), it is likely that the broad-band click will not be entirely replaced by these newer stimulation techniques, but will instead be used in combination.

Jos J. Eggermont

11 Audiologic Disorders

Any application of the outcome of psychophysical or electrophysiologic measurements to clinical problems requires the quantification of the clinical problem as well. In this respect, it will be helpful to aim at a quantification of hearing disorders before describing the use of auditory evoked potentials in this particular field. Auditory evoked potentials form just one representation of a hearing disorder, and several subsets of evoked potentials are currently in use (see Chapter 6). Among these, electrocochleography (ECochG) and the brain-stem evoked responses (BSER) are competing for a place in the diagnostic routine. This chapter will emphasize their simultaneous use and thereby provide some material about the weak and strong points of both test methods. Several schools of thought exist with respect to how these tests should be performed, either from the point of the recording or from the point of stimulus choice. The latter point often is concurrent with a stronger emphasis for on- or off-line evaluation of the patient's hearing. It is, therefore, not surprising that various methods exist, especially at first reading. The aim of the present writing is to unify most of these concepts and to evaluate individual merits of the numerous variations, keeping in mind the particular needs of audiologists and otologists.

QUANTIFYING HEARING DISORDERS

In current clinical practice a hearing disorder is indexed by three main features, i.e., *hearing sensitivity*, *dynamic range*, and *frequency selectivity*. Since this may sound somewhat unfamiliar, let us investigate this more closely on the basis of the empirical facts: (1) Measurement of hearing sensitivity is usually accomplished by octave audiometry both for air- and bone-conducted sound. This offers an additional feature in discriminating conductive from sensorineural hearing loss. (2) The dynamic range of hearing is routinely measured with the Alternate Binaural Loudness Balance test (ABLB, or Fowler test). This requires a normal reference ear and is therefore restricted to unilateral hearing losses (e.g., patients with Ménière's disease). The Short Increment Sensitivity Index (SISI-test) also relates to the dynamic range of hearing but only in an indirect way; the test offers a measure for the slope of the loudness-intensity function at a point 20 dB above threshold. An objective test can be based on measurements of the stapedius reflex threshold using an impedance meter. The distance (in dB) between the hearing threshold and the reflex threshold will be greatly reduced in patients with recruitment. (3) Frequency selectivity is generally not directly measured in clinical audiometry; an impression can be inferred, however, from the speech discrimination score. More recent psychophysical tests as measurement of the critical bandwidth (Bonding, 1979a, 1979b; 1979c; de Boer and Bouwmeester, 1979), the determination of psychoacoustic tuning curves (Leshowitz and Lindstrom, 1977, Durrant, Gabriel, and Walter, 1981), or masking with comb-filtered wide-band noise (Pick, et al., 1977) seem to be promising but are rather time-consuming and not always easy to perform.

In most clinical audiometry settings, a minimum test battery will contain one test out of each group, e.g., the audiogram (air- and bone-conducted stimuli), the stapedius reflex threshold measurement, and a speech discrimination test.

A quantification of hearing loss by electrophysiologic tests therefore requires the following: (1) The electroaudiometric test should provide an octave audiogram for at least the speech frequencies (500, 1000, and 2000 Hz), preferably extended to 4000 and 8000 Hz. (2) The test should provide an index for the dynamic range of hearing to be correlated with the presence or absence of loudness recruitment. (3) The method should quantify the frequency selectivity for relevant parts of the audiogram. It is expected (Evans, 1975) that items 2 and 3 are not independent for most types of hearing disorders.

Emphasis has already been placed upon the site-of-lesion testing that in routine audiometry can be done for conductive vs sensorineural loss (comparison of air- and bone-conduction audiograms, tympanometry) and for cochlear vs rectrocochlear loss (stapedius reflex threshold and decay). This also sets the stage for the minimum requirements pertaining to electroaudiometric methods with respect to site-of-lesion testing; the method should differentiate conductive from sensorineural hearing loss as well as various types of cochlear losses, and cochlear losses from retrocochlear hearing loss.

POTENTIAL USE OF ECochG AND BSER

During various symposia (Naunton and Fernandez, 1978), strong competition has emerged in favor of one test as opposed to the other, the basis therefore being either resentment against aggressive procedures in electrode placement (as in transtympanic electrocochleography) or aversion against the intrinsic variability of a response recovered from low signal-to-noise recording situations. Let us consider both recording techniques on their own merits. First, a redefinition of both methods is instructive.

Electrocochleography (ECochG) (transtympanic or extratympanic) is the recording of cochlear [cochlear microphonic (CM) and summating potential (SP)] and auditory nerve [action potential (AP)] evoked activity with an electrode configuration that provides a high common-mode rejection for brainstem evoked potentials. Brain-stem evoked responses (BSER) are the evoked potentials from auditory structures in the brain stem as recorded with surface electrodes (usually vertex vs mastoid or earlobe) and arising within 10 msec after stimulus presentation.

By definition, ECochG is a monaural technique, as the application does not require masking of the contralateral ear. BSER is sensitive to binaural stimulation. When large differences in sensitivity between the ears are expected, masking of the contralateral ear is required (see Chapter 10). Whether contralateral masking affects the response to the ipsilateral stimulus remains unclear; enhancement, depression as well as no effect have been found (Don and Eggermont, unpublished results; see also Chapter 9). By way of the electrode placement (promontory or ear canal), ECochG is by far more sensitive to cochlear- and auditory-nerve-generated potentials (Eggermont and Odenthal, 1974a; Elberling, 1976b); BSER provides (only at moderate-to-high sound intensities) a wave I (AP), and only at the highest intensities a discernible CM (Moore, 1971; Thornton, 1975a).

With ECochG the possibility of detailed objective audiometry (based on the AP threshold) has been amply demonstrated (Eggermont, Odenthal, and Schmidt, et al., 1974; Eggermont, 1976a; Spoor and Eggermont, 1976; Naunton and Zerlin, 1976a; Yoshie, 1973). For the BSER to date, only the potentiality has been shown (based on wave V threshold) (Don, et al., 1979; Kodera, et al., 1977; Terkildsen, et al., 1975b).

The slope of the AP amplitude vs intensity function has proven to be a good indicator for the presence of loudness recruitment (Eggermont, 1977b). When tone bursts are used as stimuli, this indication can be given for each frequency under study. Using BSER, claims have been made that the wave V latency versus intensity function could be used in this way, but it appears that it mainly distinguishes flat pure conductive losses from flat sensorineural hearing losses (Galambos and Hecox, 1977).

This feature, that the latency-intensity function for the AP as well as wave V tends to shift parallel to the normal function in ears with a pure conductive hearing loss, has frequently been used in discriminating middle- from inner-ear disturbances (Berlin, et al., 1974; Galambos and Hecox, 1977). The form of the latency-intensity function, however, does not unambiguously relate to the type of hearing loss.

Differentiation of cochlear lesions on the basis of CM and SP measurements is only possible with ECochG (Eggermont, 1976c, 1979a).

It appears that the main diagnostic potentiality of the BSER is in its excellence in site-of-lesion testing within brain-stem structures. With ECochG, attempts to discriminate between cochlear and retrocochlear hearing loss generally reveal poor results (Brackmann and Selters, 1976; Clemis and Mitchell, 1977), although more optimistic conclusions have been made (Eggermont, 1976a; Gibson and Beagley, 1976a, 1976b; Morrison, et al., 1976; Odenthal and Eggermont, 1976).

From this short survey, the following emphases become clear: (1) The electrode positions tend to favor the application of BSER. The test is less invasive than ECochG and electrode application does not require a medical license. (2) The better signal-to-noise ratio in (especially transtympanic) ECochG recording offers a greatly reduced recording time for each specific test, especially since duplication of the recordings, as is often necessary in BSER, is not needed. (3) For site-of-lesion testing, both methods are potentially powerful; the emphasis on ECochG is on differentiation of cochlear disorders (otology), and the strength of BSER is in differentiating pontine angle and brain-stem disorders (neurology). (4) Threshold measurements seem to be possible for BSER with about the same reliability as has been demonstrated for ECochG. Measurement of a complete (five-frequency) audiogram with ECochG requires 45 minutes; a conservative estimate for BSER is at least twice this amount of time. (5) Since the advent of ECochG and BSER (1967, in both cases), much more quantitative information has become available on ECochG and its use in quantifying hearing disorders than for BSER. Thus, a perfect balance of their respective merits is presently impossible.

If one is required to make a determination as to the use of both tests, one is inclined to supply ECochG to the otologist and BSER to the audiologist, neurologist, and pediatrician. However, it might well be that in making such a determination, potentially important features which may result from the combination of both techniques are discarded. It is my intention to demonstrate this in the following sections.

EVALUATION OF ELECTROAUDIOMETRIC AUDIOGRAM DETERMINATION

An objective audiogram can be basically estimated in three different ways: (1) By using frequency-specific stimuli (tone bursts, filtered clicks) and determining the threshold intensities for the particular response (generally the AP and wave V). (2) By using a wide-band stimulus (usually a short click) and deducing from the response parameters (amplitude, latency, waveform) — either by using a computer program or by a mental conversion, based on some model of auditory functions — an estimate of the audiogram. (3) By using place-specific stimuli, i.e., combining a wide-band stimulus (e.g., a click) with various types of masking (e.g., high-pass noise), so as to derive narrow-band responses. The threshold intensities within each narrow band constitute an estimate of the audiogram.

Frequency-Specific Stimuli

The basic problem with frequency-specific stimuli is that the measurement of evoked responses from the auditory nerve or brain stem structures requires stimuli with a more or less transient onset. This transient onset causes spectral broadening of the stimulus. Caution is thus required when comparing the results with subjective audiometry based on relatively long tones with a very gradual onset.

The spectral broadening of tone bursts having two cycles of rise time is acceptable in that, in general, a good correspondence with the subjective audiogram is found (Spoor and Eggermont, 1976). When using 1/3 octave filtered clicks (Zerlin and Naunton, 1976), this also seems well suited for most audiograms.

Comparison with the results from subjective audiometry is based on the calibration of the tone bursts or filtered clicks used. When a biological calibration is used (as has been for the standards for subjective audiometry), i.e., judgment by a panel of "normal" listeners, the differences in duration subjectively affect the threshold, but may not do so with respect to the AP threshold, amplitude, or wave V amplitude (Hecox, et al., 1976). If the calibration is performed mainly on the basis of physical characteristics of the stimulus (e.g., spectral level), then this particular bias is of minor importance (see Spoor and Eggermont, 1976). Continuous tones can be used to evaluate the frequency-following response (FFR) (at times considered to be a repetitive wave V, see Kruidenier, 1979, and Chapter 15). This can be a distinct advantage, but the procedure is restricted to the lower frequencies (Campbell, et al., 1977).

The most elaborate studies on audiogram determination with frequency-specific stimuli have been performed with ECochG (Yoshie, 1973; Eggermont, Odenthal, and Schmidt, et al., 1974; Spoor and Eggermont, 1976) and have been reviewed by Eggermont (1976a). Correlation coefficients have been calculated between the AP threshold at the various tone-burst frequencies and the corresponding subjective audiometric threshold for 500, 1000, 2000, 4000, and 8000 Hz. Values from 0.82-0.92 were obtained. The slope of the regression lines were close to 1.0. Subjective audiometry thresholds from 0 to 90 dB HL were included. Histograms of the threshold difference between ECochG and subjective audiometry at each of the five frequencies showed mean values of 0-5 dB and standard deviations from 7-10 dB. It was concluded that the technique is reliable as well as accurate.

Since that review appeared, Naunton and Zerlin (1976a), Davis (1976a), and Mouney, et al. (1976) have offered sufficient additional material to suggest useful application in the field of clinical audiology. Figures 11-1A and B show estimation of a subjective audiogram by means of ⅓ octave filtered clicks (Naunton and Zerlin, 1976a), and by means of short tone bursts (Eggermont, Odenthal, and Schmidt, et al., 1974), to indicate its applicability.

Results of audiogram estimations with BSER are scarce; they have only very recently appeared in the literature (Kodera, et al., 1977; Terkildsen, et al., 1978, Zöllner and Pedersen, 1980). Kodera, et al., using 5 msec rise-decay time tone pips at 500, 1000, and 2000 Hz, found mean threshold dif-

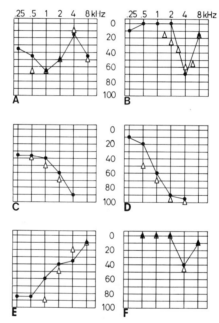

Figure 11-1. Audiogram estimation by various electro-audiometric techniques. The dots indicate the subjective hearing threshold and the triangles indicate the threshold as estimated from the evoked responses. Electrocochleography has been used in Figures 1A and B with frequency-specific stimuli as ⅓ octave filtered clicks (1A, Naunton and Zerlin, 1976a) or short tone bursts (1B, Eggermont, Odenthal, and Schmidt, et al., 1974). Use of the brain-stem evoked response combined with frequency-specific stimuli resulted in Figure 1C (Kodera, et al., 1977) and Figure 1D (Terkildsen, et al., 1978). The combination of a middle-frequency transient and a computer model was used by Elberling and Salomon (1976); a result is shown in Figure 1E. Finally, place-specific stimulation (see text) combined with BSER recording resulted in Figure 1F (Don, et al., 1979).

ferences with subjective audiograms of about 11 dB (a matter of calibration, since the difference proved to be frequency-independent) and standard deviation around 7 dB (fully comparable to the ECochG results). Terkildsen, et al. (1978), elaborating on the use of tone burst in normals (Terkildsen, et al., 1974b), reported audiograms based on FFR for 500 Hz and wave V for the higher frequencies. Two audiograms measured by each group are shown in Figures 11-1C and D.

At this writing, the material is too preliminary to deduce any differences between the two methods (ECochG vs BSER) but, in our opinion, it points to a somewhat reduced sensitivity for BSER (leading to a pessimistic estimate of the audiogram, if no correction is applied), while its variability (indicated by the standard deviations) is in the same range as reported for ECochG (Spoor and Eggermont, 1976) and the late vertex response (Salomon, 1974).

Wide-Band Stimulation

The click has been much more frequently used than frequency-specific stimuli in both ECochG and BSER. This is not surprising, since both the AP and BSER are onset responses, and their recovery from background noise by averaging depends on the close time relationship between stimulus onset and response. The results have proved best for the click. Therefore, the first clinical reports on ECochG as well as BSER (Portmann, et al., 1967; Yoshie, Ohashi, and Suzuki, 1967; Sohmer and Feinmesser, 1967; Spreng and Keidel, 1967) were based on click stimuli. There have been numerous reports dealing with the relation of click AP threshold, latency, and waveform to the shape of the audiogram (see Aran, Pelerin, and Lenoir, et al., 1971; Yoshie, 1973). The major conclusion is that click AP threshold corresponds best with the audiometric threshold in the middle frequencies (in particular, 2000 Hz). The correlation coefficients are usually low (< 0.6). Bergholtz, Arlinger, and Kyler, et al. (1977) reported correlations between free-field threshold for difficult-to-test children at 2 and 4 kHz with click AP threshold of 0.77 and 0.62, respectively. The slope of the regression line, however, was 0.6 and 0.5, respectively, indicating that ECochG generally overestimated the degree of hearing loss when used with clicks as stimuli.

The best correspondence between click threshold and 2 kHz audiometric threshold can be understood if one takes into account the external ear canal effect (about a 10 dB enhancement effect at 3.5 kHz, Shaw, 1974); and the middle-ear resonance around 1.5 kHz (Møller, 1974) on the initially flat click spectrum. Additional features, with respect to the shape of the audiogram, can be drawn from the AP latency–intensity function and the AP waveform (Aran, Pelerin, and Lenoir, et al., 1971).

Nearly all BSER studies deal with clicks as stimuli. Some investigators evaluate the effect of audiogram shape on the response parameters (Coats and Martin, 1977); some use it as a crude but clinically convincing indicator for hearing loss in infants and adults (Sohmer, et al., 1972; Hecox and Galambos, 1974; Galambos and Hecox, 1977; Mokotoff, et al., 1977,

Galambos, 1978). The basic concepts do not substantially differ from those originally used by Aran, et al. (1971), and will therefore have the same merits and drawbacks. The emergent overview indicates that click stimuli offer a quick, and for most clinical purposes, sufficient indication of the overall level of hearing loss. No detailed audiometric evidence, however, can be obtained.

The studies mentioned above employ a mental conversion from AP or wave V data to the estimate of the audiogram; the methods therefore require a considerable amount of skill. A more "hard-core" version has been advanced by Elberling (1976a; 1976b). On the basis of a physiologic model for the synthesis of the AP (convolution of the unit contribution with the latency distribution function) used in reverse, it has proved possible to derive, by deconvolution of the recorded APs with the unit contribution, the excitation pattern along the cochlear partition. This can be processed to give an audiogram estimate (Fig. 11-1E). On the basis of the results with a half-cycle 2-kHz click, basically good approximations were obtained. The need was felt to have additional high frequency stimuli because, among others, the model fell short in discriminating pure conductive hearing loss from severe high-frequency hearing loss (Elberling and Salomon, 1976). This limitation is also inherent in methods which do not use computer models; it will be discussed again in the section "Differentiating Conductive, Sensorineural, and Mixed Hearing Losses."

Place-Specific Stimulation

It is appropriate to begin with a discussion about the significant difference between frequency-specific stimulation and place-specific stimulation. At low intensities, a short tone burst evokes neural activity from a restricted part of the cochlear partition (Dallos and Cheatham, 1976; Eggermont, 1976b, 1977a) and can therefore be said to be a place-specific stimulus. When the tone burst intensity is increased, more and more fibers innervating parts basal to the most sensitive area are recruited into action (Rose, et al., 1971; Kiang, Moxon, and Kahn, 1976; Eggermont, 1976b) and the tone burst is no longer a place-specific stimulus. In this situation, the amplitude and latency of the AP and the respective BSER waves is predominantly determined by fibers innervating the basal part of the cochlea (Eggermont, 1976b; Don and Eggermont, 1978). This is true for tone bursts as well as for clicks (Elberling, 1974).

A stimulus configuration which restricts the extension of the activity pattern to basal locations consists of a click or tone burst combined with high-pass filtered noise. When the slope of the filter is steep enough ($\cong 100$ dB/octave), a rather sharp boundary of the click or tone burst-excited part is obtained. Subtracting APs or BSERs recorded in the presence of high-pass noise filtered for cut-off frequencies differing by, e.g., one or ½ an octave, yields narrow-band responses (Teas, et al., 1962; Elberling, 1974; Eggermont, 1976b, Don and Eggermont, 1978; Parker and Thornton, 1978a,

1978b, 1978c, 1978d). Measurement of click thresholds in each of the narrow bands results in accurate audiogram estimates (Don, et al., 1979) (Fig. 11-1F), comparable to the results with tone bursts. However, since the click appears to synchronize the responding nerve fibers better than the tone burst (especially low-frequency ones), thereby providing larger responses, a somewhat more sensitive threshold estimator may be obtained in this way.

Conclusion

One is inclined to state that tone burst (or ⅓ octave filtered click) stimulation or click stimulation combined with high-pass filtered noise-masking provide adequate potential for BSER to be as useful in determining audiograms as has been shown for ECochG. Extensive studies with ECochG offer guidance in interpreting the results. The fact that the amplitude of wave V in the BSER seems to be less sensitive to an increase in stimulus repetition rate than AP (Terkildsen, et al., 1975a; Thornton and Coleman, 1975) compensates, to some extent, for the fact that BSER evaluation requires more averages and a repeated trial in most cases. Under favorable signal-to-noise ratios (low noise, sedated, or relaxed patients), BSER recording times may be about the same as in ECochG, giving perhaps the same accuracy as in the average ECochG.

RECRUITMENT AND FREQUENCY SELECTIVITY

The current model linking recruitment and frequency selectivity has been expressed by Evans (1975), as

". . . the essential lesion in cochlear deafness is damage to the second filter with consequent loss of sharp tuning, [this] offers a simple explanation for the phenomenon of loudness recruitment characteristic of cochlear deafness of various etiologies, and the degradation experienced by these patients in the perception of speech."

Both phenomena will first be discussed separately (especially since both have their specific tests); later, the concepts will be integrated.

Loudness Recruitment

The phenomenon of loudness recruitment is thought to be characteristic of cochlear deafness. As a consequence, it must be measurable by ECochG and/or BSER. One of the first things to be aware of is the relation between the (psychologic) sensation of loudness and the underlying (physiologic) neural correlate. The hypothesis that loudness is related to the driven spike rate of all the fibers in the auditory nerve (Fletcher and Munson, 1933; Howes, 1974) has been theoretically investigated by Goldstein (1974). According to this theory, the loudness–intensity relationship above 40 dB HL is mainly determined by the recruitment of fibers with a characteristic frequency (CF) above the tone frequency. As Goldstein points out, loudness should therefore be influenced by moderately masking these high-CF fibers, a theory which is neither supported by psychoacoustic masking studies nor by findings in pathological cochleas (e.g., severe high-frequency sensorineural hearing loss). Hellman and Hellman (1975) evaluated a relation between loudness, $\psi(I)$, at intensity, I, and the single-unit-driven rate–intensity function, R_d (I), as

$$\psi(I) = c\, R_D\, (I)^{S(I)}$$

in which the exponent S(I) ranges from 1 (I near threshold up to 40 dB HL), about 2 at 80 dB HL, to 2.32 at 100 dB HL. This is interpreted by Hellman and Hellman (1975) as:

> "This implies that only a few neural units might be necessary to account for the growth of the loudness function over a range of at least 100 dB. In fact 2-3 neurons may be needed. The neural output can be described as the multiplicative effect over a small number of units rather than the summation over a large number of units."

In a later paper (Hellman, 1978), it is stated that "the available loudness data strongly suggest that the entire loudness growth range can be produced even when the frequency distribution of excitation is confined to a relatively narrow band."

In utilizing compound AP or BSER to predict loudness recruitment, the next issue is the relation between onset neural activity and sustained neural activity. Loudness depends on the duration of the stimulus while AP or BSER amplitude (e.g., wave V) do not (Hecox and Galambos, 1974). Smith and Zwislocki (1975) have demonstrated that the ratio between onset neural activity and steady-state (adapted) neural activity is constant over a wide intensity range. Thus, qualitatively, loudness (related to steady-state neural function, especially in conventional audiometric procedures using long tones) may be related to AP amplitude (onset neural activity).

Findings in Hearing Loss with Recruitment

Portmann, et al. (1973) characterized recruiting ears by a diphasic AP waveform, a rapid increase of AP amplitude with intensity, without a plateau in the input/output curve, and a latency of less than 2 msec at threshold. Yoshie and Ohashi (1969), however, regularly found an abrupt increase in latency for levels close to the subjective threshold. Eggermont (1977b) showed that latency at threshold depends on the audiogram configuration, as well as on the type of stimulus used. The same is generally true for the AP waveform, while the steepness of the amplitude–intensity function increases with increasing threshold level. Statistically, one could quite accurately predict the AP parameters from a given audiogram, provided that the type of hearing loss is known. Working the other way around (e.g. Elberling and Salomon, 1976), of course, may lead to audiogram prediction but uncertainty as to the type of pathology. For practical purposes, the slope of the amplitude–intensity function has been proposed (Eggermont and Odenthal, 1977).

The AP amplitude increase with stimulus intensity is mainly dominated by the extension of the excitation profile toward more basal parts of the cochlea (fibers with higher CF). Linking the steepness of the AP amplitude–intensity function to loudness recruitment should then be subject to the same criticism as the loudness model based on that phenomenon. Nevertheless, it has been demonstrated (Eggermont, 1977b) that in recruiting ears, the great majority ($\cong 80$ percent) have an input–output curve which is steeper than that found in normal ears (Figs. 11-2A, 11-3B). So that although the relationship between growth of loudness and growth of AP amplitude is unclear, the correspondence is clinically very useful.

An additional ECochG procedure is related to the SISI-test and measures the AP response to an intensity increment upon a continuous tone pedestal (Schmidt, et al., 1974). In patients with cochlear hearing loss, increments of 1.0dB above a 20 dB SL pedestal give a suprathreshold AP response (and are audible); in normal ears no AP can be measured (there is, likewise, no sensation).

Using narrow-band derived responses, it can be demonstrated (Fig. 11-2B) that the sum of narrow-band AP amplitudes in response to tone bursts (each representing a weighted summation over fibers innervating at $2\frac{1}{2}$–3 mm area along the cochlear partition) as a function of intensity parallels the driven neural rate curve calculated for the whole nerve (Goldstein, 1974), while the AP amplitude (a weighted summation over the narrow-band AP responses) follows a different course (Davis, 1976a). The summated onset activity for the whole nerve thus closely parallels the steady-state neural rate curve for the whole nerve. Both seem to be related to loudness in the case of simple stimuli, and can be used as such. Eggermont (1978) showed that if the excitation pattern is confined to a $\frac{1}{2}$-octave narrow-band, the steepness of the input–output curve was far greater for a recruiting ear than for a normal ear (Fig. 11-2C). This seems to agree with the psychoacoustic observations of Hellman (1978). In some studies, inferences about recruitment are made on the basis of latency–intensity functions (Yoshie and Ohashi, 1969; Berlin, et al., 1974; Galambos and Hecox, 1977). With a pure cochlear loss, latency (AP, or its delayed version, wave V) is a function of the intensity of the stimulus; latency is a function of the sensation level of the stimulus for a pure conductive loss. Latency measurements, therefore, do not seem to relate to recruitment per se, but mainly to the audiogram (Bergholtz, Hooper, and Mehta, 1977; Eggermont, 1977b) and the status of the middle ear.

Single-cell studies in the anteroventral cochlear nucleus (AVCN) have shown that for a certain class of cells (dominant in the AVCN), the latency of

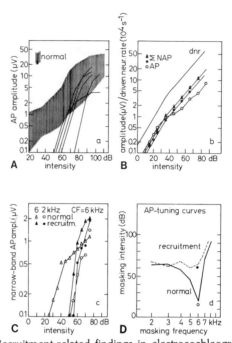

Figure 11-2. Recruitment-related findings in electrocochleography. A. Individual AP amplitude–intensity functions for recruiting ears for high stimulus levels to normal values despite the threshold elevation of around 60 dB. The shaded area is the absolute range of amplitude values observed in normal ears (data from Eggermont, 1977b). B. Loudness seems to be related to the driven neural rate of the whole auditory nerve (Goldstein, 1974), which is plotted as a function of intensity (dnr curve). The AP amplitude–intensity function (open circles) definitely follows a different course. The summated amplitude values of the narrow-band responses at each intensity, however, lead to curves (dots and triangles) which closely parallel the dnr curve. This suggests that the total onset activity of the whole nerve is simply related to the driven neural rate and, thereby, possibly to loudness. The fact that the AP curve differs from the Σ NAP curve (0 and ● refer to the same case) is due to the diphasic nature of the unit contribution which tends to cancel part of the response. C. Narrow-band AP amplitude–intensity functions for a center frequency (CF) of 6 kHz at two tone burst frequencies (2 and 6 kHz) in a normal and a recruiting ear. When the tone burst frequency equals that of the center frequency, the intensity function in the recruiting ear is much steeper than for the normal ear. This indicates that the recruitment phenomenon has already taken place within the restricted half-octave narrow-band, and does not require the contribution from more basally located nerve fibers. At 2 kHz stimulation, the curves for the normal and recruiting ear tend to be the same. D. AP-tuning curves for 6 kHz tonebursts in a normal and a recruiting ear. The open and filled circles indicate the test tone level and frequency for the normal and the recruiting ear. The sharp two-segment tuning curve found in the normal ear changes to a rather broad one in the recruiting ear (from Eggermont, 1978).

298

the initial discharge is inversely related to the average discharge rate (Kitzes, et al., 1978). The latency depends strongly on stimulus level (about 6-7 msec change over a 40 dB range was noted) as well as on stimulus duration. It appears, therefore, that onset latency measures also can be related to neural rates, and therefore, to loudness.

It can be seen that the use of the latency–intensity function for clicks (in ECochG and BSER) is not without pitfalls. Interpretation is straightforward in cases of a flat, pure conductive loss (parallel shifted curve) and flat, pure cochlear loss (latency curve within the normal range), but offers serious problems when dealing with mixed losses or with high-frequency sensorineural hearing loss (McGee and Clemis, 1980). The latency–intensity function for tone bursts may eliminate some of these problems.

Frequency Selectivity

Measurements of frequency selectivity have been established in ECochG (Eggermont, 1977a). Following Dallos and Cheatham (1976), short tone bursts are presented at 10 dB above threshold and the compound AP is recorded. A simultaneous or nonsimultaneous (e.g., forward-masking) masking tone is adjusted in frequency and intensity so that the AP to the test tone has a preset amount of amplitude decrease (e.g., 50 percent). The geometrical figure of intensity–frequency combinations of the masking tone that produce this decrease in AP amplitude is called an *AP tuning curve* (Eggermont, 1977a). A characteristic finding in normal ears is that of two segments (Fig. 11-2D): at low masker intensities and masker frequencies close to the tone-burst frequency, the tuning curve is rather sharp. At higher (>60 dB SPL) masking intensities, a broadly tuned portion, determined by the low-frequency tail, is noted. As most basilar membrane tuning curves (Kohllöffel, 1972; Rhode, 1971; Wilson and Johnstone, 1975) resemble the broadly tuned part of the single nerve fiber or AP tuning curve, the sharply tuned part had been attributed to a second filter (Evans, 1975). The sharpness of tuning for single nerve fibers (Kiang, Watanabe, and Thomas, et al., 1965), psychoacoustic tuning curves (Leshowitz and Lindstrom, 1978), and AP tuning curves is quite comparable (Eggermont, 1978a), for normal hearing.

In cochlear hearing loss, AP tuning curves lose their sharply tuned part and become broadly tuned (Eggermont, 1977a), just as has been found for single-fiber tuning curves (Kiang, et al., 1970; Evans, 1975) (Fig. 11-2D). Another way of measuring the cochlear frequency selectivity is by measurement of the response area of short tone bursts, using the narrow-band response technique (Eggermont, 1976b). The response area can be interpreted as a tuning curve with the frequency axis reversed. This method has been used to relate the increase in AP amplitude as a function of intensity to the extension of the response area to the high-frequency side. This connects steep input-output curves with the abnormally large amount of newly recruited nerve fibers with CF above the tone frequency at a particular SL of the tone burst (Eggermont, 1977b).

When using clicks instead of tone bursts, a larger part of the cochlea can be activated. The AP latencies for a particular click level (90 dB pe SPL) increase as the central frequency of the narrow bands becomes lower (Elberling, 1974; Eggermont, 1976b, 1978). This increase in latency is partially due to travelling wave delay, and partially to impulse response times of the sharply tuned cochlear filter. It has been found that click-stimulated single nerve fibers have latencies which are related in a reasonably simple manner to the sharpness of their tuning curves (Goldstein, Baer, and Kiang, 1971). One expects, therefore, that in the case of a cochlear hearing loss, where broader tuning curves are obtained, that the narrow-band AP latencies become shorter than for the normal ear. This has indeed been found for a particular class of pathological cochleas (but not in others) and does not seem to be related to the amount of hearing loss or the presence of recruitment, and (in a simple way) to the sharpness of tuning (Eggermont, 1979b).

Since the method of derived narrow-band responses is readily applicable to BSER (Don and Eggermont, 1978; Parker and Thornton, 1978a, 1978b, 1978c), this offers an opportunity to determine under which conditions (etiology of the hearing disorder, audiometric results) abnormally short narrow-band response latencies can be found.

In summary, it has been demonstrated that both steep input-output curves and broad AP tuning curves are present in recruiting ears; both are directly related to each other. Attempts to correlate the value of the slope of the input-output curve to the amount of loudness recruitment have failed, a fact which becomes more obvious when the different conditions are compared. A relation between sharpness of AP tuning and speech discrimination has not yet been established. Prediction of recruitment, however, may very well be possible (based on either the slope of the input-output curve or on basis of the latency-intensity function), although the theoretical basis seems to be weak.

DIFFERENTIATING CONDUCTIVE, SENSORINEURAL, AND MIXED HEARING LOSSES

Following conventional audiometric procedures, the use of bone-conducted sound vs air-conducted sound is a major issue in electroaudiometry concerned with topical diagnosis. The electroaudiometric application of bone conductors offers numerous serious problems centered around the vibratory inertia of most bone conductors (Yoshie, 1973; Arlinger and Kylén, 1977). This prevents the application of transient stimuli unless a Bruel and Kjaer Mini-Shaker (Copenhagen, Denmark) is used (Berlin, et al., 1977; Arlinger and Kylén, 1977; Harder, et al., 1980). The current practical application has been very limited; one study provides significant data on the use of the Mini-Shaker during temporal bone surgery (Kylen, et al., 1977; Harder, et al., 1980). Another approach has been to evoke the BSER while masking the ear with bone-conducted stimuli (Hicks, 1980).

Most emphasis has been placed upon the attenuating effects of an impaired middle ear upon the AP and BSER parameters as a function of stimulus intensity. The expectation is that amplitude–intensity and latency–intensity curves shift to higher intensity values, with the number of dB representing the loss in the middle ear (Yoshie and Ohashi, 1969; Aran, Pelerin, and Lenoir, et al., 1971; Berlin, et al., 1974, Odenthal and Eggermont, 1974; Eggermont and Odenthal, 1977). The latency-intensity function has attracted special attention and has subsequently been used in BSER-audiometry (Galambos and Hecox, 1977; Gerull, et al., 1979). There are, however, limits in employing this method. It is observed that the width of the latency–intensity range for normal ears at each particular latency value is about 20 dB (Fig. 11-3A) (Eggermont, 1976a). The implication is that the minimum pure conductive hearing loss that can be detected on this basis will be about 20 dB, and, in addition, the inaccuracy in the amount of conductive hearing loss that has been estimated will also be about 20 dB. The same impression is gained from the data presented by Berlin, et al. (1974).

An additional complication arises when the wave V latency–intensity function is used, but wave I is absent. In such cases, there is no control upon the amount of wave V delay attributable to an increased central conduction time that is thought to result from brain stem or pontine angle lesions (Starr and Hamilton, 1976). This could lead to a serious overestimation of the amount of conductive hearing loss, which is especially important in children having the quite common combination of conductive hearing loss and retardation in development (Mair, et al., 1979). Both factors cause wave V delay, irrespective of stimulus intensity (Mokotoff, et al., 1977; Starr, 1977). Separation of the effects can only be made on the basis of additional ECochG testing or a clear recording of wave I

The use of the shift to the AP amplitude–intensity function (Yoshie and Ohashi, 1969; Aran, Pelerin, and Lenoir, et al., 1971; Odenthal and Eggermont, 1974; Eggermont and Odenthal, 1977) yields the same basic problem as the latency–intensity function. The normal range of amplitude–intensity curves has, for the lower amplitude values, a width of about 30 dB (Eggermont, 1976a) (Fig. 11-2A). The same spread has to be assumed in conductive loss. Because amplitude values are negatively correlated $(r \cong 0.8)$ to latency values as expressed in the amplitude latency scattergrams (Eggermont, Odenthal, and Schmidt, et al., 1974; Eggermont, 1976a), the combined use will generally not yield a better result than one criterion alone.

In sensorineural hearing loss, the slope of the amplitude–intensity curve (especially when using frequency-specific stimuli) is elevated, with respect to

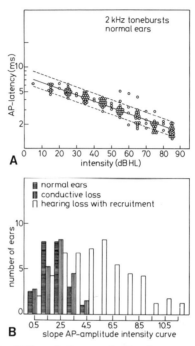

Figure 11-3. Differentiating conductive from sensorineural hearing loss. A. On the basis of the normal latency-intensity function, data from normal human ears for 2 kHz tone burst stimulation are shown together with the regression line and one standard-deviation boundary. A given latency value will occur for a range of intensities roughly 20 dB wide. This will be the consequent uncertainty in estimating the amount of conductive hearing loss by this method. B. On the basis of the steepness of the AP amplitude-intensity function, data are compared from normal ears, ears with conductive loss, and recruiting ears. While the normal and conductive-loss ears are indistinguishable, their slopes overlap considerably with the values from the recruiting ears. Taking this criterion for recruitment, for example, at 4.5, results in 5 percent false-positives (normal or conductive-loss ears detected as recruitment) and nearly 40 percent false-negatives (recruiting ears undetected). Fortunately, testing at five frequencies also gives relative slope values for the ear itself and generally leads to scores around 15-20 percent false-negatives.

those for normal hearing and conductive hearing loss (Eggermont, 1976a, for a review). In Figure 11-3B, a histogram of slope value is given for 22 normal ears, 25 conductive-loss ears, and 55 ears with recruitment. The distribution is nearly identical for normal ears ($\mu = 2.1$; sd $= 0.7$), and ears with conductive loss ($\mu = 2.4$; sd $= 1.3$). In contrast, there is very broad range of slope values (partially overlapping the normal and conduction loss distribution) found in recruiting ears ($\mu = 5.2$, sd $= 2.6$). The problems in using these data for the diagnosis of the individual patient's ear are obvious.

The latency-intensity functions for the AP in recruiting ears either fall within the normal range or show slightly elevated latencies, especially at or near threshold values. When using clicks or low frequency (0.5, 1, and 2 kHz) tone bursts, the influence of the audiogram shape is considerable (Coats, 1978). Claims have been made that mixed hearing losses are characterized by normal latencies (for click AP) at high intensities and progressively deviated (increasing difference) latencies for lower intensities (Berlin, et al., 1974). The same shift, however, is observed in pure high-frequency sensorineural hearing loss for high frequencies, when the audiogram has a slope steeper than 30 dB/octave (Yoshie and Ohashi, 1969; Aran and Negrevergne, 1973). Differentiating mixed hearing losses of up to 50-60 dB into a conductive and sensorineural component on the basis of click stimuli seems to be mainly based on wishful thinking. Generally, neither the conductive nor the sensorineural component will show a flat loss across frequency; one may obtain a far better estimate by using frequency-specific stimuli and judging, at each frequency used, the dominant feature. When one is able to say, for example, that the ear under study has a predominantly conductive-type hearing loss at lower frequencies and prominent sensorineural loss for the higher frequencies (judged together with the objective audiogram) a quite reasonable estimate of the status of the ear is possible.

The general "recipe" to distinguish, with some success, between conductive, sensorineural, and mixed hearing loss is: (1) use frequency-specific stimuli; (2) determine the slope and shift of the AP (or wave V) amplitude-intensity function referred to a normal group result; (3) determine the slope and shift of the AP (or wave V) latency-intensity function referred to a normal group result (when dealing with wave V, be sure to eliminate any delay due to a more central dysfunction; and (4) be aware of the confidence region around the estimated values, due to the considerable overlap of the various response criteria.

DIFFERENTIATION OF VARIOUS TYPES
OF SENSORINEURAL HEARING LOSS

It is standard practice to subdivide sensorineural hearing loss into cochlear vs retrocochlear losses. The cochlear types may be distinguished into sensory and neural losses. With respect to retrocochlear hearing loss, we tend to restrict ourselves to those caused by pontine angle tumors and only briefly address the problem of pseudohypacusis.

Differentiation of Cochlear Hearing Loss

Audiometrically, a cochlear hearing loss is, at times, diagnosed by the presence of loudness recruitment. The relationship between loudness recruitment and deterioration in frequency selectivity has been indicated. From experiments on single nerve fibers, it has become clear that a very large number of ototoxic agents result in the same change in tuning curves, i.e., the loss of the sharply tuned portion (Evans, 1975). Among these ototoxic agents are drugs such as Kanamycin (Kiang, et al., 1970), furosemide (Evans, 1975), and other physical agents such as noise (Kiang, Liberman, and Levine, 1976), hypoxia (Robertson and Manley, 1974), removal of perilymph (Robertson, 1974), or stimulation of the olivocochlear bundle (Wiederhold and Kiang, 1970).

Some of these agents result in irreversible damage to the cochlea accompanied by hair cell loss, which is generally more dominant for the outer hair cells. Other agents (e.g., temporary hypoxia (Nishida, et al., 1981), olivocochlear bundle stimulation, removal of perilymph, and temporary threshold shift (TTS)) produce a reversible change in the tuning curve, generally without damage to the hair cells. From a clinical point of view, it could be worthwhile to have an indication of potential reversibility of a hearing loss, as in sudden deafness (Morrison, et al., 1980). This can only be based on a test of the integrity of the hair cells, and not on recruitment, since it appears in all situations. For this test, both potentials generated by the hair cells—cochlear microphonics (CM) and summating potential (SP)—are the obvious candidates. The large majority (95-99 percent) of the recordable CM and SP in normal ears is produced by the outer hair cells (Dallos, 1973). By recording from the promontory, one may expect a dominant contribution from hair cells in the basal turn of the cochlea, as can be demonstrated using the narrow-band response technique. By saturating the SP in given parts of the cochlea with masking noise and subtracting responses, one obtains the contributions of various parts of the cochlea to the click-evoked SP (Fig. 11-4). This figure shows a decrease in amplitude of about 6 dB/octave, i.e., about 1 dB/mm, restricting the recording distance from the promontory to the region basally from 2 kHz. (Note that the narrow-band AP contribution decreases under the same conditions with only 3 dB/octave.) One may thus demonstrate outer hair cell activity in the basal turn of the cochlea. If those hair cells are affected, one can expect a decrease in the CM or SP amplitude. Using tone bursts as stimuli may indicate frequency-dependent effects and therefore localize, to some extent, certain hair cell lesions.

CM and SP amplitude at a fixed intensity level is extremely variable, even among normal hearing subjects (Aran and Charlet de Sauvage, 1976; Eggermont, 1976c), and may even be influenced by electrode placement (Eggermont, 1976a). Aran and Charlet de Sauvage (1976) concluded that the CM amplitude at 95 dB HL (click) was significantly different between Ménière's ears and other ears with cochlear hearing loss (e.g., noise trauma, ototoxic drugs). Both types of hearing loss showed recruitment, but the Ménière's ears showed fairly normal CM. A comparable conclusion was obtained for the SP in Ménière's ears as compared to other cochlear-loss ears

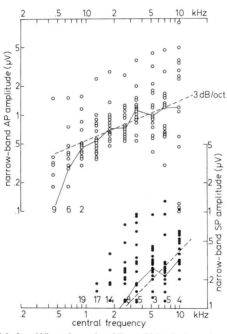

Figure 11-4. What does the SP or CM tell about hair cell lesions? As the SP and CM are mainly generated by the outer hair cells in the basal turn of the cochlea, the interest focuses upon the part of the cochlea that contributes to the promontory recorded SP or CM. Since the SP seems to be more reliable than the CM, the following holds strictly for the SP. On the basis of narrow-band SP responses, as a function of central frequency, one deduces that (for normal ears) the median values decrease by about 6 dB/octave towards lower central frequencies. In contrast, the narrow-band AP responses in the same group of ears decreases by only 3 dB/octave. The effective recording range with respect to click-evoked SPs seems to be the basal turn down to 2-3 kHz, that is, about 15 mm from the stapes.

(Schmidt, et al., 1974; Eggermont, 1976a); the Ménière ears exhibited fairly normal SP values, significantly larger than for the "hair-cell-loss" group.

Eggermont (1979a) described SP behavior in 112 patients with Ménière's disease and compared the SPs with those for normal ears. Two major conclusions were drawn: (1) In patients with Ménière's disease (with up to about 50 dB hearing loss), the SP amplitude values for 85 dB tone burst stimulation (2, 4, and 8 kHz) cannot be discerned from normal. (2) The amplitude distributions for SP amplitude found in normal ears and Ménière's ears are so wide (χ^2-shape) that only SP amplitudes $< 0.7\mu V$ indicate abnormal hair cell function. This holds for the normal form of SP, the negative SP⁻.

Positive SP⁺ (Eggermont, Odenthal, and Schmidt, et al., 1974; Yoshie, 1973) seem to point to nearly complete and sharply demarcated losses in the very base of the cochlea with near-normal hair cell populations in other parts (Rietema, 1979). As Nishida, et al. (1976) have pointed out, the absence of SP, or the presence of SP⁺ in patients with sudden deafness, indicates a poor prognosis, while normal SP⁻ generally reflect reversible hearing loss (Coats, 1981b). This seems to be true for other fluctuating hearing losses as well; for example, in Ménière's disease (Eggermont, 1979a), where the SP is affected by the status of the hydrops such that glycerin administration may show a decrease in SP (Booth, 1980). This decrease in SP is a favorable prognosis for the results of saccus surgery (Moffat, et al., 1977; Morrison, et al., 1980). From the discussion of the role of SP in differentiating cochlear hearing loss, it is obvious that a very minor role for BSER is available. Although it has been shown that CM can be recorded from surface electrodes (Moore, 1971; Thornton, 1976), group studies reflecting the distribution of surface-recorded CM amplitude and its value in diagnosis so far are lacking. SP has occasionally been observed to be present in the BSER recording as a vertex positive shoulder, appearing shortly before wave I (Eggermont, unpublished results, 1977), but has not yet been systematically explored.

Neural losses can be defined as those not having an end-organ lesion. This would place Ménière's disease in the neural loss group, which may be incorrect. A true neural lesion might be represented in some tumor cases.

Differentiation of Retrocochlear Hearing Loss due to Pontine Angle Tumors

In the differentiation of retrocochlear hearing loss due to pontine angles tumors, BSER results can be conclusive on their own. ECochG results are difficult to interpret, and generally are inconclusive. The combination of BSER and ECochG, however, will result in the smallest number of false-positives and false-negatives in diagnosis. Both methods will be independently discussed and later they will be integrated.

ECochG in Tumor Diagnosis

The promoters of ECochG in the field of pontine angle tumor detection (Gibson and Beagley, 1976a, 1976b; Morrison, et al., 1976), following the earlier findings by Portmann and Aran (1972), described a series of 89 patients with confirmed retrocochlear lesions, and claimed detection scores as high as 89 percent (i.e., 11 percent false-negatives, with about 20 percent false-positives). The particular criteria adapted for the click-evoked AP were broadening of the waveform, preservation of a clear CM, and the observation of APs for stimulus levels below the hearing threshold. Although broad waveforms and CM preservation are characteristic in Ménière's disease (e.g. Eggermont, 1979a), and the AP threshold was more than 15 dB better than the subjective hearing threshold in only 27 percent of the cases, the authors reached their conclusions by combining all of the scores (presuming that the features are independent).

On the other hand, Brackman and Selters (1976) tested 25 patients with confirmed acoustic neuroma, but were much more reluctant to claim the usefulness of ECochG in the diagnosis of VIIIth nerve tumors based on the same features. In a series of 23 confirmed acoustic neuromas, Clemis and Mitchell (1977) considered latency, amplitude, and waveform of the click-evoked AP as diagnostic indicators, and concluded that ECochG is of little value in the differential diagnosis of these tumors. In contrast, Eggermont (1976a) concluded that ECochG with additional criteria (the latency–intensity function for tone-burst stimuli, and the waveform of the derived narrow-band response) was quite promising in differentiating acoustic neuromas. The monophasic narrow-band AP waveform, found in acoustic neuromas, contrasted with either the diphasic or triphasic narrow-band waveform found in Ménière's disease, seemed to be a measure by which to differentiate broad AP waveforms. In an attempt to test most of the proposed criteria on a reasonably large group of patients, Eggermont, Don, and Brackman (1980) studied (32 patients with confirmed acoustic neuromas) the AP and SP for 2, 4, and 8 kHz tone-burst stimulation, and the narrow-band APs for click stimuli. This was a parametric study and, therefore, they considered the slope of the amplitude–intensity function, the course of the latency–intensity function, the amplitude–latency function, the width–latency function (Eggermont, Odenthal, and Schmidt, et al., 1974), the difference between AP and subjective threshold, and the waveform of the narrow-band AP, as well as the SP amplitude at 85 dB HL. Abnormality of these parameters was judged against a group of 27 normal ears and a group of 79 Ménière ears. A response parameter was abnormal when it was clearly distinct (outside 2σ-boundaries) from the data in the two control groups, taking the audiogram into account.

It appeared that in only three ears (9 percent), the peripheral threshold was 20 dB better than the subjective one. The amplitude–latency relationships all were within normal limits (and within the range for Ménière ears, see Schmidt, et al., 1974). The width-latency relationship was abnormal in 10 cases (30 percent); the latency-intensity relationship showed an abnormal course in 17 cases (53 percent); the slope of the AP amplitude-intensity function, considered with respect to the amount of hearing loss, was abnormal in 9 cases (28 percent); the narrowband AP was monophasic in 7 cases (22 percent); and the SP amplitude was below the range found for Ménière's disease in 18 cases (56 percent).

A correlation analysis (Table 11-1) shows that most of these criteria were uncorrelated or very weakly correlated (slope of amplitude-intensity function with latency-intensity function, $r = 0.29$; latency-intensity function and narrow-band AP waveform, $r = 0.39$; and width-latency relationship with NAP waveform, $r = 0.27$). In no case were all criteria abnormal; in 90 percent of the cases, one abnormal finding was noted; in 70 percent of the cases, two abnormal findings; in 25 percent of the cases, three abnormal findings were noted; and only in 10 percent of the cases were four abnormal parameters found. Considering three abnormal findings the minimum for certain diagnosis, we tentatively arrive at a 25 percent score, which is consistently lower than that of Gibson and Beagley (1976a, 1976b). We note that CM and SP data generally provided identical information (Eggermont, 1979a).

Recently Elberling and Salomon (personal communication, 1979) studied 58 patients with confirmed acoustic neurinoma and considered, in the ECochG part of the investigation, the AP waveforms (70 percent were abnormal, but not substantially differing from those of Ménière's disease); the threshold of the AP (in 30 percent of the cases, a lower AP threshold than was subjectively found, based on a 17.5 dB difference) (Gibson and Beagley, 1976a, 1976b); and the CM/AP ratio (which was found to be abnormal, > 2.5, in 28 percent of the cases).

The picture emerging from these investigations is that ECochG is likely to give a reliable prediction of the presence of a tumor in 25-35 percent of cases, which rules out the method as a single test in tumor-diagnosis.

Table 11-1
Correlation Matrix for Diagnostic Features in the ECochG with Respect to Differentiating Acoustic Neuromas from Sensorineural Hearing Loss.

	Δ	τ	A	SP	NAP
Width-Latency (Δ)	1	0.14	0.07	-0.02	0.27
Latency-Intensity		1	0.29	0.18	0.39
Amplitude-Intensity (A)			1	0.17	-0.14
Summating Potential (SP)				1	0.10
Narrow-band AP (NAP)					1

BSER in Tumor Diagnosis

Some large series of pontine angle tumor patients have been evaluated by BSER in order to deduce its merits in differentiating acoustic neuroma. Rosenhammer (1977) described findings in 29 patients, Clemis and Mitchell (1977) in 23 patients, Selters and Brackmann (1977) in 46 patients, Thomsen, et al. (1978) in 27 patients, and Josey, Jackson, and Glasscock (1980) in 52 patients.

While Rosenhammer paid attention to the general morphology and reproducibility of the response, Selters and Brackman elaborated on a quantitative detection criterion. This was based on the latency difference between waves V recorded from the tumor ear and the other ear (IT_s). An experimentally obtained correction factor for large differences in the audiograms was found to be necessary, and a corrected IT_s exceeding 0.4 msec resulted in 9 percent false-negatives (91 percent score) and 10 percent false-positives.

Clemis and Mitchell (1977), pointing to the adverse effects of small conductive losses either in the test ear (false-positives) or the reference ear (false-negatives), which prolongs the wave V latency, arrived at 10 percent false-negatives and 36 percent false-positives. They arrived at a diagnostic efficiency in a real-life situation of about 76 percent, resembling that from stapedius reflex testing. In a subsequent paper, Clemis and McGee (1979) reported further criteria in studying a group of 27 tumor patients and a group of 115 non-tumor patients. They considered latency differences (absolute wave V latency) of more than 2σ from the normal mean, IT_s-values exceeding 0.3 msec, and the absence of wave V as criteria and arrived at a 7.4 percent false-negatives (92.6 percent score). The non-tumor group resulted in 33 percent false-positives, expressing caution in the use of criteria due especially to the effect of small conductive hearing losses.

Thomsen, et al. (1978) described findings in 27 patients with surgically confirmed auditory nerve tumors, mainly on the basis of IT_s. Their distribution of IT_s-values for 70 Ménière's patients and 27 tumor patients leads to zero percent false-positives and 15 percent false negatives for $IT_s > 1.0$ msec. At the $IT_s \geq 0.5$ msec level, 11 percent false-positives and 4 percent false-negatives (one case) can be calculated; at the commonly used $IT_s \geq 0.3$ msec one arrives at 23 percent false-positives and 4 percent false-negatives. These data compare favorably to Clemis and Mitchell (1977) and Clemis and McGee (1979).

The large influence of conductive and high-frequency sensorineural losses upon the wave V latency caused Eggermont, Don, and Brackman (1980) to consider the wave I–wave V delay as the test value against the IT_s in a group of 43 surgically proven pontine angle tumor patients. Regarding the normative values for 70 normal ears (mean I-V delay = 4.01 msec, $\sigma = 0.16$ msec), and considering that, in 43 ears with unilateral Ménière's disease, the mean difference between the wave I-V values for the normal and pathologic ear was -0.02 msec with a $\sigma = 0.19$ msec, the following criteria were adopted. A I-V delay increasing beyond $\mu + 2\sigma$ ($= 4.33$ msec) will result in 5 percent false-positives and 5 percent false-negatives. A criterion taken at $\mu + 3\sigma$ (4.49 msec) will result in 0.3 percent false-positives and 9.3 percent false-negatives. Considered abnormal were, of course, all cases where a clear wave I was present in the BSER but all subsequent activity was absent (15 cases, 34 percent). *In cases where wave I was absent* (14 cases, 32 percent), *we took as the criterion AP-V delay from the simultaneously recorded transtympanic ECochG.*

The IT_s criterion applied. to this material (43 unilateral Ménière's, 43 acoustic neuromas) resulted, at $IT_s > 0.4$ msec, in 2 percent false-positives and 9 percent false-negatives.

Elberling and Salomon (personal communication, 1979) also considered the AP-V delay, because they found in 47 percent of the 58 cases that wave I was absent in the BSER. Assuming a criterion value of 4.3 msec, they arrived at 22 percent false-positives and 7 percent false-negatives; for a criterion value of 4.5 msec, at 0 percent false-positives and 15 percent false-negatives (Eggermont, Don, and Brackman, 1980). Considering that wave V identification is a serious problem in BSERs from tumor patients (e.g., how to identify wave V when all the earlier waves are missing?), Elberling (1978, 1979a, 1979b) considered two promising objective means for estimating the amount of abnormality in the response. The first method (Elberling, 1979b) comprises cross-correlating the BSER waveform with a template, based on the responses obtained at the same stimulus level from normal and sensorineural hearing loss ears. This results in a maximum cross-correlation coefficient and a group delay for the BSER as a whole. For normal and sensorineural loss ears, a standard 2.5σ ellipse in the correlation coefficient-delay plane was established. Data from tumor patients were compared with this normal area; the 2.5σ criterion resulted in 0 percent false-positives and 11 false-negatives, in effect, as good as the AP-V method, but completely *objective.*

A second criterion requires again the *combined measurement* of the AP and the BSER. Considering the AP as the input to the brain stem, Elberling (1978) computes the so-called compound-impulse response (CIR) by deconvolution of the BSER with the AP. In this series of tumor patients (Elberling and Salomon, personal communication, 1979), the latency of the third peak in the CIR was evaluated according to the criterion > 2.56 msec and resulted in no false-positives (based on a set of sensorineural loss ears) and 17 percent false negatives. In addition, since the delay calculated from the cross-correlation procedure and the latency of the third peak in the CIR are uncorrelated, both criteria were combined. This resulted in the very promising 0 percent false positives and 4 percent false negatives; this evaluation is performed in a truly objective manner (Fig. 11-5).

The conclusions from these recent studies (Eggermont, Don, and Brackman, 1980; Salomon, et al., 1979; and Elberling and Salomon, personal communication, 1979) point to the overall impression that if the AP-latency measurement (by ECochG) is added to the BSER, a quite dramatic reduction in the number of false-positives [from 35 percent in both Clemis and Mitchell (1977) and Clemis and McGee (1979), to 0 percent] can be obtained. This arises because any effect peripheral to the generation of the BSER (conduc-

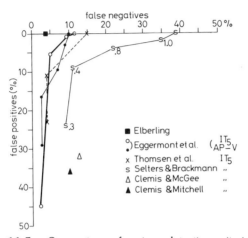

Figure 11-5. Comparison of various detection criteria and scores in acoustic neuroma detection, on the basis of receiver-operating curves (ROC). The percentage of false-positives (non-tumor ears diagnosed as having tumors) is plotted against the percentage of false-negatives (undetected tumors). Clearly, a technique is better when a small number is found for both false scores, therefore the curves that approach the left upper corner are based on good criteria. Shown are the uncorrected IT_s results as derived from the material published by various investigators, one AP-wave V delay criterion (Eggermont, open circles) and one objective method (Elberling, 1976b). The curves obtained, however, do not only reflect the value of the criterion per se but are also determined by the composition of the control group. When this group contains a large number of conductive-loss ears the performance will be poor with respect to the percentage of false-positives when an IT_s criterion is used. If the same patient population is used for IT_s or AP-V criteria, there is a marginal difference when the reference group does not contain conductive-loss ears.

The figures drawn along the s-curve indicate the various IT_s-values and their diagnostic result, for example, at 0.4 msec there are about 10 percent false-positives and 10 percent false-negatives.

tive hearing loss, high-frequency sensorineural hearing loss) is, effectively, taken out of the diagnostic criterion. In all cases reported, the number of false-negatives (missed tumors) is acceptably small (<7 percent), and retests within a few months often showed abnormalities in these ears (Eggermont, Don, and Brackman, 1980).

Effects of Tumor Size on the BSER

Selters and Brackmann (1977) suggest a more or less linear relation between IT_s and tumor sizes; from their data one may calculate

$$IT_s(msec) = 0.14 + 0.55S(cm)$$

with $r = 0.72$, for the 18 tumors in which a wave V could be detected. The non-response tumors (28), however, ranged in size from 1 to 4.5 cm with $\mu = 2.75$ cm and $\sigma = 1.0$ cm.

Clemis and McGee (1979) show data from which one may calculate

$$IT_s(msec) = 0.87 + 0.54S(cm)$$

with $r = 0.46$, for 22 tumors (3 tumor ears did not produce a wave V). Thomsen, et al. (1978), describing 27 tumors, stated that they were unable to find any correlation between IT_s and tumor size. These data lead to

$$IT_s(msec) = 1.43 + 0.12S(cm)$$

with $r = 0.19$. Eggermont, Don, and Brackman (1980) attempted an exponential curve fit between the I-V delay and tumor size:

$$I\text{-}V(msec) = 4.2 \exp [0.13S(cm)]$$

with $r = 0.7$. However, 15 tumors ranging in size from 1 to 4.5 cm gave no wave V response. Elberling and Saloman (personal communication, 1979) could not demonstrate any significant correlation between the delay computed with the cross-correlation function and tumor size.

This indicates that the composition of the various tumor groups, the identification of wave V, and the omission of patterns which cannot be interpreted greatly influence the results. Even as a rule of thumb, a 3 msec delay (either I-V or IT_s) may not be seen as an indication for a tumor the size of a small orange. In such a case, one would expect involvement of the contralateral evoked BSER. Selters and Brackmann (1977) indicated the influence of large tumors pressing against the brain stem on the contralateral wave III-wave V latency difference (see also Shanon, et al., 1981). This was found to be prolonged, resulting in an increased wave V latency at the reference ear and thereby again decreasing the IT_s, indicating another weak point of this measure.

In sum, BSER with additional AP-latency information is an excellent test in differentiating retrocochlear hearing loss. In practice, an augmentation of wave I may be sufficient; this can be obtained by moving the mastoid or earlobe electrode into the external ear canal. The closer the electrode is to the tympanic membrane the larger the AP (wave I) amplitude (see Chapter 8).

Electroaudiometry and Pseudohypacusis

Electroaudiometry and pseudohypacusis may become an important topic when legal assessment cases have to be objective. First of all, one must understand that no electroaudiometry test, ECochG, BSER, middle latency, or cortical responses, is a test of *hearing*. Electroaudiometry tests the capability of the auditory nervous system to produce click or tone burst synchronous (or time-locked) evoked potentials. The very fact that in a large number of patients with VIIIth nerve tumors no wave V can be detected while the stimulus is clearly audible to them illustrates this fact. The tumor produces desynchronization of individual fiber firing patterns; they do not add up to a detectable onset response, and one could conclude that the patient does not "hear" the stimulus.

The only case where electroaudiometry is helpful in establishing an indicated amount of hearing loss is when the etiology points to a peripheral cause (e.g., noise trauma). In all other cases, only the confirmation of the amount of hearing loss is of value (Berlin, 1980).

Combined use of all electroaudiometry tests, however, may give some indication about very occult types of hearing loss, for example, when ECochG, BSER, and middle responses are clearly present in a patient who is deaf and did not give a slow vertex response (Eggermont, unpublished observation, 1977).

ECochG OR BSER:
A PROBLEM-ORIENTED CHOICE?

Electroaudiometry can be performed at various levels of sophistication, arbitrarily arranged within three subgroups: (1) the economic level, (2) the audiometric level, and (3) the physiologic level.

On the economic level, the ease and speed of test performance competes heavily with the amount of information derived from the test. At the audiometric level, the weight is placed more towards requirements in the test result and generally involves a longer test session. On the physiologic level, electroaudiometry is performed either to compare electrophysiology with psychoacoustics or to study a particular disease in large groups of patients. In these cases, one attempts to obtain as complete a picture as possible, whether or not the approach is very time consuming.

The Economic Test Level

In these situations, usually a click stimulus is used. The answer to be provided by the test is simple and straightforward; has the patient normal hearing, a moderate hearing loss, or a severe hearing loss? What is the nature of the hearing loss (conductive or sensorineural)? Are there any brain-stem abnormalities? The recorded click-evoked AP or BSER as a function of stimulus level may optionally be complemented by computer analysis to obtain more accurate estimation of the audiogram or normalcy of the brain stem.

The Audiometric Level

The answer from the test at this stage has to include a detailed audiogram with indications for the presence of recruitment at each frequency studied. This requires the use of filtered clicks, tone bursts, or (most probably) clicks combined with high-pass filtered masking noise. Recording times are longer but the test result is directly comparable to standard subjective audiometry.

The Physiologic Level

In this approach, the investigator pays attention to CM, SP, AP, and BSER, usually applying frequency- or place-specific stimuli. The object is to create a complete (and probably redundant), picture of the input-output properties and frequency-selectivity at various stages along the auditory nervous system.

Once the test level is specified, either by clinician demands or by the composition of the patient population in a given clinic, one should decide ECochG *or* BSER vs ECochG *and* BSER. I think most investigators in the field will make a decision on the basis of the following question: *What is the particular information to be gained from ECochG that is not obtained from the BSER?*

We have seen that audiogram estimation (either click or tone burst based) can be as accurate in BSER as in ECochG. In the latter, the more favorable signal-to-noise ratio results in a shorter recording session. If the objective is simply to obtain a click input-output series, BSER gives nearly all of the information needed. At the economic level of testing, ECochG is definitely out of the picture.

If one desires more information from the test, recall that with BSER (as with ECochG) generally some idea can be obtained about the nature of the hearing loss, especially in pure conductive or sensorineural hearing loss. Testing for recruitment using the BSER is, however, not yet well established. And what should be done in the 1-to-4-year-old child? In ECochG, one uses general anesthesia if the condition of the child allows it; in BSER, a sedation could be sufficient, but is not always possible in the anxious child who may fight off the sedative action for hours. This generally does not allow tight testing schedules. At the audiometric level, ECochG is valuable to obtain a complete and reliable audiogram in a limited amount of time.

As to additional information to be gained from ECochG, the CM and the SP unquestionably provide important information in case of inner-ear disorders, as in Ménière's disease, and in establishing a prognosis for sudden deafness. The favorable signal-to-noise ratio allows for the measurement of tuning curves and detailed narrow-band analysis. The latency of AP measurement is of considerable value when combined with BSER information in the differentiation of cochlear from retrocochlear hearing loss, and quite substantially reduces the number of false-positives in tumor diagnosis. Performing electroaudiometry at the physiologic level is only possible with the inclusion of ECochG.

In conclusion, ECochG without BSER is only of value when the patient material excludes brain stem disorders. BSER is to be used on its own account without ECochG when the test level is directed more towards a screening for the amount of hearing loss, or the presence of brain stem disorders. BSER should always be combined with ECochG when studying hearing disorders, especially those of cochlear origin, and when detailed audiogram information and conclusive evidence about the site of the lesion is to be obtained (Ryerson and Beagley, 1981). BSER will suffice for charting development in children.

In order to quantify hearing disorders as outlined above, the combination of ECochG and BSER is definitely indicated, but the weight of both methods on the test result is heavily dependent on the patient, as well as on the particular information that is needed.

Harvey (Haim) Sohmer

12 Neurologic Disorders

The recording of the auditory BSER in patients with suspected neurologic disorders has been shown to be a valuable functional test of the peripheral and central nervous system. The test complements the clinical neurologic examination, aids laboratory tests, and assists in the interpretation of several radiologic studies, including the pneumoencephalogram, angiography, and computerized axial tomography scan. We have been instructed in previous chapters that an intense, rapid-onset auditory stimulus elicits electrical responses in successive portions of the auditory pathway, beginning with the receptor (hair) cells within the cochlea, progressing to the auditory nerve, traversing the brain-stem auditory pathway, and coursing to the cerebral cortex and associated cerebral structures. The rationale for the use of the BSER in the diagnosis of neurologic disorders is that a relatively large volume of neural tissue is devoted to the transmission and processing of auditory information. In other words, an appropriate sound stimulus generates electrical activity at many levels of the brain, so that there is a relatively high probability that a lesion in a particular region of the brain will affect the functional electrical activity of one or more levels of the auditory pathway. It follows that this may give rise to abnormalities in one or more of the BSER waves.

A diagram of the family of auditory evoked potentials and their assumed

Supported in part by a grant from the Chief Scientist's Office, Ministry of Health, Israel. The author wishes to express his sincere gratitude to each of his colleagues, assistants, and students who participated in various aspects of the research, discussions, and preparation of the manuscript.

sites of generation are shown in Figure 12-1, and are summarized in Table 12-1. In the literature, several of these evoked responses have different names and, for clarity, these also are listed in the table (see also Chapter 6). The responses, which have been developed for use in audiologic disorders, are also candidates for use in diagnosis of neurologic disorders. However, all of the auditory evoked responses (AER) cannot contribute equally to an appropriate diagnosis. Following are several criteria for the incorporation of a particular AER into a neurologic test battery:

1. *Replicability*. The response should be highly repeatable within the same subject and across subjects. Repeated testing should generate responses which are similar in their waveform, amplitude, and latency.
2. *Source*. In order to contribute to lesion localization, the site of generation of the response in the brain should be known. There would be little contribution to neurologic lesion localization in a patient if a particular component, whose source was unknown, was absent.
3. *Correlation with Pathology*. A particular AER would be more helpful in diagnosis if a specific AER response pattern abnormality were always associated with a specific neurologic disorder.

We shall soon see, then, that the majority of the auditory BSERs fulfill these criteria. They are thus the potentials of choice in most laboratories involved in AER-based neurologic diagnoses.

We shall also see that, in general, the responses which are generated with short latencies (and therefore more peripherally generated) can "withstand" high-stimulus repetition rates and have most of their response energy at higher frequencies. On the other hand, the later-appearing more central responses, require lower stimulus repetition rates, and their response waveform is lower in frequency (see Chapter 13). Sedation is required with the uncooperative patient and one must be aware of the possible effects of the sedating drug on the later AER responses. It has been shown that the auditory BSER is not, for the most part, affected by sedative drugs (Sohmer, Fahn, and Amit, et al., 1978).

In studying the response traces for signs of abnormality, we pay particular attention to the presence or absence of particular waves, to wave amplitudes and latencies, and to overall waveform structure. All of these attributes are compared to the normal response configuration that is recorded in subjects who are devoid of any pathology (Kaga and Tanaka, 1980). In considering latency and/or amplitude parameters, it may be useful to develop a BSER profile, since multiple parameters are in existence (Lolas, Hoeppner, and Morrell, 1979).

The following discussion will consider some of the fundamental observations noted in other chapters (Chapters 9, 10, and 11). We repeat them here so as to extend the continuity evident throughout this volume.

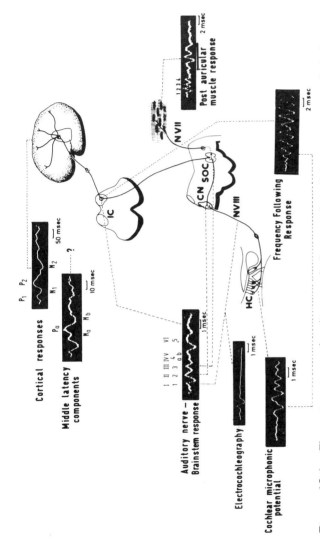

Figure 12-1. The various types of auditory evoked potentials and the structures in which they are thought to be generated. Wave I is generated in the auditory nerve; waves II and III are thought to be generated in the more caudal regions of the brain stem auditory pathway while waves 4a (IV), 4b (V), and 5 (VI) are thought to be generated in the more rostral regions of the brain stem (see also Chapter 7).

319

Table 12-1
Types of AER, Their Latencies, Sources, Stimuli, and Recording Conditions

Type of AER	Synonyms	Latencies (msec)	Source	Stimulus Type	Rate/Sec	Electrode Sites	Filter Bandpass (Hz)	Average Window (msec)
Cochlear microphonic	CM	0	Cochlear hair cells	Single sinusoid	10-80	Lobe (vertex)	100-4000	10
Auditory nerve brain-stem	Far-field ECochG short latency evoked	3-6	Auditory nerve Cochlear nucleus Superior olivary complex Lateral lemniscus Inferior colliculus	Clicks & tone bursts	10-20	Lobe (mastoid)-vertex	200-5000	10
Electrocochleography (cochlear microphonic, summating potential, auditory nerve)	ECochG transtympanic ECochG	0-2	Cochlear hair cells and auditory nerve	Clicks & tone bursts	10-20	Promontorium (earlobe)	100-4000	10
Middle-latency components		10-100	Medial geniculate body(?) Primary auditory cortex(?)	Clicks & tone bursts	10	Earlobe (mastoid)-vertex	10-200	100

Cortical responses	Late components	50–300	Cerebral cortex	Clicks & tone bursts	1	Earlobe (mastoid)–vertex	0.2–40	500
Frequency following response	FFR	0–Duration of tone burst	Cochlear hair cells Inferior colliculus	Tone bursts	5	Earlobe (mastoid)–vertex	100–5000	20
Post auricular muscle	PAM, crossed acoustic response	10–30	Postauricular muscle, mediated by cochlea	Clicks, filtered clicks & tone bursts	4–10	Mastoid–vertex Mastoid–neck below earlobe Mastoid–temple	20–4000	20–30
Event-related potentials	CNV, expectancy wave, ER	250–3000	Secondary auditory cortex, association cortex, frontal cortex	Lights and tones	1/5 sec	Vertex–mastoid	DC–5000	3000

THE AUDITORY BSER

The electrical response of the auditory nerve and of a large portion of the brain-stem auditory pathway to click stimuli can be recorded as the potential difference between electrodes on the earlobe (or mastoid) and on the vertex. In this array, both electrodes of the pair detect electrical activity which originates in these neural structures, the auditory nerve and the brain stem. The earlobe (or mastoid) electrode records waves which are progressing away from this site as negative-going waves, while the vertex electrode detects these same waves as approaching the vertex, and records the same waves as positive-going waves. One can thus refer to the same waves as either earlobe-negative waves or vertex-positive waves (see Sohmer and Feinmesser, 1973, and Chapter 6).

The series of waves originating from the auditory nerve and brain stem (Figs. 12-1 through 12-4) are recorded in the same response trace in normal subjects. They appear as five to seven (designated waves I-VII) distinct waves. The first earlobe-negative wave (N_1 or I) appears with a latency of about 1.4 msec following the arrival of the acoustic stimulus at the tympanic membrane. The second (II) wave appears with a latency of 2.6 msec, while the third (III) displays a latency of 3.6 msec. The fourth (V) wave appears in about 72 percent of the normal population as two independent waves, and as one prominent wave in about 28 percent of the normal population. In 42 percent of the subjects, there were different wave patterns in the two ears (Chiappa and Gladstone, 1978). Examples can be seen in Figure 12-2. Therefore, some workers refer to the IV-V double peak as waves 4a and 4b respectively, while others refer to the same waves as IV and V (Jewett and Williston, 1971).

In this chapter, we shall adhere to both systems. Wave 4b (i.e., wave V) has a latency of about 5.5 msec and the fifth wave (or, alternatively, wave VI) has a latency of about 7.1 msec. It is also convenient to specify the earlobe-positive (vertex-negative) wave following wave 4b (V) (Sohmer and Student, 1978). Some refer to this as wave P_4 (Shanon, Gold, and Himmelfarb, et al., 1979) and FFP_7 (Terkildsen, Osterhammel, and Huis in't veld, 1974a) (Fig. 12-2). Note that the latencies cited for these waves are in response to click stimuli at high intensities, and at repetition rates no greater than about 20 stimuli/sec.

As stimulus intensity is decreased, the latencies of each of the waves increase to more or less the same extent while the amplitudes decrease, although the amplitude of wave 4b (V) will decrease the least. As the repetition rate of the click stimulus is increased, the latency of the waves increase and the amplitude will decrease. Here again, the amplitude of wave 4b (V) will decrease to the least extent (see Figure 12-3). The stability of wave 4b (V) is probably responsible for the fact that in certain conditions (when one employs very high intensity stimuli), it is the only wave apparent in the response trace.

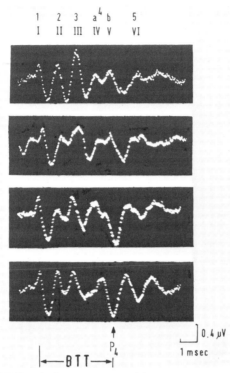

Figure 12-2. Auditory nerve and brain-stem responses in four different normal subjects of the same age (10 years). Note the variability in the amplitude of waves II and 5 (VI) and the different patterns of wave 4 (IV-V). The waves are labelled with both systems, P_4 is indicated and the measure of brain-stem transmission time (BTT) is defined.

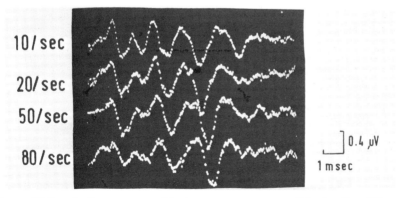

Figure 12-3. Auditory nerve and brain-stem responses to click stimuli at different repetition rates. Note that as repetition rate increases, BTT also increases.

The auditory BSER is used in neurologic diagnosis more than other AERs for several reasons. First of all, BSERs are relatively easy to record, not requiring surgical intervention (in comparison to transtympanic ECochG). In addition, BSERs are highly replicable, both in the same subject and across subjects (von Deuster and Seiley, 1979). Figure 12-2 shows BSER recordings in several normal subjects; the recording traces are qualitatively similar. Figure 12-4 shows a series of response traces from the same subject over a span of 6 years—here too, the responses are seen to be similar. Note that long latency cortical responses are not as replicable (see Chapter 13). The BSER's high replicability has led to the generation of normative data for amplitude and latencies across several age spans, and even for both sexes.

Responses

The absolute latencies of the auditory BSER to high-intensity stimuli (60-80 dB HL) in the normal adult population are very stable. The differences in latencies found in different laboratories are at least partially due to differences in coupling between the earphone and the ear (see Chapter 8). In general, the standard deviation of the latencies within any particular research group is about 0.2 msec. Some recommend the use of two standard deviations from the mean latency (Cox, et al., 1981).

Women between the ages of 20 and 80 years have been found to have slightly shorter latencies than men of the same age; this difference is signifi-

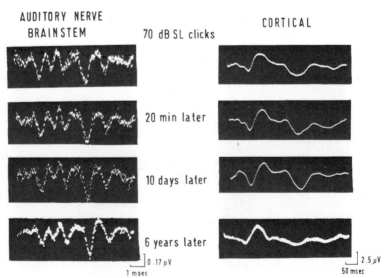

Figure 12-4. Auditory nerve, brain-stem, and cortical responses to click stimuli in the same subject over a period of 6 years. Note the great similarity of the auditory BSER and the relative variability of the cortical response.

cant (Beagley and Sheldrake, 1978). In this laboratory (Goldman, Sohmer, Godfrey, et al., 1981), a similar difference has been found in 10-year-old boys and girls, and is on the order of 0.05-0.14 msec. These values are statistically significant. The difference may be due to the fact that females generally have smaller head circumferences, the internuclear segments of the axons generating these responses may thus be shorter.

The relationship between subject age (in adults) and response latency is problematic. Beagley and Sheldrake (1978), studying patients by age groups (grouped in decades, from 20 years to 80 years), found no increase in latency with age. On the other hand, Rowe (1978) comparing a group of 17-33-year-old subjects to a group of 51-74-year-old subjects, found the older group to have latencies 0.30-0.50 msec longer than those of the younger group.

In young infants, all workers agree that latencies are prolonged; more prolonged in premature neonates (Cox, Hack, and Metz, 1981; Morgon and Salle, 1980; Schulman-Galambos and Galambos, 1975), and gradually decreasing, reaching adult values at the age of 12-18 months (Hecox and Galambos, 1974), or 2.5 years (Salamy, McKean, and Buda, 1975). This decrement of latency during early infancy has been ascribed to more rapid axonal propagation, probably due to increased myelinization of axonal properties (Leiberman, Sohmer, and Szabo, 1973).

Factors other than age and neurologic disorders affect absolute latencies of the BSER, including the presence of a conductive hearing loss due to an external- or middle-ear condition (Dobie and Berlin, 1979a; Sohmer and Cohen, 1976). Additional factors which give rise to longer latencies are low-stimulus intensity (Pratt and Sohmer, 1976; Leiberman, Sohmer, and Szabo, 1973b), and high-stimulus repetition rates (Hyde, Stephens, and Thornton, 1976; Pratt and Sohmer, 1976). In order to overcome these possibly confusing problems (conductive hearing loss and low-stimulus intensities), a different latency measure has been suggested: the time interval between brainstem waves.

In our laboratory, we use the time interval between the earlobe-negative peak of the auditory nerve response (wave I—considered the "input" to the brain stem) and the trough of the earlobe-positive wave following wave 4b (V) or P_4 (the clearest, most prominent response from more rostral parts of the brain stem). We call this interval brainstem transmission time (BTT) (Fabiani, Sohmer, and Tait, et al., 1979). This is shown in Figure 12-2. Normal adults show BTT values of 4.5 ± 0.2 msec. We do not use the term "conduction time," since, in an audiologic-otologic context, "conduction" refers to the transfer of sound vibrations through the middle ear. However, we have no quarrels with Stockard and Stockard (Chapter 10), since it is too early to attempt to standardize terminology and techniques.

Other groups consider other time intervals; for instance, the time interval between waves 4b (V) to 2 (II), calling it "central transmission" (Salamy,

McKean and Buda, 1975; Salamy and McKean, 1976), or the time between 4b and 1 (V-I), calling it "central conduction time" (Starr, 1977; Rowe, 1978). We have preferred using, as an end point of this time interval measurement, the downward-going trough following wave 4 (IV-V) (P_4) since, as stated above, wave 4 often appears as two peaks. In several normal cases, wave 4b (V) is smaller in amplitude than wave 4a (IV). At times, only one of the two waves is present (see Fig. 12-2, botton two traces) (Chiappa and Gladstone, 1978). This possible source of confusion is thus overcome by using instead the downward trough, P_4, the latency of which is not dependent on the form that wave 4 (IV-V) takes. Such measures of latency difference are independent of stimulus intensity, stimulus frequency, and the presence of a conductive hearing loss (Fabiani, Sohmer, and Tait, et al., 1979).

Amplitude

The amplitudes of the auditory BSER show greater variability; attempts have therefore been made to overcome this problem by defining a relative amplitude measure, for example, by using the ratio of the amplitude of wave 4b (V) to that of wave I (Starr and Achor, 1975). This ratio in normal subjects is reported to be greater than 1.0 (Starr and Achor, 1975; Rowe, 1978).

Abnormal Traces

The auditory BSER reflects disorders affecting the posterior cranial fossa, including conditions such as space-occupying lesions, degenerative lesions, increased intracranial pressure, aminoglycoside treatment (Bernard, Pechere, and Hebert, 1980; Ramsden, Wilson, and Gibson, 1980), and vascular disturbances. The particular pattern of abnormality of the BSER trace will depend greatly on the location, nature, and degree of the disorder.

Prolonged Brain-Stem Transmission Time (BTT)

Prolonged BTT is found in several neurologic conditions, among which are cerebellopontine angle tumors and multiple sclerosis. (These will be discussed in greater detail below.) BTT is found to be prolonged also in hypothyroidism (Lakritz, 1979), in barbiturate overdoses (Brinkman and Ebner, 1977), in several children with psychopathology (Sohmer and Student, 1978), conditions of hypothermia (Stockard, Rossiter, and Wiederholt, et al., 1976), and in alcohol intoxication. BTT appears to return to normal with alcohol withdrawal (Chu, Squires, and Starr, 1978). We have also seen this in diffuse cerebral sclerosis (Schilder's disease), which is a progressive demyelinating disease seen in children (see Fig. 12-5). On the other hand, comparisons of BTT in a group of narcoleptics and primary insomniac showed no significant differences for these sleep disorders (Hellekson, Allen, and Greeley, et al., 1979).

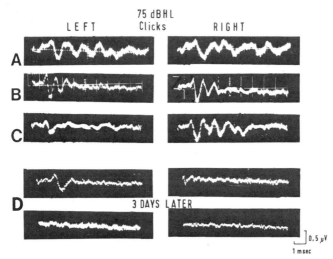

Figure 12-5. Abnormal auditory nerve and brain-stem response patterns. A. BTT is prolonged (5.5 msec instead the normal value of 4.5 msec for this age). B. Waves 4 (IV-V) and 5 (VI) are absent. C. The brain-stem responses are absent on the left. D. Wave I and a very small wave II can initially be seen on the left (no response from the right). Three days later, no response can be recorded.

Findings of prolonged BTT in certain neurologic disorders warrant further study, since BTT is made up of several internuclear segments and of two components of neural delay, axonal propagation and synaptic-dendritic delays (see Chapters 4 and 7). It would be interesting to try to differentiate between these two possible contributing factors in normal BTT and prolonged BTT. This might be studied by comparing BTT values in neurologic conditions known to affect axonal propagation as opposed to those conditions thought to affect synaptic transmission. It would be helpful in such an endeavor to use stimuli which stress or force the system out of equilibrium. This is another argument for the use of slow (e.g., 10/sec) and rapid (e.g., 30/sec) click repetition rates (Fujita, Hosoki, and Miyazaki, 1981). Such strategies may expose abnormal response patterns not otherwise apparent. Figure 12-3 shows the effect of various click repetition rates on the responses in a normal subject.

Such a strategy has been tested on neurologic patients by Chiappa, Gladstone, and Young (1979). There was no case in which the response to 60 dB SL stimuli was normal at 10/sec and abnormal at 30/sec. The increased rate of 70/sec was also not useful for evoking abnormalities. However, the amplitude of wave V is already saturated at 60 dB SL (i.e., wave V amplitude reaches its maximum at click intensities below 60 dB SL), so that the loss of a few incoming fibers going to the inferior colliculus due to the use of high click repetition rates may not affect the amplitude of this wave. Perhaps a more successful strategy would be to use a lower click intensity and to systematically study, in addition, the amplitudes and latencies of the other brain-stem response waves.

Absence of Waves 4 and 5 (IV/V and VI)

Since these waves are generated in the upper brain stem, their absence is usually correlated with conditions affecting the pons, such as head trauma affecting this region (Sohmer, Fahn, Amit, et al., 1978), pontine glioma (Fig. 12-5B), stenosis or occlusion of the basilar artery, and intrapontine hemorrhage (Fahn, 1979). Starr and Hamilton (1976) report a similar response pattern in the case of a pineal gland germinoma involving hemorrhage of the upper brain stem.

Absence of Waves 3, 4 and 5 (III, IV/V, and VI)

Such a pattern is observed in diffuse brain-stem lesions and in cerebellopontine angle tumors which probably do not originate within the interna auditory meatus (Fahn, 1979; Starr and Hamilton, 1976). Stockard and Rossiter (1977) report the same pattern in a case of caudal pontine tegmentum infarct. A case of congenital hypothyroidism has been reported with the presence only of waves I and II. Following the thyroxine treatment, waves 3, 4, and 5 (III, IV, V, VI) that originally were absent, subsequently appeared (Mendel and Robinson, 1978). The mechanism whereby low hormone levels could interfere with the generation of the response waves is not clear.

Absence of All Brain-Stem Components (II–VI) with Sparing of the Auditory Nerve Response (I)

This is seen in widespread diffuse brain-stem damage, such as arachnoiditis; severe psychomotor retardation in infants with enlarged ventricles (including the third and fourth ventricles) (Sohmer and Feinmesser, 1974; Sohmer, Feinmesser, and Szabo, 1974); herniation of the cerebellar tonsils; cerebellopontine angle tumors (Sohmer, Feinmesser, and Szabo, 1974; Fahn, 1979); in posterior fossa tumors (irrespective of their histologies) (Sohmer, Feinmesser, and Szabo, 1974); in brain death due to severe, prolonged anoxia (Feinmesser and Sohmer, 1976; Fahn, 1979; Starr and Hamilton, 1976; Uziel and Benezech, 1978); and in one case of lateral pontomedullary junction infarct (Stockard and Rossiter, 1977). Figure 12-5C shows the absence of the brain-stem responses with the preservation of the auditory nerve response in a patient with a large posterior fossa meningioma on the left side.

Absence of All Brain-Stem Responses

Complete absence of all response components is seen in cases of widespread brain-stem damage accompanied by brain-stem edema, retro-cochlear conditions which lead to loss of the auditory nerve response (see cerebellopontine angle tumor section), and in brain death. Worthington and Peters (1980) recently reported four cases in which the BSER was absent, although no neurologic deficits could be demonstrated. Such findings are in need of further substantiation. One instance of brain death is seen in Figure 12-5D. Initially, the only response present was that of the left auditory nerve; 3 days later, this response was absent. At autopsy, herniation of the cerebellar tonsils was found. Ahmed (1980) has observed similar findings. Experimental studies conducted on cats reveal a high correlation with work on humans (Nagao, Roccaforte, and Moody, 1979; 1980).

This pattern of "progressive" brain death beginning rostrally (centrally) and progressing caudally (peripherally) is a common finding. This is demonstrated in Figure 12-6, showing brain death in a cat. At first BTT is pro-longed, followed by disappearance of the later brain-stem components. With time, earlier brain-stem responses disappear leaving only the auditory nerve responses. Eventually, this is also lost.

In using auditory BSER in vital decisions (e.g., confirmation of brain death), it is essential to be absolutely certain that the patient has not suffered a fracture of the petrous part of the temporal bone, that blood clots or other debris is not blocking the external auditory meatus, and that normal hearing was present prior to the present disorder. In addition, one must absolutely make certain that the recording equipment is functioning properly. Therefore, in order to confirm the equipment's integrity, when no responses are obtained from a suspected brain-death patient, recordings should be taken from a known normal subject at the patient's bedside.

BSER APPLICATIONS

Pediatric Neurology

Several of the examples presented above of abnormal auditory BSER came from pediatric cases. These point out that BSER testing can contribute to diagnosis not only in adults but also in children (Crowell, Pang-Ching, and Anderson et al., 1980), where the clinical examination is sometimes difficult. The use of the high-risk register is still a good approach (Sarno and Clemis, 1980). Many congenital, perinatal, and neonatal insults, such as genetic-inborn errors of metabolism (e.g., phenylketonuria), rubella in pregnancy, perinatal asphyxia, ototoxicity (Schwent, Williston and Jewett, 1980), and neonatal hyperbilirubinemia (Kaga, Kitazumi, and Kodama, 1979) can in-

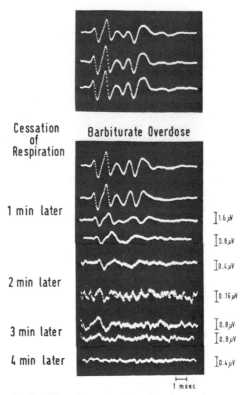

Cessation
of
Respiration   Barbiturate Overdose

1 min later   ]1.6 µV

                                                               ]0.8 µV

                                                               ]0.4 µV

2 min later   ]0.16 µV

                                                               ]0.8 µV
3 min later   ]0.8 µV

4 min later   ]0.4 µV

                              ⊢─┤
                              1 msec

Figure 12-6. The changes induced in the auditory nerve and brain-stem responses accompanying brain death in a cat. Initially, response latency (BTT) is prolonged, followed by the absence of the later brain-stem responses. Gradually, shorter latency responses are also absent, leaving only the response from the auditory nerve. Eventually this too is lost.

duce structural and biochemical changes in the developing brain. Following a clinically silent period of varying durations, these changes can give rise to various developmental disorders, such as psychomotor retardation, failure to thrive, and convulsions.

BSER recordings can assist in the detection of structural changes in the developing brain and thus contribute to diagnosis and lesion localization (Charachon and Dumas, 1980; Charachon, Dumas, and Richard, 1979). Such an approach may also lead to the early identification (during the clinically silent period), of these changes prior to the clinical manifestation of the developmental disorder. It can be posited, then, that the BSER can serve as a predictor of pediatric neurologic dysfunction (Galambos and Despland, 1980; Despland and Galambos, 1980; Sohmer, Gafni, and Tannenbaum, et al., 1979). Furthermore, the discovery of a new wave, the binaural interaction (BI) potential, may add additional power to the standard BSER test. This potential is more fully explained in Chapter 10. Additional discovery of "new" early waves such as the SN 10 (Hawes and Greenberg, 1981) and a 40 Hz response (Galambos, Makeig, and Talmachoff, 1981) will undoubtedly add further dimensions to this procedure.

Cerebellopontine Angle Tumors

Since the AERs have been mainly developed within an otologic-audiologic framework, one of the first neurologic disorders to be studied in detail via the AER was cerebellopontine angle tumor, since it invariably causes hearing loss (Portmann, Cazals, and Negrevergne, et al., 1980). These tumors mainly include the acoustic neuroma (occasionally called acoustic tumor, neurilemmoma, and vestibular schwannoma) and occasional meningioma of the angle. An acoustic tumor originates from migration of neurilemmal cells of the vestibular portion of the VIIIth nerve and may be located within the internal auditory canal or outside the canal, within the cerebellopontine angle. The symptoms of the patient are generally due to pressure on the cranial nerves and brain structures situated in the cerebellopontine angle. The main presenting symptoms include hearing loss, tinnitus, dizziness, decreased corneal reflex, and decreased facial sensation.

With the advent of ECochG and BSER testing, one of the first reported response patterns in cases of cerebellopontine angle tumors was the presence of a response from the auditory nerve (wave I), but the complete absence of other BSER waves (Sohmer, Feinmesser, and Szabo, 1974). We see an example in Figure 12-7B. The patient's chief complaint was intense tinnitus. The audiogram was generally normal except for a 20 dB loss at 4 kHz. This is of course consistent with the presence of a space-occupying lesion, located within a narrowly confined region, causing pressure on the auditory nerve and preventing propagation of impulses beyond the point of pressure (MacKay, Hosobuchi, and Williston, et al., 1980). This often gives rise to the seemingly paradoxical finding that the patient is suffering from a total hearing loss in that ear while a response from the auditory nerve, generated peripherally to the site of the tumor, is still present (an example can be found in Sohmer, Feinmesser, and Szabo, 1974). The preservation of the auditory nerve response in the absence of brain-stem responses in cases of cerebellopontine angle tumor has also been reported by other workers (Sagales, Gimeno, and Vallet, et al., 1977; Starr and Hamilton, 1976; Stockard and Rossiter, 1977). An additional response pattern seen in cerebellopontine-angle-tumor patients is the complete absence of all auditory nerve brain-stem responses (Selters and Brackmann, 1977; Clemis and McGee, 1979).

Several groups have reported finding prolonged BSER latencies in confirmed cases of acoustic tumors. They suggest paying particular attention to the absolute latency of wave 4B (V) in the suspected ear and comparing its

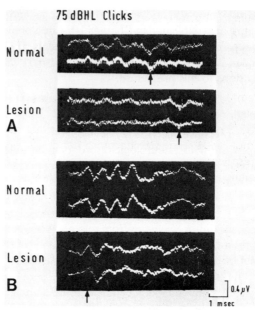

Figure 12-7. Auditory nerve and brain-stem response patterns seen in cerebellopontine angle tumors. A. The only response which can be seen on the side with the tumor is a long latency response from the region of the inferior colliculus. There were no signs of a conductive hearing loss. B. Taken from the tumor side of a second patient; only the auditory nerve response can be seen.

latency to that in the normal ear. In this way, the normal ear serves as a control for the ear with the suspected lesion. An interaural latency difference greater than 0.4 msec is considered confirmatory (Selters and Brackmann, 1977; Thomsen, Terkildsen, and Osterhammel, 1978; Clemis and Mitchell, 1977). However, the absolute latency of the brain-stem responses may be prolonged by many factors which are unrelated to cerebellopontine angle tumors, such as a conductive hearing loss. Therefore, it would be more advisable to use a relative latency measure—that is, the time interval between response waves, such as BTT (Fabiani, Sohmer, and Tait, et al., 1979). Such relative latency values have been found to be prolonged in several cases of acoustic neurinomas (Eggermont, 1977a). An example of prolonged latency in a case of cerebellopontine angle tumor is shown in Figure 12-7A, in which only wave 4-P_4(IV-V) can be seen; its latency is prolonged. Other workers report that occasionally acoustic stimulation of the normal contralateral ear also elicits a prolonged BTT (Selters and Brackmann, 1977; Rosenhamer, 1977; Shanon, Gold, and Himelfarb, 1981). BTT in the ipsilateral (tumor) ear was even more prolonged, so that there was still an interaural latency difference.

Continuing along these lines, one can see in Figure 12-5C, recordings in a patient with a large posterior fossa meningioma on the left. From the tumor side, only the first wave can be visualized, while stimulation of the normal ear elicits a distorted response from the region of the inferior colliculus (diminution of wave IV/V). This condition was thought to be due to an axial shift of the brain stem, induced by the large tumor; this was confirmed at surgery. A similar situation can be seen in an earlier article (Sohmer, Feinmesser, and Szabo, 1974). At that time, the prolonged BTT in the ear contralateral to the tumor was not recognized. On the other hand, the presence of all of the brain-stem responses with normal amplitude and latency is evidence against a cerebellopontine angle tumor.

In general, then, four different auditory nerve/brain-stem response patterns have been reported in cerebellopontine angle tumors: (1) prolonged response latency (BTT) on the lesion side, (2) prolonged response latency (BTT) occasionally on the contralateral side, (3) absence of BSER with preservation of the response from the auditory nerve, and (4) the complete absence of any response. These different response patterns probably represent different degrees of tumor growth and different tumor locations. During its early development, a tumor situated within the cerebellopontine angle would be expected to cause pressure on the nerve and cause a decrease of nerve conduction velocity, giving rise to the response pattern with prolonged latencies. A large tumor, or a tumor which develops within the internal auditory canal, may cause dysynchrony of nerve impulses or may be expected to completely block propagation in the nerve fibers, leaving only the auditory nerve compound action potential from the more peripheral segment of the auditory nerve fibers. Such a tumor may cause sufficient brain-stem distortion so as to cause decreased propagation in contralateral pathways. At a later stage, the pressure may cause retrograde degeneration of the auditory nerve fibers, or the pressure induced by the tumor may cause stenosis of the internal auditory artery. This may lead to cochlear ischemia and loss of the cochlear microphonic (CM) and the auditory nerve response. The preservation of a CM in such an ear may constitute evidence that the artery is still patent.

In conclusion, it seems that there is no single, consistent auditory BSER response pattern in cerebellopontine angle tumors. Rather, the pattern seems to depend on the functional changes induced by the size and location of the tumor.

Multiple Sclerosis

Multiple sclerosis (MS) is a demyelinating disease which has also been studied by evoked-response testing. The diagnosis of MS is particularly difficult, since it is mainly based on various clinical signs, reflecting the sites of some of the demyelinated plaques.

Laboratory examination of cerebrospinal fluid for particular constituents has been found to be helpful. It was hoped that the introduction of evoked-response testing would be able to provide objective evidence of lesions which are still clinically silent (Parving, Elberling, and Smith, 1981). The visual evoked response (see Chapter 14) has been found to be prolonged in latency even in the absence of visual complaints (Halliday, McDonald, and Mushin, 1973). Similarly, clinically silent plaques have been detected in the spinal pathways using somatosensory evoked-response techniques (Small, Matthews, and Small, 1978; see also Chapter 14).

Using the BSER, Robinson and Rudge (1977) and Stockard, Stockard, and Sharbrough (1977) have demonstrated prolonged latencies and diminished amplitudes of wave 4b (V) in cases of MS, even in patients lacking clinical auditory signs. Latency deviation was a more reliable indicator of abnormality than amplitude. This finding of a prolonged absolute latency of wave 4b (V) in MS has been more clearly defined as a prolonged BTT, which would be consistent with a slower nerve conduction velocity due to the demyelinization process. Waves II or 5 (VI) were also found to be diminished in amplitude or absent (Shanon, Gold, and Himmelfarb, et al., 1979).

Robinson and Rudge (1978) conducted serial brain-stem recordings on the same MS patients over periods of 9 to 30 months. In those patients who were clinically stable over this period, the BSERs were highly consistent. However, those MS patients who had clinical relapses during the serial study showed variations of the latency of wave 4b (V). Lacquaniti, Benna, and Gilli, et al., (1979) seem to have observed similar response variations over shorter periods of time. They report that for several patients, repeated, consecutive response traces could not be superimposed, indicating large, short-term, intertrial variability.

Examples of auditory BSER in MS are shown in Figure 12-8. Neither

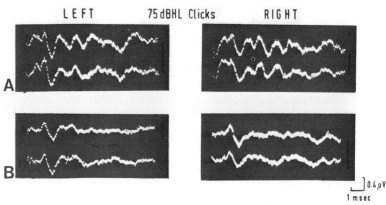

Figure 12-8. Auditory nerve and brain-stem responses in MS. None of these patients had auditory complaints. A. Note the prolonged BTT. B. Only the first three waves can be seen (on the left). On the right, the first wave is the clearest response present.

subject had any auditory complaints; more sophisticated audiologic testing would perhaps be required in order to expose an auditory dysfunction. Patient B was tested with a modified rapid alternating speech perception test. While normal subjects are able to correctly repeat 90-100 percent of the sentences, this patient was able to repeat only 4 percent, even though she had a normal pure tone audiogram for both ears (see also Bergman and Matathias, 1979).

Robinson and Rudge (1977) also recorded the middle-latency and cortical evoked responses to sound stimuli (see Chapter 13). About half of their patients showed prolonged latencies in several of the components. Prolonged latency in one of the cortical response components was observed only in a small number of patients.

The ability to detect central nervous system lesions in suspected MS patients even in the absence of clinical complaints in the sensory modality tested is very helpful, since two or more central lesions must be demonstrated in order to confirm a diagnosis of MS. When an additional lesion can be demonstrated in these patients by such a noninvasive technique, one can avoid the use of other hazardous procedures (e.g., myelography, angiography), which would otherwise be needed in order to exclude other disorders (Stockard, Stockard, and Sharbrough, 1977).

Effects of Coma

It is often difficult to diagnose the site-of-lesion which gives rise to a comatose state. The comatose condition prevents the use of the complete battery of sensory and motor function tests (e.g., behavioral testing of auditory, visual, and cutaneous sensation and voluntary motor responses). AER recordings in comatose patients can be particularly helpful. In our laboratory, auditory BSERs were recorded in 40 comatose patients very close to admission or soon after the patient had become comatose. These 40 patients were selected from a larger coma sample because there was additional supportive evidence for the site of the lesion.

The presumed etiology of the coma in these patients included head trauma incurred in road accidents, infectious states (meningitis or encephalitis), and anoxic-ischemic episodes (generally due to cerebrovascular accidents, or strokes). In one patient, the cause was the neurotoxin of a scorpion, and in others, barbiturate overdose. The patients' families reported that they had normal hearing prior to their comatose state. In most cases, the BSER was able to corroborate the suspected site of lesion as suggested by the clinical and laboratory findings. When one or more of the brain stem responses were absent, the clinical, radiologic, and morphologic findings also indicated a brain stem lesion. When all of the brain stem responses were present with normal amplitudes and latencies, clinical findings suggested a cerebral lesion.

Figure 12-9 shows examples of response traces obtained in several comatose patients. Trace A is from a 9-year-old girl in coma following a head injury in a road accident. She regained consciousness 7 days later. Trace B is from a 6-year-old boy in coma following meningoencephalitis. There was very gradual improvement in his condition; after 4 months, he was alert but quadriparetic. Note that in these two patients who regained consciousness, all of the response components were present. The final trace is from a 19-year-old male in coma who suffered from promyelocytic leukemia. Only the first two waves can be seen. This patient died 12 hours after admission. At autopsy, massive intracranial bleeding, probably due to leukemia infiltration, filling the ventricles was found. Starr and Hamilton (1976) and Uziel and Benezech (1978) have also used auditory BSER in the diagnosis of comatose patients.

It is interesting to note that these recordings contributed not only to the diagnosis of the coma in these patients, but also to their prognosis. Other workers have observed similar findings (Seales, Rossiter, and Weinstein, 1979). All of our patients in whom one or more of the brain-stem response components were absent either did not survive or remained in a chronic vegetative state. At the time of recording during the early stages of hospitalization, the initial clinical examination often could not indicate the exact site of the lesion. A brain-stem lesion, as indicated by the BSERs, was usually confirmed by later tests or at autopsy. Even more important, most patients in whom all the response components were present regained consciousness.

From the material presented in other studies, one can draw a similar conclusion concerning the poor prognosis when brain-stem waves are absent (Starr and Hamilton, 1976). In practice, the regaining of consciousness when all response components are present seems to be a common finding (Starr and Achor, 1975; Starr, 1976; Brinkmann and Ebner, 1977).

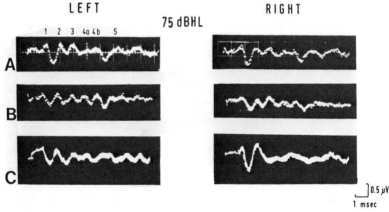

Figure 12-9. Auditory nerve and brain-stem responses in three comatose patients. Patients A and B, in whom each of the auditory nerve/brain stem responses could be recorded, regained consciousness. Patient C, lacking the later brain-stem response components, passed away shortly after the recordings were made.

BSER recording has been shown to have significant prognostic value in comatose patients with relatively normal hearing prior to the comatose state and who had not suffered a fracture of the petrous part of the temporal bone. Furthermore, when all brain-stem responses are present, there is reason to believe that the patient will regain consciousness. In contrast, if several or all of the brain-stem responses are absent, the patient's prognosis is not good (Amit, 1978). Somewhat similar findings have been reported by Greenberg, Becker, and Miller, et al., (1977b).

Role of Other Types of AER

Very little use has been made of the cortical response to auditory stimuli so as to understand neurological disorders. This is probably due to the greater variability of the cortical response (see Fig. 12-4), and to the absence of clarity as to the pathway (lemniscal, extralemniscal, or both) (David and Sohmer, 1972) involved, and as to the site of generation of the responses as the primary auditory cortex (Vaughn and Ritter, 1970) or other widespread cortical areas (Celesia and Puletti, 1969).

In a patient with a suspected neurologic disorder, in whom normal auditory BSERs are recorded, it should be worthwhile to record the cortical response to sound stimuli. For example, the latency of cortical late component N_1 was found to be prolonged in 4.5 percent of MS patients studied (Robinson and Rudge, 1977).

Compared to the paucity of the use of auditory-cortical responses, much greater use has been made of the somatosensory and visual (Halliday, McDonald, and Mushin, 1973; Celesia, 1978) cortical responses in the diagnosis of neurologic disorders (see Chapter 14).

Similarly, the middle-latency auditory evoked responses (see Chapter 13) have rarely been used to detect neurologic disorders, probably reflecting the uncertainties as to the neural generators of these potentials. Clarification of the sources, as has been undertaken (Hinnan, Buchwald, and Brown, et al., 1978), may lead to the increased use of middle-latency components in neurology.

With respect to both the middle- and long-latency responses, care must be taken to differentiate between myogenic and neurogenic sound-evoked contributions to the recorded waveforms (Bickford, Jacobson, and Cody, 1964). These muscle responses to sound stimuli are also known as sono-motor responses, and represent reflex muscle responses to sound stimuli activated by a brain-stem reflex pathway. The postauricular muscle response (PAR) has received recent attention in auditory diagnosis and in facial nerve palsy; responses could be recorded only in those cases with extracranial facial nerve damage, while the response was absent in patients with intracranial involvement (Bochenek and Bochenek, 1976).

As already indicated, the preservation of the cochlear microphonic response in a patient in whom the auditory BSERs are absent would be indicative of a functioning cochlear transduction system and a patent internal auditory artery. However, CM responses cannot always be recorded in normal elderly patients using surface electrodes and, therefore, if a unilateral lesion is suspected, one should attempt recording CM responses from the normal ear as well. One may draw conclusions from the absence of CM on the side of the lesion only if CM responses can be recorded from the normal ear.

Attempts have also been made to use ECochG (Portmann, et al., 1980) (see Chapter 11) in neurologic diagnosis, particularly in the diagnosis of cerebellopontine angle tumors. Recall that ECochG is defined as recording the electrical activity of the cochlea (AP, CM, SP) via a needle electrode which penetrates the tympanic membrane and makes contact with the promontorium near the round window of the cochlea (transtympanic ECochG). Several groups (Brackmann and Selters, 1976; Gibson and Beagley, 1976a, 1976b; Odenthal and Eggermont, 1976) report that a typical ECochG finding in patients with acoustic tumors was widening of the AP waveform. It is not completely clear how pressure on the auditory nerve would cause a widening of the waveform of the more peripheral segments of the auditory nerve. although attempts have been made to explain this phenomenon (Beagley, Legouix, and Teas, et al., 1977). However, these same workers also found such a widened waveform in Ménière's disease (a condition characterized by episodes of vertigo, tinnitus, and fluctuating hearing loss, thought to be due to labyrinthine hydrops causing increased hydrostatic pressure in scala media). In many patients with large tumors, no auditory nerve action potential could be recorded, but preservation of the CM response was taken as evidence that the blood supply to the cochlea was at least intact (Gibson and Beagley, 1976a).

Precautions

An absent response wave generally is a positive sign of abnormality. There is no sense, however, in using auditory AERs for diagnosis of a suspected neurologic legion in a patient with a profound hearing loss extant prior to the appearance of the suspected lesion. Also, in traumatic head injuries, one must make certain that the trauma has not caused fracture of the petrous part of the temporal bone. If responses are not recorded in both of these conditions, their absence cannot be taken as signs of a neurologic lesion. On the other hand, if a hearing loss is suspected to be due to a cerebellopontine angle tumor, this is ample evidence to record the auditory BSER since, as previously shown, a response from the auditory nerve may still be apparent, and its presence contributory to diagnosis.

Prolonged auditory BSER latencies can be problematic, since they are encountered in situations which do not involve neurologic disorders, such as excessive filtering, conductive hearing loss, lower stimulus intensities, low-stimulus frequencies, very high-stimulus repetition rates, severe sloping high-frequency hearing loss, hypothermia, and a unilateral profound hearing loss with acoustic crossover to the normal ear. Therefore, in order to properly evaluate suspected neurologic disorders by means of response latency, one must be able to clearly delineate between these factors (Chapter 10). When both wave I and wave V can be recorded, then their difference (as previously described) yields the BTT, which is independent of excessive filtering, conductive hearing loss, stimulus intensity, stimulus frequency, low- and moderate-stimulus repetition rates, high-frequency hearing loss, and acoustic crossover to the normal ear from an ear with a profound hearing loss. The situation becomes difficult when only wave V alone can be observed. This problem may be minimized by recording the electrocochleogram simultaneously from the external auditory meatus and the BSER from the vertex and mastoid (see Coats and Martin, 1977).

In those cases where recording the auditory nerve response from the ear canal is not desirable (e.g., patients with ear canal atresia), not feasible, or does not give better resolution of the auditory nerve response, other techniques must be used. Conductive hearing loss can usually be diagnosed by otoscopic examination, by air and bone conduction audiometry, and by tympanometry. High-frequency hearing loss can of course be determined in cooperative, adult patients by standard, pure tone audiometry. Such tests become problematic in uncooperative patients (e.g., infants, mentally retarded patients, comatose patients). Excitation of pathways originating in the normal ear by acoustic crossover from the ear with a profound hearing loss can be prevented by presenting, simultaneously, white noise masking to the normal ear. Examples of several of these situations are shown in Figure 12-10. Trace A is in response to 75 dB HL clicks; the second is from the same ear in response to 10 dB HL clicks. Note the prolonged latency of wave 4-P_4(V). Trace B shows recordings from an ear in response to 10/sec (upper) and 80/sec (lower) clicks. Here, too, the latencies are prolonged. These two situations are due to stimulus variables and can be controlled by the experimenter (see Chapter 9). Trace C shows recordings from the normal ear (upper) and from an ear with a conductive hearing loss (atresia of external ear canal) (lower) in an infant. One can clearly see waves I, III, and 4 (IV-V). Their latencies are prolonged. The recordings in D are from the normal ear (upper) and from the other ear with a high-frequency hearing loss. Note the small latency prolongation. The lower trace in E was recorded while stimulating and recording from an ear with a total hearing loss. A long latency wave 4 P_4(V) can still be seen, but this response disappeared when white noise masking was simultaneously presented to the normal ear. (Recordings from the normal ear are shown in the upper trace of E.) This procedure indicates that the response recorded from the totally deaf ear is actually due to the "leakage" of acoustic energy around the head, crossing over, and stimulating the normal ear. The final set of traces is from an ear with a cerebellopontine angle tumor, showing a prolonged response latency. Of all six sets of records

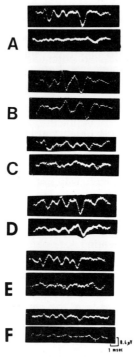

Figure 12-10. Examples of abnormally prolonged brain-stem response latencies. A. Responses in the same ear to two different click intensities. B. Responses to two different click repetition rates. C. Recordings from the two ears of an infant with a unilateral conductive hearing loss (congenital atresia of the external ear canal). D. Recordings from the normal ear and from the ear with a high frequency hearing loss. E. Recordings taken from a patient with a unilateral total hearing loss. Stimulation of that ear elicits a response due to the crossing over of acoustic energy to the normal ear. F. These recordings are the only ones in this Figure from a patient with a neurologic disorder—acoustic neuroma (there were no signs of a conductive hearing loss, only an average 45 dB loss).

showing prolonged latencies, the final trace is the only one due to a neurologic disorder. Each of these factors should be considered when interpreting response traces obtained in a patient.

DISCUSSION

In conclusion, auditory evoked potentials make great contributions to neurologic diagnosis in spite of the fact that they are generally not pathognomonic for any specific neurologic disorder. These contributions are offered in conjunction with any complementary clinical examination, other labatory tests and radiological studies. Nevertheless, in certain conditions, such as cerebellopontine angle tumors and MS, the auditory nerve/brain-stem trace may lead to an earlier diagnosis (Stockard, Sharbrough, and Westmoreland, et al., 1978). With a better understanding of several of the problems discussed above, auditory BSER tests will probably be making even greater contributions in the future.

Other types of sensory electrical potentials, such as visual and somatosensory responses in conjunction with auditory BSERs (Goldie, Chiappa, and Young, et al., 1981), are also being used in neurologic diagnosis (see Chapter 14). These techniques are undergoing further elucidation as well. For example, somatosensory evoked responses, presumably generated in peripheral nerve, dorsal column nuclei, medial lemniscus, and primary somatosensory cortex, have been recorded with surface electrodes in humans (Cracco and Cracco, 1976); natural stimuli were used to evoke these responses in humans (Pratt, Amlie, and Starr, 1979); and short latency visual responses have been investigated in humans (Cracco and Cracco, 1978). Together, these auditory, somatosensory, and visual evoked responses are being developed into a comprehensive, sensory evoked response diagnostic test battery (Greenberg, Mayer, and Becker, et al., 1977a), thus complementing the clinical and laboratory tests leading to earlier and more conclusive neurologic diagnosis and monitoring (Poland, Wells, and Ferlauto, 1980).

IV OTHER EVOKED RESPONSES AND UTILIZATION

John M. Polich
Arnold Starr

13 Middle-, Late-, and Long-Latency Auditory Evoked Potentials

This chapter surveys middle-, late-, and long-latency components (Fig. 13-1 and Table 13-1). Emphasis will be placed on normative data and the influence of exogenous and endogenous factors. The relevant applications will then be examined with attention to age differences, states of consciousness, and the diagnostic utility of the components in each latency range. The latter goal is made difficult by the fact that the neuroanatomic origins of these waveforms are not well known. Moreover, the late- and long-latency portions of the auditory evoked response (AER) are relatively variable, because the subject's psychological state can have strong effects on component latency, amplitude, and overall morphology. Several recent studies, however, have begun to explore the application of the middle-, late-, and long-latency components to clinical problems, and serve to illustrate their clinical possibilities in conjunction with the short-latency BSER.

MIDDLE-LATENCY COMPONENTS

Middle-latency AER components occur at a latency of 10-50 msec and have amplitudes ranging from 0.5 to 3.0 μV. They are generally denoted by the labels No, Po, Pa, and Nb, although Pb and Nc are occasionally seen with

The writing of this Chapter was supported in part by Grant R01 NS 11876-07, from the National Institute of Neurological and Communicative Disorders and Stroke, awarded to A. Starr.

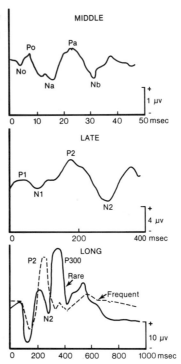

Figure 13-1. Examples of middle-, late-, and long-latency auditory evoked responses.

Table 13-1

Characteristics of Middle-, Late-,
and Long-Latency Auditory Evoked Potentials

Latency Class	Main Components	Latency Range (msec)	Amplitude Range (μV)	Exogenous Effects	Endogenous Effects
Middle	No	8–10	0.5– 3.0	Moderate to large	Very small
	Po	11–13			
	Na	16–25			
	Pa	25–35			
	Nb	35–45			
Late	P1	50–80	3.0–15.0	Moderate	Moderate to large
	N1	80–120			
	P2	160–200			
	N2	200–250			
Long	P3 or P300 (CNV, sustained potential, slow wave)	250–400	5.0–20	Small	Large

somewhat longer time bases (e.g., 10-80 msec). When the middle-latency components were initially reported (Geisler, Frishkopf, and Rosenblith, 1958) they were called the "early" AER responses, but have more recently been termed the middle-latency responses (Picton, Hillyard, and Krausz, et al., 1974; Davis, 1976b), due to the definition and increased interest in the auditory brain-stem response which occurs before the middle-latency group (Jewett and Williston, 1971; Skinner and Glattke, 1977; Starr, Sohmer, and Celesia, 1978).

The earlier middle-latency components (No, Po, Na) might arise from the medial geniculate and polysensory nuclei of the thalamus, while the later portions of the waveforms are found over wide areas of association cortex (Geisler, et al., 1958; Picton, Hillyard, and Krausz, et al., 1974; Davis, 1976b). Recordings from electrodes placed on the superior surface of the temporal lobe during intracranial surgery have yielded a large, positive wave similar to Pa in this latency range, quite similar to those obtained from the vertex of the scalp (Celesia and Puletti, 1969; Celesia, 1976). Several reports have noted that sound-evoked activity from scalp muscles occur at these same latencies, especially when the stimulus is relatively intense (Bickford, Jacobson, and Cody, 1964; Bickford, 1972; Picton, Hillyard, and Krausz, et al., 1974). While there is still debate over the neurogenic vs myogenic origins for middle-latency components, careful measurements of the relative contribution of scalp muscles (Picton, Hillyard, and Krausz, et al., 1974) and comprehensive scalp distribution studies of the middle-latency range (Goff, Matsumaiya, and Allison, et al., 1977; Goff, Allison, and Lyons, et al., 1977) suggest that these responses are primarily neural in origin, especially for stimuli of low-to-moderate intensities and when the electrode is not overlying the inion (Mast, 1963; 1965; Picton, Woods, and Baribeau-Braun, et al., 1977). However, recent clinical evidence with bilateral auditory cortical damage suggests that these responses do not arise from primary auditory cortex (Parving, Salomon, and Elberling, et al., 1980).

Normative Data

The maximal response for middle-latency components is obtained at the vertex and is symmetrical around this point (Peters and Mendel, 1974; Picton, Hillyard, and Krausz, et al., 1974). Middle-latency components are usually recorded from the vertex (Cz) referenced to a mastoid or earlobe, with a narrow band-pass filter of 25-200 Hz. As intensity is increased, latency (Fig. 13-2A) slightly decreases, whereas amplitude (Fig. 13-2B) substantially increases (Madell and Goldstein, 1972; Picton, et al., 1977; Thornton, Mendel, and Anderson, 1977). While click stimuli tend to evoke somewhat longer latencies and greater amplitude changes compared to tone bursts (Zerlin and Naunton, 1974; Zerlin, Naunton, and Mowry, 1973), tonal stimuli have been found to provide reasonably sensitive frequency-specific responses (Moushegian, Rubert, and Stillman, 1973; Kupperman and Men-

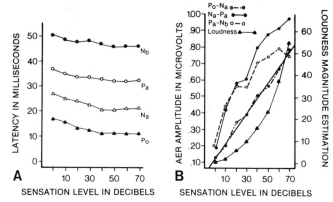

Figure 13-2. Effects of increases in intensity on the latency (A) and amplitude compared to behavioral measures of loudness (B) of middle latency components. (Reprinted with permission from Madell, J. R., and Goldstein, R. Relation between loudness and the amplitude of the early components of the average electroencephalic response. *Journal of Speech and Hearing Research*, 1972, 15: 134-141.)

del, 1974; McFarland, Vivion, and Goldstein, 1977; Thornton, et al., 1977). Stimulus onset, or rise time, also affects amplitude, whereas stimulus duration, or spectrum, has little influence (Lane, Kupperman, and Goldstein, 1971; Skinner and Antinoro, 1971).

Stimulus rates (Fig. 13-3) of 1 to 10 stimuli/second demonstrate little effect on amplitude, although higher rates do produce some overall amplitude decline (Goldstein, Rodman, and Karlovich, 1972; McFarland, Vivion, and Wolf, et al., 1975). A rapid adaptation of middle-latency responses may occur, since substantial decreases in overall component amplitudes are found with the first 500 stimulus presentations, and greater numbers of stimuli produce no significant amplitude reduction (Goldstein, et al., 1972; McFarland, et al., 1975; Vivion, Goldstein, and Wolf, et al., 1977). Presentation of a contralateral masking stimulus of moderate intensity does not appear to affect component amplitudes (Gutnick and Goldstein, 1978). Similarly, binaural stimulus presentation also shows little effect on the waveform at low-to-moderate levels of intensity (Peters and Mendel, 1974), but does produce an overall decrease in component amplitudes when intensities are greater than 70 dB nHL (Dobie and Norton, 1980).

Some reports indicate difficulty in obtaining reasonable waveforms in neonates (Engel, 1971; Davis, Hirsh, and Shelnutt, et al., 1974; Skinner and Glattke, 1977). Other studies, however, have been relatively successful, and note little difference between adult and infant morphology for middle components as a function of intensity, or rate of stimulus presentation (McRandle, Smith, and Goldstein, 1974; Goldstein and McRandle, 1976; Mendel, Adkinson, and Harker, 1977). The major differences between these populations are that neonates demonstrate slightly shorter latencies and smaller

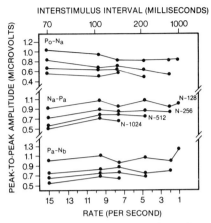

Figure 13-3. Effects of stimulus rate and number of trials on the middle-latency components of the auditory evoked response. (Reprinted with permission from Goldstein, R., Rodnan, L. B., and Karlovish, R. S. Effects of stimulus rate and number on the early components of the averaged electroencephalic response. *Journal of Speech and Hearing Research*, 1972, *15*:559-566.)

amplitudes than do adults, no significant activity is observed beyond 50 msec (Pb, Nc) as is often seen in adult waveforms, and ipsilateral stimulation produces more well defined waveforms than contralateral stimulation (Goldstein and McRandle, 1976; Mendel, Adkinson, and Harker, 1977; Wolf and Goldstein, 1978; 1980). Only the Pa component appears to increase in amplitude with an increase in neonatal age from 1 to 8 months (Mendel, Adkinson, and Harker, 1977). When these differences are taken into account, several researchers have noted the promise of middle-latency components as an auditory diagnostic tool for very young children (Davis, 1976a; Mendel, 1977; Vivion, 1980; Wolf and Goldstein, 1980).

The effects of endogenous factors on middle-latency components are minimal. They remain essentially unchanged with attention to the stimulus train, ignoring the stimulus as in reading a book, or sitting with eyes open or closed (Picton and Hillyard, 1974; Mendel and Goldstein, 1969a). The various stages of natural sleep (Mendel and Goldstein, 1971; Mendel, 1974; Mendel and Kupperman, 1974) or sleep deprivation (Mendel and Goldstein, 1969b) have little effect on the middle-latency responses. Similarly, light sedation does not diminish the overall response (Kupperman and Mendel, 1974; Mendel and Hosick, 1975; Mendel, Hosick, and Windman, et al., 1975), nor does skeletal muscle paralysis (Harker, Hosick, and Voots, et al., 1977). However, when complete anesthesia is attained, middle-latency responses are eliminated (Goff, Allison, and Lyons, et al., 1977), even when recordings are taken from the surface of the cortex (Celesia and Puletti, 1971).

Clinical Utility

Although the effects of many different parametric manipulations on middle-latency responses have been reported in the literature, there have been only a few studies of these components in clinical situations (Vivion, Hirsch, and Frye-Osier, et al., 1980). The main attempt has been to correlate middle-latency AER responses to behavioral measures of auditory threshold. For normal-hearing subjects, estimates of sound thresholds obtained with middle-latency measures range from 10 to 30 dB nHL of behavioral measures (Madell and Goldstein, 1972; Mendel, Hosick, and Windman, et al., 1975; McFarland, Vivion, and Goldstein, 1977; Skinner and Glattke, 1977; Vivion, Wolf, and Goldstein, et al., 1979). When hearing-impaired individuals are similarly compared, however, the studies that have been done find few systematic and reliable differences in the middle-latency waveforms compared to normals at the same suprathreshold intensity levels (McFarland, et al., 1977; Vivion, et al., 1979). The major problem with this approach seems to be the large intersubject variability obtained for the AER measures of threshold relative to behavioral indices. Thus, despite the frequency-specific sensitivity of the middle-latency components and their attractiveness as an audiometric tool (Davis, 1976b, Picton, et al., 1977), more refinement of the procedures is apparently necessary before they can be employed as an objective measurement technique for hearing evaluation. However, recent work by Galambos and his associates (Galambos, Makeig, and Talmachoff, 1981) has defined a series of middle-latency components obtained with 40 stimulus presentations/second. This "40 Hz evoked potential" appears to reflect the number and basilar membrane location of the auditory nerve fibers a given tone excites. Such an auditorially sensitive measure is a promising new approach for the clinical application of middle-latency components.

Middle-latency components of the AER have also been used in conjunction with brain-stem responses to study patients with multiple sclerosis (MS). An early study (Robinson and Rudge, 1975) noted latency and amplitude changes in the middle-latency AEPs for MS patients. When the auditory BSER and middle-latency responses from this patient population were later compared, 12 percent of the patients demonstrated significant latency abnormalities of the middle-latency components while obtaining normal brain-stem responses (Robinson and Rudge, 1977). Serial recordings of these patients indicated that abnormalities in the middle-latency responses could distinguish between active and quiescent disease states (Robinson and Rudge, 1978). This type of work points the way toward promising neurologic applications of the middle-latency components for assessing patients with brain lesions (Cohen and Rapin, 1978).

LATE-LATENCY COMPONENTS

The series of components occurring in the 50–250 msec range are called late components and are described in the middle row of Table 13-1. They consist of the P1, N1, P2, and N2 waves, and are relatively large in amplitude, ranging from 3 to 15 or more μV. The example provided in the middle portion of Figure 13-1 is illustrative of their morphology. Unlike the middle-latency components, the late-latency responses change in amplitude and latency as a function of endogenous variables related to the subject's psychological state. They are widely distributed over the frontal cortex, with the greatest amplitude at the vertex (Davis and Zerlin, 1966; Kooi, Tipton, and Marshall, 1971; Picton, Hillyard, and Krausz, et al., 1974), and have been called the V (or vertex) potentials (Davis, Mast, and Yoshie, et al., 1966). In addition to their frontal and central scalp distribution, there is also evidence that auditory stimulation contralateral to a temporally placed electrode produces larger waveforms than ipsilateral stimulation for these late components (Taub, Tanguay, and Doubleday, et al., 1976; Mononen and Seitz, 1972; Tanguay, Taub, and Doubleday, et al., 1977; Wolpaw and Penry, 1977).

The sources of the late components are unknown, although they can be obtained from the scalp with visual and somatosensory stimuli (Walter, 1964; Hay and Davis, 1971; Davis, Osterhammel, and Weir, et al., 1972; Chapter 14). On the basis of their frontal-central maximal distribution in the AER, it has been suggested that they originate from the frontal cortex (Picton, Hillyard, and Krausz, et al., 1974). Extensive recordings over the scalp and with depth electrodes indicate that a polarity reversal occurs for the N1-P2 waves across the Sylvian fissure (Vaughan and Ritter, 1970; Goff, 1978; Goff, Allison, and Vaughan, 1978), which implies some form of auditory cortex association. A recent comparison of patients with frontal or temporal cortex lesions demonstrated little effect on the amplitudes of the N1 or P2 components for frontal lesions. Extensive lesions of the temporal-parietal cortex, however, virtually eliminated the N1 component, although the P2 showed the same amplitude and refractory period as age-matched controls (Knight, Hillyard, and Woods, et al., 1980). Such data suggest involvement of the posterior-superior temporal plane and adjacent cortex of the parietal lobe in generation of the N1, with no support for contributions by the frontal cortical areas for at least the early portion of the late components.

Stimulus Variables

The comparatively large amplitudes of this portion of the AEP make definition of late-latency components relatively easy, with only 30 to 50 stimulus repetitions required to produce a clear waveform. The components have gradual slopes and are broad in duration. The usual filter settings employed are DC, or 1 to 30 or 100 Hz. Latency (Fig. 13-4A) of the N1-P2 components generally decreases as intensity is increased (Beagley and Knight, 1967; Onishi and Davis, 1968; McCandless and Lentz, 1968; Picton, et al., 1977), with click stimuli producing less of an effect than tones (Rapin, Schimmel, and Tourk, et al., 1966). Component latencies will also increase if the rise time of the stimulus tone exceeds 30 msec (Onishi and Davis, 1968). In general, latency changes due to stimulus intensity are quite variable close

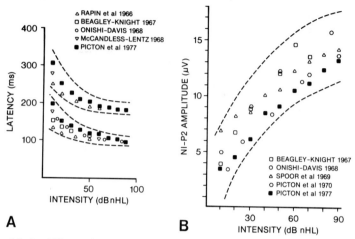

Figure 13-4.   Effects of intensity increases on the latency (A) and amplitude (B) of the late-latency components. (Reprinted with permission from Picton, T. W., Woods, D. L., and Baribeau-Braun, J., et al. Evoked potential audiometry. *Journal Otolaryngology*, 1977, 6:90-118.)

to threshold, but stabilize with signals 30 to 50 dB nHL more intense (Davis 1976b; Picton, et al., 1977).

Amplitude (Fig. 13-4B) increases with increases in stimulus intensity. The increase in amplitude from threshold to 20 dB nHL is steep; it then only gradually increases further up to about 80 to 100 dB nHL (Davis and Zerlin, 1966; Beagley and Knight, 1967; Onishi and Davis, 1968; Spoor, Timmer, and Odenthal, 1969; Picton, et al., 1977). Some individuals demonstrate a saturation or flattening of amplitude with stimulus intensities above 80 dB nHL. This effect is also influenced by the higher frequency tones (Nelson and Lassman, 1968; Antinoro, Skinner, and Jones, 1969; Moore and Rose, 1969; Khechinashvili, Kevanishvili, and Kajaia, 1973) and short inter-stimulus intervals (Picton, Goodman, and Bryce, 1970). Stimulus durations of 30 msec (Onishi and Davis, 1968) and rise-fall times of 20 msec yield good amplitudes (Skinner and Jones, 1968; Onishi and Davis, 1968; Ruhm and Jansen, 1969). The largest responses are also obtained to tone frequencies between 1000 and 2000 Hz (Evans and Deatherage, 1969; Rothman, 1970; Henderson, 1972). A sudden change in the stimulus parameters (e.g., frequency, intensity, etc.) will also produce large amplitude late components (Butler, 1968; McCandless and Rose, 1970; Picton, Hillyard, and Galambos, 1976; Tietze, 1979).

Increasing interstimulus intervals, or the refractory period (Fig. 13-5), causes an increase in N1-P2 amplitudes (Davis, Mast, and Yoshie, et al., 1966; Milner, 1969; Davis, et al., 1972), up to rates of about ten stimuli/ second when little further significant change in amplitude is observed (Ritter, Vaughan, and Costa, 1969; Fruhstorfer and Bergstrom, 1969; Fruhstorfer,

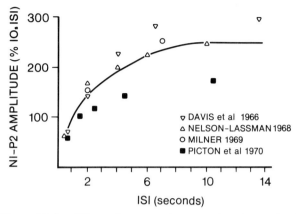

Figure 13-5. Effects of interstimulus interval on the amplitude of the N1 and P2 components. (Reprinted with permission from Picton, T. W., Woods, D. L., and Baribeau-Braun, J., et al. Evoked potential audimetry. *Journal of Otolaryngology*, 1977, 6: 90-119.)

Soveri, and Jarvilehto, 1970). Stimulus rate interacts with stimulus intensity and tone frequency (Picton, et al., 1970; Nelson and Lassman, 1968). Varying stimulus presentation rates between 0.5 and 4 seconds but keeping the average rate constant produces a slight increase in amplitude changes (Roth, Krainz, and Ford, et al., 1976). For most purposes, intervals of 1 to 2 seconds are recommended to obtain the optimum amplitude in a reasonable amount of recording time (Davis, 1976b; Picton, et al., 1977).

Subject Variables

The variability of the late component's amplitude with respect to changes in the rate of stimulation or variations in stimulus parameters reflects the sensitivity of these components to changes in the psychological state of the subject. The N1-P2 waves of the AER show a marked and systematic decrease in amplitude for repeated presentations of stimuli (Davis, Mast, and Yoshie, et al., 1966; Rothman, et al., 1970; Ohman and Lader, 1972), with the maximum decrease observed within 30 minutes after stimulus onset (Roeser and Price, 1969). Normal amplitudes can be immediately restored with slight changes in the stimulus parameters (Fruhstorfer, 1971; Salamy and McKean, 1977), or if the subject falls asleep (Firth, 1973; Townsend, House, and Johnson, 1976). Such findings seem to indicate the operation of habituation and dishabituation processes rather than sensory adaptation (see Picton, et al., 1976).

Another major influence on the late components arises from fluctuations in the direction of the subject's attention (see Hillyard, Picton, and Regan, 1978; Sabat, 1978; Picton, Campbell, and Baribeau-Braun, et al., 1978;

Näätänen and Michie, 1979). Many studies have found that the N1-P2 amplitude increases substantially when the subject focuses attention toward the
eliciting stimulus (Davis, 1964; Wilkinson and Morlock, 1967; Keating and
Ruhm, 1971; Picton, Hillyard, and Galambos, et al., 1971; Hillyard, Hink,
and Schwent, et al., 1973; Picton and Hillyard, 1974; Roth, et al., 1976;
Okita and Ohtani, 1977; Okita, 1979). The N1 component has been extensively studied in this context and found to increase 30-50 percent in
amplitude when attention is directed toward a specific pitch, locale, intensity,
or delivery rate (Fig. 13-6A) (Schwent and Hillyard, 1975; Schwent, Hillyard, and Galambos, 1976a, 1976b; Hink and Hillyard, 1976; Schwent,
Snyder, and Hillyard, 1976; Hink, VanVoorhis, and Hillyard, 1977; Hink,
Fenton, and Pfefferbaum, et al., 1978; Parasuraman, 1978). More recently,
the effect on N1 amplitude has been shown to result from an overall negative
displacement of the AER reflecting attentional instructions (Näätänen,
Gaillard, and Mantysalo, 1978; Chesney, Michie, and Donchin, 1980). This
negative displacement seems to imply that a simple gating mechanism for
human selective attention is not tenable (Hansen and Hillyard, 1980).

Waveform morphology, amplitude, and latency of the late components
generally become more variable in deep sleep (Williams, Tepas, and Morlock, 1962; Weitzman and Kremen, 1965; Rapin, Schimmel, and Cohen,

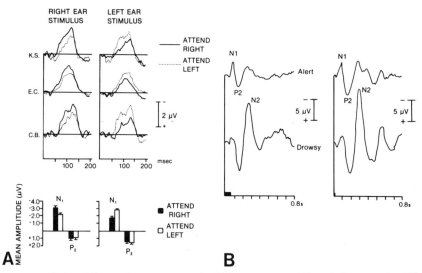

Figure 13-6. Effects of attention on the N1 component (A) and sleep on the N2
component (B) of the late-latency auditory evoked response. (A is reprinted with permission from Hillyard, S. A., et al. Electric signs of selective attention in the human
brain. *Science*, 1973, *182*:177-180. Copyright 1973 by the American Association for
the Advancement of Science. B is reprinted with permission from Picton, T. W., Hillyard, S. A., and Galambos, R. Habituation and attention in the auditory system. In
W. D. Keidel and W. D. Neff (Eds.), *Handbook of Sensory Physiology. Vol. V. Auditory Systems, part 3.* Heidelberg:Springer-Verlag, 1976.)

1972). Intensities of 30 dB nHL are often needed to elicit the long-latency components in sleeping adults (Osterhammel, Davis, and Wier, et al., 1973; Mendel, Hosick, and Windman, 1975). The N2 component (Fig. 3-6B) has been shown to dramatically increase in amplitude with sleep onset (Ornitz, Ritvo, and Carr, et al., 1967; Picton, et al., 1974) and deep sleep (Williams, et al., 1962). During REM (rapid eye movement) sleep, N2 latency is slightly shorter, with greater variability associated with all the components compared to other sleep stages (Ornitz, Ritvo, and Carr, et al., 1967a, 1967b). The late components during sleep also show marked changes in their amplitude and latency as a function of stimulus presentation rate compared to awake subjects (Ornitz, Tanguay, and Lee, et al., 1972; Ornitz, Lee, and Tanguay, et al., 1972; Ornitz, Tanguay, and Forsythe, et al., 1974). These changes, however, appear correlated with a basic rest-activity cycle of the nervous system that influences the long-latency responses of the AER during sleep (Tanguay, Ornitz, and Forsythe, et al., 1973), rather than to changes in the background electroencephalogram (EEG) activity, which occurs during the various sleep stages (Tanguay and Ornitz, 1972). In addition, use of sedation (e.g., chloral hydrate) to induce sleep also appears to increase the variability of the waveforms (Skinner and Antinoro, 1969; Hosick and Mendel, 1975; Skinner and Shimota, 1975), and alcohol has been found to diminish N1-P2 amplitudes (Krough, Khan, and Fosuig, et al., 1977; Wolpaw and Penry, 1978).

Maturation and maturity affect the latency of these components. They decrease in latency from birth to about 10 years of age, and lengthen thereafter. The amplitude increases during childhood and then becomes stable, eventually decreasing with advanced age (Callaway and Halliday, 1973; Ellingson, Danahy, and Nelson, et al., 1974; Callaway, 1975; Dustman, Schenkenberg, and Beck, 1976; Goodin, Squires, and Henderson, et al., 1978b; Ohlrich, Barnet, and Weiss, et al., 1978; Pfefferbaum, Ford, and Roth, et al., 1980a, 1980b). For infants in the first few months of life, component latency change appears to result directly from changes in sleep patterns which includes more "quiet" sleep (Rapin and Graziani, 1967; Weitzman and Graziani, 1968; Akiyama, Schulte, and Schultz, et al., 1969; Davis and Onishi, 1969; Barnet, Ohlrich, and Weiss, et al., 1975). Similar variability in waveform morphology, amplitude, and latency observed for changes in stages of sleep is then observed as with adults (Weitzman, Fishbein, and Graziani, 1965; Ferriss, Davis, and Dorsen, et al., 1967; Suzuki and Taguchi, 1968; Taguchi, Picton, and Orpin, et al., 1969). The most significant decreases in latency for the P2 component occur within the first year, although marked individual differences in variability have been reported (Barnet and Goodwin, 1965; Ohlrich and Barnet, 1972; Barnet, et al., 1975; Ohlrich, et al., 1978).

Clinical Utility

The major use of the late AER has been to evaluate hearing thresholds. In adults, the late components have yielded threshold estimates within 10 to

30 dB nHL of behaviorally obtained thresholds (McCandless and Best, 1966; Price, Rosenblut, and Goldstein, 1966; Davis, Hirsch, and Shelnutt, et al., 1967; Beagley and Kellogg, 1969; Botte, Bujas, and Chocholle, 1975; Pratt and Sohmer, 1977; 1978). Similar results have been reported for infants (Suzuki and Origuchi, 1969; Tyberghein and Forrez, 1971), although some studies have estimated infant thresholds with late components at 40 to 80 dB nHL above those obtained from adults (Appleby, 1975; Hrbek, Hrbkova, and Lenard, 1969; Lenard, von Bernuth, and Hutt, 1969). Use of these components for the evaluation of hearing loss has obtained mixed results (Davis, et al., 1967; McCandless, 1967; Taguchi, et al., 1970; Lentz and McCandless, 1971). Taken as a whole, this set of findings cautions against the routine use of late-latency components in audiometry until a better understanding of their implications is obtained (Roeser, Price, and Hnatiow, 1971; Rose, Keating, and Hedgecock, et al., 1972), or to employ them as one of several evoked-response audiometric tools (Picton, et al., 1977; Mendel, 1977; Picton and Smith, 1978; see also Chapter 12).

The late components of the AER have been used for quantifying various types of psychopathology (see Shagass, Ornitz, and Sutton, et al., 1978; Lifshitz, Susswein, and Lee, 1979; Roth, Ford, and Pfefferbaum, et al., 1979), and cerebral or neurologic dysfunction (Dustman, Snyder, and Callner, et al., 1979). Initial investigations of hyperactive children using the N1 and other late components of the AER have demonstrated smaller amplitude changes for this population for attentional manipulations compared to normal children (Zambelli, Stamm, and Maitinsky, et al., 1977; Klorman, Salzman, and Pass, et al., 1979; Loiselle, Stamm, and Maitinsky, et al., 1980). In general, however, the overall clinical utility of this portion of the AER has not been great because of the large inter-and intrasubject variability and nescience of the specific neural generators for these components (Mendel, 1977; Starr, Sohmer, and Alesia, 1978, Cracco, 1979).

LONG-LATENCY COMPONENTS

After 250 msec, the general characteristics of the AER dramatically change from that of groups of fairly uniform responses to highly variable and subject-dependent manifestations of perceptual and cognitive activity. A variety of different types of waveforms, such as the P3, the contingent negative variation (CNV) (see Tecce, 1972; Hillyard, 1973; Reneau and Hnatinow, 1975), sustained potential (see Picton, et al., 1977; Picton, Woods, and Proulx, 1978a, 1978b), and slow waves (see Rohrbaugh, Syndulko, and Linsley, 1978, 1979; Ruchkin, Sutton, and Stega, 1980; Ruchkin, Sutton, and Kietsman, et al., 1980) can be observed. The P3 wave (also termed the P300 or sometimes the late positive component) is probably the most studied in this latency range, and is similar in form for visual and somatosensory stimuli (Snyder, Hillyard, and Galambos, 1980). It is described in the bottom row of Table 13-1 and is illustrated in the lower portion of Figure 13-1. Several comprehensive reviews are available which survey the broad spectrum of research findings from various paradigms and theoretical interpretations (see Picton, Woods, and Proulx, 1978a; Donchin, Ritter, and McCallum, 1978; Donchin, 1979; Sutton, 1979). The focus here will be to review the basic findings of the P3 and then to examine the relevant clinical data.

The P3 component can be observed with a number of stimulus presentation conditions in which the subject must process task-relevant information. The most common situation for auditory stimuli is called the "oddball" paradigm, and consists of the subject covertly counting relatively rare occurrences of a target tone embedded in a series of more frequently occurring standard tones. While the target tone is physically different from the standard tones (e.g., different frequency, intensity, etc.), it is not the physical difference which produces the large (10–20 μV), positive-going component with about a 300 μsec latency, but rather the information supplied to the subject with the occurrence of the relevant target tone (Sutton, Braren, and Zubin, 1965; Sutton, Braren, and Zubin, et al., 1967). That the information content of the target and not the change in physical stimulus is responsible for the production of the P3 component is known because the same response is also obtained by omitting a stimulus in a series of tones and having the subject count the number of omissions (Klinke, Fruhstorfer, and Finkenzeller, 1968; Picton, Hillyard, and Krausz, et al., 1974). Another method is to have the subject detect a near-threshold signal which may occur at a specific time (Ritter and Vaughan, 1969; Hillyard, Squires, and Bauer, et al., 1971; Hillyard, Hink, and Schwent, et al., 1973). In each case, a P3 component can be obtained with as few as 20 to 30 replications of the relevant target event with very low band-pass cutoffs (e.g., 0.01 Hz, Duncan-Johnson and Donchin, 1979). These observations suggest that the P3 component is associated with the detection of a task-relevant stimulus event and a memory-updating process involved with the decision that a novel event has been perceived (Donchin, et al., 1978; Picton, et al., 1976).

The P3 component amplitude is maximal in the central-parietal midline area and bilaterally symmetric for most types of auditory tasks, as well as for other modalities (Simson, Vaughan, and Ritter, 1976; 1977). Because of these findings, it was originally thought that P3 and the associated long latency potentials (e.g., P2 and N2) were cortical in origin. However, several reports employing the oddball auditory paradigm and measuring intracranial brain activity with multicontact electrodes have implicated subcortical brain structures (Goff, et al., 1978; Wood, Allison, and Goff, et al., 1978), such as the hippocampal formation and amygdala (Halgren, Squires, and Wilson, et al., 1980). Thus, the source of the brain's response to the oddball tone paradigm may involve deep brain structures not directly involved with the auditory cortex (Goff, Williamson, and VanGilder, et al., 1980).

Endogenous Effects

Implied by the use of the oddball task for the production of the P3 wave is the sensitivity of this wave to a changing stimulus environment. This sensitivity is manifested in numerous ways but is perhaps most apparent in the systematic amplitude changes as a function of the a priori probability of the target stimulus. Many studies have demonstrated that the less probable the target event (given that the subject is attending to the sequence), the greater the amplitude of the resulting P3 component (e.g., Tueting, Sutton, and Zubin, 1971; Donchin, Kubovy, and Kutas, et al., 1973; Duncan-Johnson and Donchin, 1977). A thorough analysis of this effect performed on a trial-by-trial basis has revealed that not only does the objective probability of the target stimulus affect P3 amplitude, but the subjective probability generated by expectancy contributes to amplitude difference. As the number of immediately preceding trials consisting of the standard tone increases, P3 amplitude increases, reflecting fluctuations of the subject's expectancy in conjunction with his or her short-term memory store for the preceding events (Squires, Wickens, and Squires, et al., 1976; Squires, Petuchowski, and Wickens, et al., 1977; Johnson and Donchin, 1980).

These effects require the subject to attend to the target stimulus. When this condition is not met, the P3 component will not be generated, regardless of the target event's probability (Ford, Roth, and Dirks, et al., 1973; Ford, Roth and Kopell, 1976; Squires, Donchin, and Herning, et al., 1977). If the subject is engaged in the appropriate task-relevant behavior(s), however, and attention is directed elsewhere but the subject is able to successfully perform the primary oddball counting task, P3 amplitude has been shown to decrease systematically as a result of the difficulty of the secondary task (Isreal, Chesney, and Wickens, et al., 1980; Isreal, Wickens, and Chesney, et al., 1980). Thus, overall P3 amplitude is governed by factors related to a cognitive participation in the eliciting task events.

Latency of the auditory P3 component has been found to increase as a function of task difficulty (Wilkinson and Morlock, 1967; Ritter, Simson, and Vaughan, 1972; Squires, Donchin, and Squires, et al., 1977; Ritter, Simson, and Vaughan, et al., 1979) and age of subject (Goodin, et al., 1978a; Squires, Chippendale, and Wrege, et al., 1980). The latter effect—subject age—is illustrated in Figure 13-7, for a modified oddball task wherein target and non-target stimuli were presented 20 percent of the time and the frequent stimuli presented 80 percent (Pfefferbaum, Ford, and Roth, et al., 1980a). Although the subjects manually indicated the occurrence of the target event, a P3 component was also generated to the rare non-target stimulus. Note the maximal amplitude at the central-parietal sites and the latency differences be-

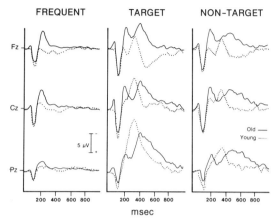

FREQUENT   TARGET   NON-TARGET

Fz

Cz

Old ——
Young ·····

5 μV

Pz

200 400 600 800   200 400 600 800   200 400 600 800

msec

Figure 13-7. Comparison of young and older subjects' P3 components from an auditory oddball paradigm with both target and non-target rare tones. (Reprinted with permission from Pfefferbaum, A. Ford, J. M., and Roth, W. T., et al. Age-related changes in auditory event-related potentials. *Electroencephalography and Clinical Neurophysiology*, 1980b, 49:266–276.)

tween young and older subjects after the N1 component, but not before (Goodin, et al., 1978a).

Because the P3 is sensitive to changes in the subject's psychological state, latency measures taken from the peak of the waveform averaged over individual trials can reflect variability often unassociated with the specific variables of interest (e.g., attention fluctuation, subjective probability). Moreover, visual analysis of the P3 peak latency can be difficult because of the variety of possible peaks associated with P3 waves obtained with auditory stimuli (Squires, Squires, and Hillyard, 1975; Snyder and Hillyard, 1976). One approach to overcoming this difficulty has been to employ an iterative correlational technique on individual target tone trials, in order to eliminate latency jitter in the final average (Woody, 1967; Ruchkin and Glaser, 1978). This technique has proven successful in examining precise latency differences in several populations of interest (Pfefferbaum, Horvath, and Roth, et al., 1979; Ford and Pfefferbaum, 1980; Michalewski, Patterson, and Thompson, et al., 1980).

Clinical Applications

Use of the P3 component to examine clinical populations is a relatively new endeavor. Most often, visual stimuli are employed in some form of cognitive task situation to investigate various forms of psychopathology (e.g., Shagass, et al., 1978; Roth, et al., 1979), attentional or memory abilities in the aged (Ford, Roth, and Mohs, et al., 1979; Pfefferbaum, et al., 1980a; Smith, Thompson, and Michalewski, 1980), as well as a host of problems in human information processing (Donchin, et al., 1978; Donchin, 1979). Some possibilities also exist for the use of the auditory P3 in audiometric evaluation (Picton, et al., 1977; Picton and Smith, 1978).

The simple auditory oddball paradigm has been applied to the evaluation of changes in cognitive functioning due to aging (Goodin, et al., 1978b; Squires, Aire, and Buchwald, et al., 1980). Capitalizing on the theoretical implications of the P3 component as reflecting short-term memory function during stimulus categorization, Goodin, Squires, and Starr (1978) measured P3 latency in normals, demented patients, and non-demented patients. The main findings are presented in Figure 13-8. While normals and non-demented patients demonstrated an increase in P3 latency as a function of age (Goodin, Squires, and Starr, 1978; Pfefferbaum, Ford, and Roth, et al., 1980b), the demented population produced P3 latencies that were generally more than two standard deviations beyond their age-matched controls. In another related study, patients were followed serially and their mental abilities

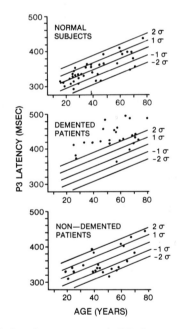

Figure 13-8. Comparison of P3 latencies for normal, demented, and hospitalized non-demented subjects as a function of age. (Reprinted with permission from Goodin, D. S., Squires, K. C., and Starr, A. Long latency event-related components of the auditory, evoked potential. *Brain*, 1978, 101:635-648.)

were measured with a standard psychometric exam over the course of their hospitalization. Their P3 component latencies decreased over time, as mental status improved (Squires, Aire, and Buchwald, et al., 1980). A recent investigation by Pfefferbaum, et al. (1979) employed the same methodology and found P3 latencies in chronic alcoholics were appreciably slower than their age-matched normal controls. The authors concluded that long-standing alcoholism produces the same type of mental disability as that associated with a demented population (Goodin, Squires, and Starr, 1978). These studies illustrate the possible applications of the P3 component derived from a task involving minimal subject cooperation.

SUMMARY

There is still considerable work needed to define the general clinical utility of the middle-, late-, and long-latency AER components. However, there is some promise for latency components to measure aural perception, or "hearing." The P3 component is particularly suited to this last categorization. Use of AERs can also have important applications to the measurement of various cognitive processes, such as the decline in mental ability associated with aging. The major problems in the application of the late- and long-latency components are their sensitivity to factors of age, attention, and the structure of the subject's task. If the precise influence of these variables can be readily understood, AERs may provide a wide range of clinical measures— from cochlear function to cognitive processing—and they should enhance the short-latency BSER diagnostic battery.

Roger Q. Cracco
Gastone G. Celesia

14 Somatosensory and Visual Evoked Potentials

It is becoming increasingly important to introduce or include other sensory modality responses within the diagnostic scheme. As such, it is incumbent upon both the audiologist and otologist to have at least a working knowledge of other sensory modality responses.

This chapter describes the possible roles and probable contributions of averaged evoked potentials other than those elicited by auditory stimulation. Several disciplines routinely employ multimodality evoked responses; for example, when direct contact is made with the neurologist or when referrals are made to neurology departments.

An entire volume could certainly have been devoted to the subjects of this chapter; nevertheless, it was not possible to include a number of tutorial topics pertinent to visual and somatosensory evoked responses. For a more detailed description and background to multimodality potentials, one should consult several of the relevant references within this chapter (listed at the end of this volume).

SOMATOSENSORY EVOKED POTENTIALS

Studies of averaged somatosensory evoked potentials (SEP) demonstrate that these noninvasive methods permit an evaluation of the human nervous system from peripheral nerves to cerebral cortex. Potentials evoked in response to peroneal nerve or tibial nerve stimulation, which arise in the cauda equina and in spinal cord afferent pathways, have thus been recorded from surface electrodes placed over the spine (Liberson, Gratzur and Zales, et

363

al., 1966; Cracco, 1973; Dimitrijevic, Larsson, Lehmkuhl, et al., 1978). Cerebral evoked potentials in response to stimulation of nerves in the lower extremities have been recorded from the scalp (Tsumato, Hirose, Nonaka, 1972; Perot, 1973). Additionally, SEPs in response to median nerve stimulation which arise in peripheral nerves, subcortical, and cortical structures have been recorded from the scalp (Dawson, 1954a, 1954b; Goff, Rosner, and Allison, 1962; Cracco and Cracco, 1976; Kritchevsky and Wiederholt, 1978).

In this section, the results of studies concerning peripheral nerve, spinal cord, subcortical, and cortical SEPs are reviewed.

Peripheral Nerve Action Potentials

Conduction velocities over peripheral segments of certain peripheral nerves can be determined without using averaging techniques; these determinations are routinely made in the electromyography laboratory. Information concerning conduction in both proximal and distal segments of motor nerve fibers can be obtained by determining F wave latencies, while H reflex studies give information concerning conduction in proximal and distal segments of both sensory and motor fibers.

Averaged evoked potentials can also be recorded from both proximal and distal segments of peripheral nerves (Liberson, et al., 1966; Cracco and Cracco, 1976). The median nerve may be stimulated at the wrist, for example, and recording electrodes (consisting of discs attached to the skin) may be placed over the course of the nerve from the point of stimulation to the spinal cord. The peripheral nerve action potential may be recorded via bipolar leads (interelectrode distance 3-4 cm) or via reference leads, where the reference electrode is placed at a distance from the nerve. Although supramaximal stimulation of the nerve is academically ideal, it is painful and usually not tolerated. The intensity of stimulation (duration 0.1-0.2 msec) is therefore adjusted to produce a good thumb twitch. Intensity should be below a level that causes discomfort. The nerve can be stimulated at rates up to 10/sec, at which the response is not affected (faster rates are usually uncomfortable for the patient). Responses elicited by 20 to 1000 stimuli may be summated; analysis times of 20 msec may be used. Since the median nerve is a mixed nerve, the potential evoked by stimulating this nerve at the wrist arises in both sensory and motor fibers. If information only concerning sensory fibers is desired, stimulating ring electrodes may be applied to the index finger; since the digital nerve is purely sensory, the potential recorded along the course of the median nerve will reflect activity arising only in sensory fibers.

The evoked response recorded along the course of the nerve typically consists of an initially positive, predominantly negative, triphasic potential (Fig. 14-1). One or both positive phases may be poorly defined at certain recording locations. The onset of the negative potential is often used to

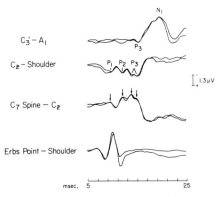

$C_3' - A_1$

C_z – Shoulder

C_7 Spine – C_z

Erbs Point – Shoulder

msec. 5   25

Figure 14-1. Somatosensory evoked potential (SEP) in response to right median nerve stimulation; 2048 responses were
summated in each recording and two recordings are superimposed in each trace. There is a 5 msec delay between the
stimulus and the sweep onset. In the C_3' ear recording, a small
positive potential (peak latency 15 msec) is followed by a negative potential (peak latency 20 msec). In the C_z noncephalic reference lead, three short-latency positive potentials are recorded,
the third of which is bilobate. In the C_7 spine-C_z lead, four
potential peaks are recorded. An initially positive, predominantly negative, triphasic potential is recorded over Erb's point.

measure response latency and to determine conduction velocity, since this is
when the fastest fibers contributing to the response pass under the recording
electrode (in reference leads) and under the electrode nearest the approaching volley (in bipolar leads) (Gilliat, Melville, and Velate, 1965). The
negative potential peak can also be used to determine response latency. The
conduction velocity along any segment of nerve may be determined by
dividing the distance between two recording locations by the difference in
response latency between those locations. These values are slow in many patients with disorders affecting peripheral nerves.

Median Nerve Evoked Potentials

Short-Latency Potentials

Stimulating electrodes are placed over the median nerves just proximal
to the wrist. These electrodes usually consist of discs that are attached to the
skin with collodion and filled with conductive jelly. The cathode is placed 2-3
cm proximal to the anode. Needle-stimulating electrodes are used in some
laboratories, and have the advantage that the effective stimulus level is lower;
the shock artifact is therefore reduced. Needle electrodes have the disadvantage that the skin must be penetrated, which causes subject discomfort.

Sterlization of needle electrodes is required. The stimulus intensity (pulse duration 0.1-0.2 msec) is adjusted to produce a clear thumb twitch. This intensity should be below the patient's threshold level for discomfort. Analysis time should be 25-40 msec, and stimulus rates of 5-10/sec are used. A large number of potentials (1000-4000) must be summated to get good definition, because of the potentials' small signal size (Cracco and Cracco, 1976). These potentials are not significantly affected at these rapid stimulus rates. A frequency response of 10-3000 Hz is commonly used.

The methods used to record these potentials have not yet been standardized. In most clinical laboratories, short-latency potentials are being recorded via leads in which a recording electrode is placed at C_3' (2 cm behind C_3, International 10-20 System) (right median nerve stimulation) and C_4' (left median nerve stimulation). These locations overlie the specific somatosensory receiving area for median nerve stimulation. An ear or frontal scalp location (F_z) serves as the reference electrode site. The short-latency components recorded using this derivation consist of positive, negative, and positive potentials with peak latencies of about 14, 19 and 25 msec (Fig. 14-1). The median nerve evoked action potential is also recorded over the brachial plexus at Erb's point, ipsilateral to the side of stimulation (Fig. 14-1). The peak latency differences between the prominent negative peak of the Erb's point potential and the scalp-recorded components are measured. In this way, the variability in latency of the scalp-recorded potentials (due to differences in arm length and temperature) are eliminated.

C_z- noncephalic reference leads are used to record short-latency SEPs in some laboratories. The shoulder, hand, or knee contralateral to the side of stimulation serves as the reference site. These recordings may be noisy, because of the noncephalic location of the reference electrode. Expert technique is required to record these potentials in this way. Patients may be sedated if necessary. Using this derivation, three positive potentials are followed by a negative potential (P_1, P_2, P_3, and N_1), with approximate peak latencies of 9, 11, 13, and 19 msec (Fig. 14-1). P_2 is not consistently recorded in all normal subjects. P_3 is often bilobate; the approximate latencies of the two peaks are 13 and 14 msec. Abnormalities of these potentials are based on the absence of consistently recorded components (P_1, P_3, N_1) and increased interpeak latency differences between components (Anziska, Cracco, Cook, et al., 1978; Anziska and Cracco, 1980a, 1980b).

P_3 and N_1 recorded in C_z-noncephalic reference leads roughly correspond to the first positive and negative potentials recorded in C_3' or C_4' ear reference leads, described above, although their peak latencies may not be identical in the two derivations. P_1 and P_2 are poorly defined or absent in scalp-ear leads, because they are similar in amplitude at all cephalic locations and undergo cancelation in scalp-ear recordings (Cracco and Cracco, 1976).

Cervical spine-scalp leads are also used to record these potentials (Jones,

1977). The cervical electrode is placed over the spine, usually at C_7 or C_2, and is linked to a scalp electrode placed at F_z or C_z. A well-defined potential with up to three inflections (peak latencies of about 11, 13, and 14 msec) is recorded using this derivation. These inflections are sometimes preceded by a small potential, peaking at about 9 msec (Fig. 14-1). Abnormalities of these potentials are judged on the basis of decreased amplitude or absence of potentials and increased duration of potentials (Small, Mathews, and Small, 1978; Chiappa, Choi and Young, 1980; Eisen, Steward, Nudleman, et al., 1979).

Generator sources. In contrast to the auditory brain-stem evoked responses, a preliminary consensus has not yet been reached concerning the neural origins of the short-latency SEPs. Based on a study of 31 patients with focal lesions of the nervous system, Anziska and Cracco (1980) have provided evidence which suggests the following origins for these potentials recorded in scalp noncephalic or scalp ear leads: P_1 originates in proximal segments of stimulated median nerve fibers as they course from the axilla to cervical spinal cord; P_2 originates in the cervical spinal cord and dorsal columns; P_3 develops from brain-stem and diencephalic pathways, with the medial lemniscus being the primary source; and N_1 originates in thalamocortical radiations and cerebral cortex. The positive potential following N_1 which peaks at 25 msec arises in specific somatosensory cortex. Subsequent potentials are thought to be cortical in origin. The generator sources of potentials arising within the first 15 msec recorded in neck-scalp leads is uncertain; it has not yet been demonstrated that components of similar latency recorded in neck-scalp and scalp-noncephalic reference leads have identical origins.

Abnormalities of these short-latency SEPs have been found in patients with peripheral nerve lesions, cervical root avulsion, focal subcortical lesions (situated along the neuraxis from cervical spinal cord to somesthetic cortex), brain death, and degenerative diseases (Anziska and Cracco, 1980; Chiappa, Choi, and Young, 1980; Cracco, Bosh, and Cracco, 1980). Several studies demonstrated abnormalities of these short-latency SEPs in a significant number of patients with multiple sclerosis (MS), even in the absence of relevant clinical signs or symptoms (Mastaglia, Black, Cala, et al., 1977; Anziska, et al., 1978; Small, et al., 1978; Eisen, et al., 1979) (Fig. 14-2). Such studies, used in combination with visual and auditory evoked potentials, will be of obvious value in demonstrating the presence of multiple lesions in MS patients, which is essential in making this diagnosis. The audiologist and otologist would do well to require these tests on certain of their patients.

Hume and Cant (1978) reported a method for measuring what they termed *central somatosensory conduction time.* SEPs to median nerve stimulation were simultaneously recorded from cervical spine-(C_7 or C_2) scalp (F_z) leads and from the scalp (C_3 or C_4), using F_z or combined ears as ref-

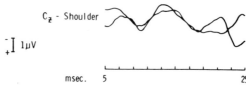

Figure 14-2. Patient with multiple sclerosis (MS) with no abnormal sensory, brain stem, or cerebellar findings on examination. Stimulation of the right median nerve elicits only a P_1 potential. (Reprinted with permission from Anziska, B., Cracco, R. Q., and Cook, A. W., et al. Somatosensory far field potentials: Studies in normal subjects and patients with multiple sclerosis. *Electroencephalography and Clinical Neurophysiology*, 1978, 45:602-610.)

erence. The peak latency difference between the first negative potential (N_1) of the scalp-recorded SEP and the major component recorded in the neck-scalp lead was thought to reflect central conduction time from caudal brain stem to cerebral cortex. Determinations of this central conduction time in a group of comatose patients at 10 and 35 days after the onset of coma were shown to significantly correlate with the patients' eventual outcome (Hume, Cant and Shaw, 1979). It can be seen that the addition of SEP to the diagnostic regimen can prove useful when auditory stimulation is contraindicated or impossible.

Short latency SEPs in response to stimulation of mechanical receptors in the finger have been recorded over the peripheral nerve and from the scalp (Pratt, Starr, Amlie, et al., 1979). Such work is important for two reasons: First, unlike electric shock, this form of stimulation is more "natural." Second, such techniques provide a method for evaluating cutaneous receptors as well as peripheral nerves and central afferent pathways. The disadvantage of this method is that the sensory elements are less synchronously depolarized, resulting in lower-amplitude evoked potentials, due to the greater temporal dispersion of impulses.

After a consensus is reached concerning the generator sources of each of the short-latency SEP components, the recording of these potentials will have greater application in the evaluation of patients with nervous system disorders. It will then be possible to define a neuraxis lesion site from cutaneous receptor to somesthetic cortex.

Longer-Latency Potentials

The methods used to record these potentials resemble those used to record the short-latency SEPs, with the following exceptions. Stimulation rates should not exceed 1-2/sec, because many of these components are significantly attenuated at rapid rates of stimulation. These potentials are greater in latency, duration, and amplitude than the short-latency potentials. Therefore, fewer (100-200) responses need to be summated, longer analysis times (100-500 msec) are required, and a frequency response of 1-1000 Hz is commonly used.

Recording electrodes are usually placed over the specific somatosensory receiving area, which is about 2 cm behind C_3 and C_4 for right and left median nerve stimulation, respectively. Ear reference recordings are usually obtained, although frontal scalp locations have also served as reference sites despite their activity in these SEPs. More scalp electrodes can be applied in topographic studies of these potentials.

Generator sources. The short-latency positive, negative, and positive potentials recorded in scalp-ear leads (described in the preceding section) are followed by a series of negative and positive components lasting several hundred msec, which are widespread in their distribution over the scalp (Goff, Matsumiya, Allison, et al., 1977; Giblin, 1964) (Fig. 14-3). These longer-latency potentials show considerable variability both within and across subjects. They are sensitive to changes in level of consciousness, as well as other ill-defined factors (Cracco, 1972). The longer-latency potentials are

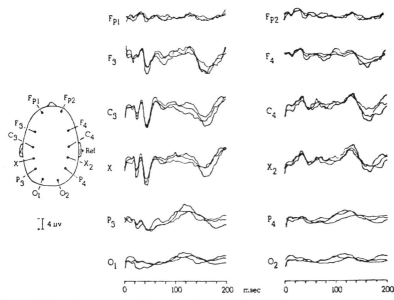

Figure 14-3. Distribution of the longer-latency scalp-recorded somatosensory evoked potentials to right median nerve stimulation in right ear reference recordings. Three recordings are superimposed in each trace. The X scalp electrode lies over somatosensory cortex. Early components are most prominent overlying somesthetic scalp regions contralateral to the side of stimulation. Later components are more generalized. (Reprinted with permission from Calmes, R. L., and Cracco, R. Q. Comparison of somatosensory and somatomotor evoked responses to median nerve and digital nerve stimulation. *Electroencephalography and Clinical Neurophysiology*, 1971, *31*:547-562.)

thought to be primarily mediated by dorsal column and lemniscal pathways (Halliday and Wakefield, 1963), and are thought to arise in cerebral cortical elements. Little is known concerning the precise generator sources of these potentials.

All components of the scalp-recorded SEPs may be increased in peak latency and duration and decreased in amplitude in patients with peripheral neuropathy (Giblin, 1964; Bergamini, Bergamasco, Fra, et al., 1965). This can be explained by the decreased number of functioning sensory nerve fibers, the reduced conduction velocity of other affected fibers, and the resultant increased temporal dispersion of impulses. This technique is, however, of limited value, since peripheral nerve function can be more directly evaluated by recording peripheral nerve action potentials.

Longer-latency SEPs are decreased in amplitude over the affected hemisphere in many patients with focal destructive cerebral lesions (Giblin, 1964; Liberson, 1965; Laget, Mamo, and Houdart, 1967; Williamson, Goff, and Allison, 1970; Kazaki, Shiota, Terada, et al., 1971). In these patients, the degree of SEP alteration generally correlates well with the severity of sensory impairment, but exceptions have been noted. Abnormal but inconsistent alterations in SEP amplitude and waveform have also been observed in epileptic patients. SEPs may be enhanced in some patients with myoclonus or epilepsy (Halliday, 1965; Broughton, Maier-Ewert, and Abe, 1969; Halliday and Halliday, 1970). These potentials may be absent in some patients with degenerative disease (Cracco, Cracco, and Stolove, 1979), and the evaluation of these potentials in severely brain-injured patients is thought to be useful in estimating prognosis (Greenberg, Becker, Miller, et al., 1977a, 1977b). SEPs in response to simultaneous bilateral median nerve stimulation have been obtained from the scalp and abnormal responses have been recorded over the affected cerebral hemisphere of patients with cerebral lesions (Yamada, Kimura, Young, et al., 1978). For the most part, however, these findings in patients with cerebral dysfunction add little to the information that can be obtained from either the clinical evaluation or the electroencephalogram (EEG). For this reason, this method has not received much enthusiasm in the neurology clinic. There are two important reasons why the recording of these later potentials have not yet found clinical application: First, they are widely variable both within and across subjects, and they are markedly affected by differences in level of arousal. It is difficult, because of this variability, to define "abnormal response." Secondly, little is known concerning the precise generator sources of these components.

Peroneal or Tibial Nerve Evoked Potentials

Evoked potentials to stimulation of nerves in the lower extremities can be recorded from surface electrodes placed over the stimulated peripheral nerves, the spine, and the scalp. Since peripheral nerve action potentials have already been discussed, the evoked potentials recorded from the scalp and spine will now be described.

Scalp-Recorded Potentials

Stimulating electrodes are usually placed over the peroneal nerves in the popliteal fossa or tibial nerves at the ankle. Stimulus intensity (duration 0.2-0.3 msec) should be sufficient to produce a good muscle contraction but below the patient's pain threshold. In many laboratories, stimulus rates of 1-2/sec are used and 100-300 responses are summated. Since these responses are smaller than evoked potentials to median nerve stimulation, both peroneal or both tibial nerves may be simultaneously stimulated. A recording electrode is usually placed at C_z or 2 cm behind C_z, since this location overlies the specific somatosensory receiving area for lower-extremity stimulation. Additional scalp-recording electrodes are often applied. The reference electrode is usually placed on an ear or at a frontal scalp location. The frequency response of the recording apparatus is usually 1-1000 Hz, and analysis times of 100-200 msec are used.

This evoked response is greater in latency but otherwise similar to the longer-latency median nerve evoked potentials to which they correspond (Tsumato, et al., 1972). These potentials are also variable within and across subjects; it is therefore difficult to precisely define "normal" or "abnormal" responses. Nevertheless, these potentials have been found to be useful in the evaluation of patients with spinal-cord trauma and other lesions of the spinal cord (Perot, 1973). The presence of a scalp-recorded response indicates that there is transmission of the ascending volley across the site of spinal-cord pathology. This provides another parameter in the estimation of the completeness of physiologic transection of the spinal cord, and is particularly useful in infants and young children (where the clinical evaluation may be difficult and unreliable), and in patients who are either unconscious or uncooperative. Abnormalities of this response, including increases in response latency, have also been found in MS patients (Namerow, 1968). This method has also been employed in monitoring patients during surgery for scoliosis or spinal-cord pathology (Nash, Lorig, Schatzinger, et al., 1977; Engler, Spielholz, Bernhard, et al., 1978). Evoked potentials to both median nerve and tibial or peroneal nerve stimulation may be recorded in these patients. SEP changes induced by anesthesia or blood pressure changes would be expected to affect SEPs to stimulation of both upper and lower extremities, whereas SEP changes induced by the spinal surgery would be expected to affect only the lower-extremity SEPs. Variations in these peroneal or tibial nerve SEPs have been observed in some patients during surgical procedures. However, significant SEP configuration changes remain to be precisely defined. Therefore, more experience with this method is required before its true value in monitoring neurosurgical procedures can be assessed.

Spinal Evoked Potentials

Evoked potentials which arise in the cauda equina and in spinal cord afferent pathways can be recorded from surface electrodes attached to the skin over the spine (Liberson, et al., 1966; Cracco, 1973). Over rostral spinal cord segments, these potentials are diminished in amplitude and are recorded at best with difficulty. Stimulating methods are the same as those used for recording potentials from the scalp, except stimulus rates of about 9/sec are used and 1000-4000 responses are summated. The analysis time should be 20-30 msec. Simultaneous stimulation of multiple nerves, such as both peroneal nerves or both tibial nerves, increases the signal size (Cracco, Cracco, and Stolove, 1979). This method is routinely employed in some laboratories.

Since recordings over the spine are often obscured by random myogenic activity, this can be minimized by recording when patients are drowsy, sedated, or sleeping; a sedative may be administered prior to the recording sessions. Recordings are performed with the patient lying prone on a bed. Recording disc electrodes filled with conductive jelly are attached to the skin over the spine with collodion. Electrode impedance is maintained between 1500 and 3000 ohms. Bipolar recordings (interelectrode distance 3-6 cm) are obtained over various spinal locations. The frequency response of the recording apparatus is 10-3000 Hz.

These spinal potentials may also be recorded in reference leads where the reference electrode is placed over the iliac crest, torso, scalp, or sacrum (Cracco and Cracco, 1976; Dimitrijevic, et al., 1978; Jones, 1977). Far fewer responses need be summated when recording potentials only over the cauda equina or caudal spinal-cord, since these potentials are much greater in amplitude than those recorded over rostral spinal-cord segments. Technically satisfactory and reliable recordings have been obtained by summating fewer than 100 responses. In these recordings, the electrocardiogram was monitored and used to trigger the stimulator so that shocks were delivered during a silent interval (Dimitrijevic, et al., 1978).

These potentials progressively increase in latency from lumbar to cervical recording locations (Cracco, 1973; Cracco, et al., 1975; Cracco, Cracco, and Stolove, 1979) (Fig. 14-4). Similar potentials have been obtained from epidural leads in the human (Magladery, Porter, Park, et al., 1951; Caccia, Ubcali, and Andreussi, 1976; Ertekin, 1976a; 1976b; Shimoji, Matsuki, and Shimizu 1977; Shimoji, Shimizu and Maruzama, 1978). In bipolar surface leads over the lumbar spine, the response consists of initially positive, triphasic potentials. This would be expected when recording an impulse traversing a nerve trunk in volume and is consistent with potentials arising in the roots of the cauda equina. In leads over the lower thoracic spine which overlie caudal spinal cord segments, the response is often greater in amplitude and duration and more complex in configuration than in more rostral or more caudal leads. In adults, this potential usually consists of an initially positive, triphasic potential, the negative component of which has several peaks or inflections (Cracco, et al., 1975) (Fig. 14-4). In infants and young children, this response usually consists of a large positive-negative diphasic potential followed by a broad negative and, at times, by a broad positive potential (Cracco, et al., 1975; Cracco, Cracco, and Stolove, 1979) (Fig. 14-5). Investigations of similar potentials recorded over caudal cord segments in cats and

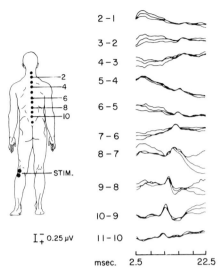

Figure 14-4. Bipolar recordings of the spinal potential evoked by left peroneal nerve stimulation (interelectrode distance, 4.5 cm). Electrode 11 is placed over the second lumbar spine and electrode 1 over the third cervical spine. Three separate averages are superimposed; 8,192 samples were averaged for each trace. The potential progressively increase in latency at more rostral recording locations. In the lead in which the caudal electrode is placed, over the ninth thoracic spine (trace 8-7), a complex potential (three negative components) is recorded. (Reprinted with permission from Cracco, R. Q. Spinal evoked response. Peripheral nerve stimulation in men. *Electroencephalography and Clinical Neurophysiology*, 1973, *35*: 379-386.)

monkeys suggest that the initial diphasic potential arises in the intramedullary continuations of dorsal root fibers; subsequent potentials reflect synaptic and post-synaptic activity that is concerned with local reflex mechanisms rather than with the propagation of the response to more rostral levels (Cracco and Evans, 1978; Feldman, Cracco, Farmer, et al., 1980).

Over rostral cord segments, the response in children and adults consists of small, initially positive, triphasic potentials with poorly defined positive phases that progressively decrease in amplitude rostrally (Cracco, 1973; Cracco, et al., 1975; Cracco, Cracco, and Stolove, 1979) (Figs. 14-4 and 14-5). This amplitude decrement probably reflects temporal dispersion and the greater distance between the skin-recording electrodes and the spinal cord at rostral thoracic and cervical recording sites. Investigations in cats and monkeys suggest that these potentials arise in multiple, rapidly conducting, afferent pathways, including the dorsolateral columns which lie primarily ipsi-

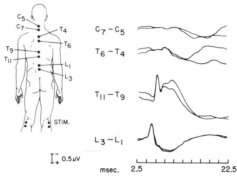

Figure 14-5. Surface bipolar recordings of the potential evoked by bilateral peroneal nerve stimulation in a 1-year-old (interelectrode distance, 5 cm). Two recordings are superimposed in each trace; 2,048 samples were averaged in each recording. Spinous process levels are indicated. The response increases in latency rostrally. The potential over the caudal thoracic spine consists of a positive-negative diphasic component, followed by a negative component, and then by a positive component. Differences between latencies of onset are greatest between adjacent leads placed over the lower and upper thoracic spine (middle two traces). (Reprinted with permission from Cracco, J. B., Cracco, R. Q., and Stolove, R. Spinal evoked potential in man. A maturational study. *Electroencephalography and Clinical Neurophysiology*, 1979, 46:58-64.)

lateral to the stimulated peripheral nerve (Sarnowski, Cracco, Vogel, et al., 1975; Cracco and Evans, 1978; Feldman, et al., 1980). These animal studies also provide evidence which suggests that the peripheral nerve fibers which mediate these potentials recorded at all spinal levels are primarily muscle-nerve rather than cutaneous-nerve afferent fibers (Sarnowski, et al., 1975).

The onset of the negative potential at each recording site may serve as the latency indicator, and can be used in determining conduction velocity, since it is thought to reflect the approximate time the fastest fibers contributing to a response pass under the recording electrode (in reference leads) or the recording electrode nearest the approaching volley (in bipolar leads) (Gilliat, et al., 1965). Latency differences are greater between equidistant leads placed over caudal spinal-cord segments than they are between leads placed over the cauda equina or rostral spinal-cord (Cracco, 1973; Cracco, Cracco, and Stolove, 1979). This indicates a decrease in the speed of conduction of the response over caudal cord segments. The slowing probably reflects the branching of dorsal root fibers and synaptic activity, since this is the region where these fibers undergo synaptic contact (in Clark's column and other nuclei).

In normal adults, the mean conduction velocity of the response from lumbar to cervical recording locations is about 70 m/sec. Segmental conduction velocities are about 65 m/sec over peripheral nerve and cauda equina (point of peripheral nerve stimulation to L_3 spine), 50 m/sec over caudal spinal cord (T_{12} to T_6 spines), and 85 m/sec over rostral spinal-cord (T_6-C_7 spines) (Cracco, Cracco, and Stolove, 1979). In the newborn, these segmental conduction velocities are about half those values obtained in the adult. They progressively increase with age. Peripheral conduction velocities are largely within the adult range by 3 years of age, whereas velocities over the spinal cord do not reach adult values until the fifth year (Cracco, Cracco, and Stolove, 1979). This suggests that maturation of rapidly conducting spinal afferent pathways proceeds at a slower rate than maturation of rapidly conducting peripheral sensory fibers. Similar findings have been obtained when recording the scalp-recorded evoked response to median nerve stimulation. Conduction velocities in the median nerve reach adult values between 12 and 18 months of age, whereas conduction velocities within central lemniscal pathways do not reach adult values until 5-7 years of age (Desmedt, Noel, Debecker, et al., 1973; Desmedt, Brunko, and Debecker, 1976). This increase in conduction speed which accompanies peripheral nerve and spinal cord maturation is probably related to the increasing fiber diameter and progressive myelination which accompanies maturation. However, explanations for the differential rate in maturation of peripheral and central afferent pathways can only be speculative at this time.

    In adult patients with clinically evident complete spinal-cord lesions, evoked potentials recorded from surface electrode caudal to the lesion are similar to those obtained in normal subjects. No response has been recorded in leads rostral to the lesion (Cracco, 1973) (Fig. 14-6). In a study of a group of infants and children with myelodysplasia on whom spinal and cerebral evoked potentials were recorded, there was good correlation between the degree of evoked potential abnormality and the clinical status of the patients (Cracco, et al., 1974; Cracco and Cracco, 1979) (Fig. 14-7). In a few of these patients, it was possible to diagnose caudal displacement of the spinal cord; the large complex spinal potentials which are normally recorded over the lower thoracic spines were recorded over lumbar spinous processes. In several children with myelomeningocele, a positive potential was recorded in leads immediately rostral to the lesion. This potential progressively decreased in amplitude but did not change in latency rostrally. This is a non-propagated volume-conducted potential, consistent with physiologic transection of the spinal cord. Similar positive potentials have been recorded rostral to spinal cord transections in cats and monkeys (killed-end effect) (Sarnowski, et al., 1975; Cracco and Evans, 1978; Feldman, et al., 1980).

    In a group of children with degenerative diseases of the central nervous system, the short- and longer-latency SEPs were recorded from the scalp; spinal evoked potentials were also obtained (Cracco, Cracco, and Stolove, 1979). Conduction velocities over peroneal nerve were normal. Responses

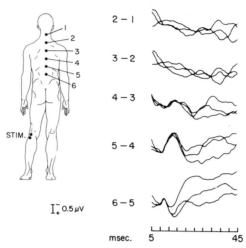

Figure 14-6. Bipolar recordings of the spinal potential evoked by left peroneal nerve stimulation in a patient with a clinically complete spinal-cord lesion at T_8. There is a 5 msec delay between the stimulus and the sweep onset. The analysis time is 40 msec, and interelectrode distance is 8 cm. Potentials caudal to the lesion (bottom three traces) are similar to those recorded in normal subjects. No potential is apparent in the lead in which the caudal electrode is placed over the sixth thoracic spine (trace 3-2) in relation to the lesion or in the more rostral lead (top trace). (Reprinted with permission from Cracco, R. Q. Spinal evoked response. Peripheral nerve stimulation in man. *Electroencephalography and Clinical Neurophysiology*, 1973, *35*: 379-386.)

were recorded over the spinal cord in most patients, but conduction velocities over the cord were slowed. The short-latency evoked potentials occurring in response to median nerve stimulation, which arise within and rostral to the brain stem, were absent in most of the patients, as were the longer-latency potentials of cerebrocortical origin. This demonstrates that these noninvasive methods permit an evaluation of the neuraxis from peripheral nerve to cerebral cortex.

Dorfman has recently devised a method by which conduction velocities within spinal cord afferent pathways may be indirectly estimated (Dorfman, 1977). He used the scalp-recorded SEPs in response to stimulation of nerves in the lower extremity and the upper extremity as latency indicators, and subtracted out the estimated peripheral conduction time by determining the F-wave latencies for the stimulated peripheral nerves. He found slowing in conduction speed within spinal-cord afferent pathways in normal elderly subjects and in some MS patients (Dorfman, Bosley, and Cummins, 1978; Dorfman and Bosley, 1979).

STIMULATION   RIGHT PERONEAL NERVE   LEFT PERONEAL NERVE

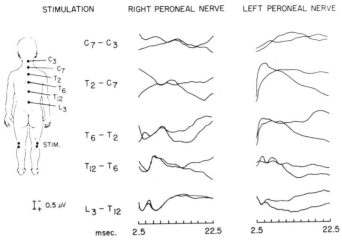

Figure 14-7. Bipolar surface recordings of the spinal potential evoked by left and right peroneal nerve stimulation in a 6-month-old infant with a lumbosacral myelomeningocele and a clinically asymmetric defect. With stimulation of the relatively normal right leg, potentials are apparent at all recording locations. With stimulation of the paralyzed left leg, small potentials are recorded only over the cauda equina and caudal spinal cord. Rostral leads yield no potential. (Reprinted with permission from Cracco, R. Q., Cracco, J. B., and Anziska, B. J. Somatosensory evoked potentials in man. Cerebral subcortical and peripheral nerve potentials. *American Journal of EEG Technology,* 1979, *19*:59-81.)

CONCLUSION

Peripheral nerve action potentials are easily recorded; this method is clinically useful, particularly in patients with disorders affecting proximal segments of peripheral nerves where more conventional methods have limited value. The longer-latency scalp-recorded SEPs occuring in response to median nerve stimulation are large in amplitude and therefore easy to record, but show considerable variability both within and across subjects. It is therefore difficult to define "abnormal response" with any precision. Little is known concerning the generator sources of these potentials. For these reasons these potentials are not in widespread clinical use.

The short-latency SEPs in response to median nerve stimulation are lower in amplitude than the longer-latency potentials, but they are much more stable. Methods to record these potentials have not yet been standardized, and a consensus has not yet been reached concerning the generator sources of each of the components. Nevertheless, abnormalities of these potentials have been found in patients with many neurologic disorders, and a consensus on recording methodology and component origin is likely to be reached in a short period of time. This method will soon have considerable diagnostic utility.

Spinal evoked potentials are also small in amplitude and, therefore, difficult to record, particularly over rostral spinal-cord segments. They are larger in infants and young children than in adults. Abnormalities of these potentials have been demonstrated in a number of patients with pathology affecting the spinal cord and cauda equina. It seems that this method provides another parameter in the evaluation of spinal cord function in the human. The scalp-recorded evoked potential to stimulation of peripheral nerves in the lower extremities has also been found useful in evaluating patients with spinal-cord dysfunction. Studies designed to determine whether these methods are useful in monitoring spinal-cord function during surgical procedures are underway in many laboratories.

The recording of SEPs provides a unique opportunity to evaluate the entire neuraxis from cutaneous receptor to cerebral cortex. Information can be obtained concerning receptors, peripheral nerves, spinal cord, brain stem, and cerebral cortex. When these methods are combined with those used in obtaining auditory and visual evoked potentials, it seems that it should be possible to obtain a reliable measure of the physiologic integrity of the somatosensory system in the human.

VISUAL EVOKED POTENTIALS

Visual evoked potentials (VEPs) are scalp-recorded electrical potentials generated in the occipital cortex as a result of photic stimulation of one or both eyes. Since the introduction (in the late 1960s) of complex visual stimuli and, more particularly, of pattern-reversal stimulation, these potentials have become increasingly useful for the detection of visual pathway lesions (Cobb, Morton and Ettlinger, 1967; Halliday and Michael, 1970; Halliday, McDonald, and Mushin, 1972; Celesia and Daly, 1977a).

This section will describe the state of the art in visual evoked potentials as they apply to the diagnosis of neurologic disorders. Two major subdivisions are discussed: (1) transient visual evoked potentials, and (2) steady-state visual evoked potentials.

Transient Visual Evoked Potentials

Transient visual evoked potentials (TVEPs) are electrical potentials resulting from the transient change of brain waves following a photic stimulus. TVEPs behave differently than those electrical events recorded during steady-state visual stimulation, as will be shown in the following pages. Conventionally, the term *transient* is omitted, but it will be retained here for clarity.

TVEPs can be evoked by various light sources; these are described elsewhere (Graham, Bartlett, Brown, et al., 1965; Regan, 1972; Armington,

1974; Celesia, 1978). Three systems have been most commonly utilized: stroboscopic xenon flash tubes, slide projector with movable mirror, and television.

Flashes can be obtained with any strobe usually available in an electroencephalography laboratory. Three major precautions need to be taken when using flashes, i.e., background luminance, intensity of the flash, and pupillary diameter must be kept constant. Changes in background luminance will interact with the flash stimulus, modifying the percentage change of intensity during stimulation and affecting TVEP amplitude. Increasing the stimulus intensity increases TVEP amplitude until a plateau is reached (Armington, 1974). The latencies of all the components of TVEP are also affected by changes in flash intensity, with latency becoming shorter as the intensity increases (Cobb and Dawson, 1960). Only when the background luminance, pupillary diameter, and stimulus intensity are matched can data from two laboratories be compared. Similarly, normative data from any laboratory can be used only when conditions of stimulation are equal. TVEPs contain both a photopic and a scotopic component. Flash stimulation is usually carried out on light-adapted eyes (photopic state). However, since the cortical representation of the fovea (cones) is so extensive compared to the cortical rod representation, the study of the scotopic (rod) component of TVEP is usually neglected.

Pattern-reversal can be produced either with commercially available television or with projectors. Pattern TVEPs are critically dependent on many parameters. Arden, Bodis-Wollner, Halliday, et al. (1977) have suggested that the following parameters be controlled and specified: (1) stimulus luminance or brightness; (2) type of pattern (checkerboard or grating, etc.); (3) size of the pattern (dimension to be specified in terms of visual angle); (4) total field size, shape, and its relation to the fixation point (to be specified in terms of visual angle and retinal eccentricity); and (5) method of presentation of the pattern (pattern reversal, brief pattern onset, or offset patterned light, etc.). The presentation rate of the pattern should also be specified. Only when these parameters are equal can TVEPs obtained from two laboratories be compared.

Different check sizes produce responses of different amplitude. Potentials of maximum amplitude are evoked by check sizes ranging from 11 to 18 min subtense (Regan and Richards, 1971). Asselman (1975) compared pattern-reversal checks of 57 min to smaller checks of 30 min, with a constant whole field of 18°, and found that the TVEPs had identical latencies but the amplitude was slightly smaller for the larger checks. TVEPs obtained with checks of less than 15 min are mostly due to stimulation of the macular region while TVEPs produced with checks larger than 15 min are the result of foveal and extrafoveal stimulation (Harter and White, 1969; Regan, 1972). The choice of check size may have to change according to the region of the visual pathway under study. In order to detect small demyelinating lesions affecting optic nerve fibers originating from ganglion cells in the foveal region (the papillomacular bundle), smaller checks with a small total field should be used. Hennerici, Weznel, and Freund (1977) have shown that a stimulus subtending 45 min of arc was more sensitive in detecting abnormalities of VEPs in MS patients than a stimulus field subtending 20° of arc at the subject's eyes. On the other hand if the aim is to detect retrochiasmatic lesions, checks larger than 15 min with fields larger than 10° may be a better choice.

Variations in recording techniques also affect TVEPs. Halliday's group (Barrett, Blumhardt, Halliday, et al., 1976; Blumhardt, Barrett, and Halliday, 1977; Halliday, Barrett, Halliday, et al., 1977) have shown that earlobe and mastoid references are not indifferent. They may pick up evoked responses themselves, especially if the field of stimulation is large. Similarly, Kuroiwa and Celesia (1981) have shown considerable waveform amplitude variation between TVEPs simultaneously recorded with bipolar and monopolar montages. Precise estimation of latency measurements for the early negative and the major positive waves requires the use of a wide band-pass filter in the recording system including the electroencephalogram (EEG) amplifiers, the averager amplifiers, and if used, the magnetic tape. Desmedt, Brunco, Debecker, et al. (1974) showed severe distortion of latencies and amplitudes for low-pass filtering below 1 KHz. Thus, TVEPs should be recorded with a bandwidth of 0.3 Hz to at least 1 KHz.

Silver–silver chloride electrodes applied to the scalp with collodion and having impedance below 3000 ohms are to be used. It is recommended that the electrode placement of Halliday's group be adopted (Barrett, et al., 1976; Halliday, 1978), because of the extensive normal data-base existing with these electrode montages. A midoccipital electrode is placed 5 cm above the inion. The lateral occipital electrodes are situated 5 cm to the right or left of the midoccipital electrode. Lateral temporal electrodes are situated 5 cm apart from the lateral occipital electrodes. The electrodes are referred to a common midfrontal electrode placed 12 cm above the nasion. Electroretinograms (ERGs) should be monitored. In neurologic practice, it is sufficient to record ERGs from skin electrodes. Well-formed ERGs in response to flashes can be obtained by placing silver–silver chloride electrodes around the eyes (Fig. 14-8). One electrode is placed in the middle of the infraorbital ridge just below the eye and referred to an electrode placed 2 cm laterally to the outer canthus of the same eye. Contact-lens electrodes allow the recording of larger and more detailed ERGs (Armington, 1974). One-hundred-fifty to 200 samples are usually averaged over 200 to 250 msec following the stimulus.

TVEPs to flashes presented at a frequency of less than 1/sec consist of seven positive-negative deflections within the first 250 msec following the stimulus. The responses are greatly variable, imposing some limitation on their clinical application (Ciganek, 1975). For further details of VEPs to flashes, we refer the reader to the work of Kooi and Bagchi (1964). In con-

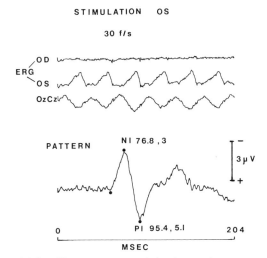

Figure 14-8. The upper part of the figure shows a normal response to a train of flashes at the frequency of 30 flashes/sec presented to the left eye. The lower part of the figure illustrates a normal transient visual evoked potential (TVEP) to pattern stimulation. Note that positive polarity is a downward deflection for scalp recording but an upward deflection for the ERG. Key: OD = right eye; OS = left eye.

trast to the potentials evoked by flashes, TVEPs evoked by pattern-reversal (checks of 15.5 min, field of 9.3°, reversing every 600 msec, luminance of 34 foot-lamberts (ft-L)) are reliable and constant; they consist of two major waves (Fig. 14-8). A major negative wave (N_1) with a peak latency ranging from 62.2 to 90.4 msec (mean, 73.4 ± 5.4) is followed by a major positive wave (P_1) with a peak latency ranging from 84.6 to 118 msec (mean, 97.8 ± 6.8). The amplitude of N_1 varies from 0.2 to 15 μV. P_1 amplitudes range from 1 to 30 μV. Wave N_1 is frequently preceded by a small positive wave. The difference in latency between the right and left eye for wave N_1 ranges from 0 to 5.6 msec (mean, 1.6 ± 1.3), and the latency difference for wave P_1 ranges from 0 to 6 msec (mean, 1.7 ± 1.6).

Peak latencies of TVEPs are influenced by age. With advancing age, there is an increase in peak latency for both N_1 and P_1 (Celesia and Daly, 1977b). This increase in latency probably reflects a slowing of conduction velocity in the optic nerve and/or optic pathway. Aging is a variable that must be considered when establishing the boundary of normality. It is suggested that the boundaries of normal be placed 2.5 times above the standard deviation of the regression line; 99.5 percent of normal subjects will have scores below this line (Celesia and Daly, 1977b). The effects of aging on the latency differences between the right and left eyes are too small to be considered significant. The limit of normal for latency differences for N_1 is (mean + 2.5

sd) 5 msec; for latency differences of P1, 6 msec. Assuming a normal distribution for these parameters, the use of the mean ± sd reduces the overlap between normal and abnormal values to 0.5 percent. A similarly strict criterion of defining abnormal values as those responses with latencies falling beyond two-and-a-half times the standard deviation of the mean was used by Halliday, et al. (1973); Asselman, Chadwick, and Marsden, (1975) used the mean ± 3 sd as limit of normal. The utilization of these rigid statistical criteria from three different laboratories indicates the reliability of the VEP to pattern reversal. The statement of Ciganek (1975), that boundaries between the normal and the pathologic are uncertain, only applies to flash-produced TVEPs. The normal limits of TVEP latencies to pattern stimulation are now clearly defined.

Some controversy has arisen about the topography of pattern TVEPs to full- and half-field stimulation, and the reliability of measuring amplitude asymmetries to detect retrochiasmatic lesions (Halliday, 1978; Starr, Sohmer, and Celesia, 1978; Holder, 1978). Most discrepancies result from the utilization of different electrode montages and stimulation parameters. Pattern stimulation with checks subtending 40 min of arc at the subject's eye and whole field subtending 18° (luminance 34 ft-L, pattern reversing every 600 msec) results in symmetrical TVEP distribution over both occipital regions. In contrast to this symmetry, half-field stimulation (field of 9°) results in TVEPs with the largest amplitude over the lateral occipital scalp (Fig. 14-9) ipsilateral

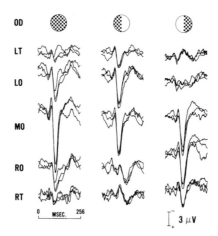

Figure 14-9. TVEPs amplitude distribution during full- and half-field stimulation in a normal subject. The superimposition of three TVEPs obtained in three subsequent trials demonstrates the reliability of the responses. Note the ipsilateral preponderance of the responses to half-field stimulation. Key: LT = left temporal; LO = left occipital; MO = midoccipital; RO = right occipital; RT = right temporal.

to the half-field that is stimulated (Kuroiwa and Celesia, 1981). These find-ings are in agreement with the data of Barrett, et al. (1976) and Blumhardt, et al. (1977) who suggested that this paradoxical lateralization of the major positive TVEP wave is related to the mesial location of the potential gener-ators on the hemisphere contralateral to the field stimulated. The location of ipsilateral electrodes is optimal to record a potential from the posteromedial aspect of the contralateral occipital lobe. Celesia (1982) propose the utili-zation of amplitude ratios to normalize the intersubject variations and permit statistical quantification of the data. The lateral occipital ratio, defined as the TVEP amplitude (in microvolts) at occipital scalp contralateral to the hemifield stimulated, divided by the TVEP amplitude at occiptal scalp ipsilateral to the hemifield stimulated, was found to be useful. The mean normal value of this ratio is 0.61 ± 0.30. The boundary of normal for the lateral occipital ratio is 1.36 (mean + 2.5 sd).

Steady-State Visual Evoked Potentials

Steady-state potentials are electrical events evoked by rapid, repetitive sensory stimulation. Rapid and continuous stimulation produces evoked re-sponses of constant amplitude and frequency; each potential overlaps one another so that no individual response can be related to any particular stimu-lus cycle (Regan, 1972; 1975). It is presumed that the brain has achieved a "steady state" of excitability.

Steady-state visual evoked potentials (SVEPs) are utilized for the deter-mination of *critical frequency of photic driving* (CFPD). CFPD is defined as the highest frequency of photic driving response in flashes/sec. Flash stimula-tion begins at low frequencies of flashes and gradually increases until no photic driving can be obtained (Celesia and Daly, 1977a, 1977b). Two-hundred to 300 samples are summated for each frequency tested. CFPD is simultaneously recorded with ERGs at the retinal level (*retinal* CFPD) and at the occipital scalp level (*cortical* CFPD). The responses to flashes of high fre-quency consist of sinusoidal waves following the stimulus (Fig. 14-8). Subhar-monic waves are often seen, particularly at a lower frequency of flashes, at both the retinal and cortical level. Retinal and cortical CFPD values relate to the intensity of the flash as well as to the brightness of the background illumin-ation and the pupillary size. They are also influenced by age, decreasing as age progresses (Celesia and Daly, 1977b). In normals, retinal and cortical CFPD have similar values. Using a Grass photic stimulator (Grass Instrument Co., Quincy, Massachusetts) Model PS-2 set at intensity 1, with the strobo-scope placed 45 cm in front of the eye to be stimulated, background lumi-nance of 0.01 ft-L and the pupil dilated by homoatropine (1 percent ophthal-mic solution), CFPD had the following mean values: 72 flashes/sec (age 20 to 30); 69 flashes/sec (age 30 to 60); and 60 flashes/sec (above age 60). Under these stimulation condition, differences between retinal and cortical

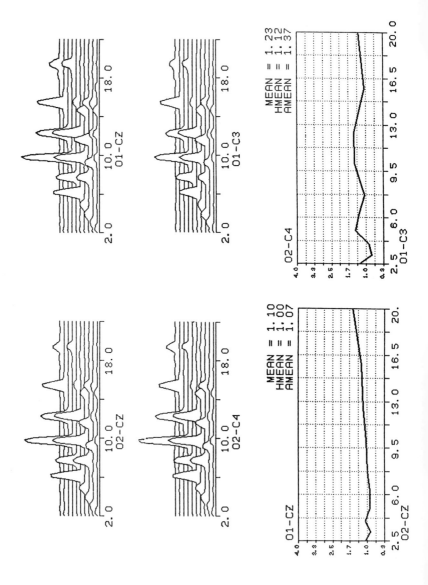

Figure 14-10. The upper portion of the figure shows a visual evoked spectrum array (VESA) in a normal subject. Each line represents averaged spectrum array of two 4-sec EEG epochs. The major peaks indicate responses to flashes. Additional peaks represent second and third harmonic responses. Abscissa represent peak energy; ordinate, frequency in Hz. Note the similarity between VESA obtained from bipolar (O_2-C_4/O_1-C_3) and referential (O_2-C_z/O_1-C_z) recordings. The lower half of the figure shows the VESA ratio plots and the numerical values of the VESA ratios. Mean indicates the average ratio for all 10 frequencies of stimulation, H mean indicates the average ratio for frequencies above 6.0 Hz, and A mean indicates the average ratio for frequencies of 7 to 12.5 Hz. Note that all ratios have values below 2.

CFPD had to be higher than 10 flashes/sec to be considered abnormal. Cortical CFPD never exceeds retinal CFPD.

Regan (1972) was the first to obtain a precise description of SVEPs to harmonically simple light, via Fourier analysis. He studied SVEP phase and amplitude. The method was effective in detecting retrobulbar neuritis (Regan and Heron, 1969; Heron, Regan and Milner, 1974; Regan 1975); SVEPs were delayed and had low amplitude with monocular stimulation of the affected eye. Celesia, Soni, and Rhode (1978) introduced the test method of visual evoked spectrum array. The test consists of analyzing EEG activity during trains of flashes of increasing frequency by the technique of compressed spectrum array (Bickford, Fleming, and Billinger, 1971). Visual stimulation consists of 8-sec trains of flashes. Average compressed arrays are computed using the fast Fourier transform. Each array consists of the summation of two 4-sec EEG epochs during a specific steady frequency of stimulation. As shown in Figure 14-10, the bottom line of each display represents the visual evoked spectrum array at the stimulation frequency of 2.5 flashes/sec. Each succeeding line represents the spectrum at a higher frequency of stimulation, with the top line representing the spectrum at 20 flashes/sec.

Quantification was achieved by calculating the ratios of spectral energy at each 10 frequencies for homologous regions of the right and left hemisphere. If the two hemispheres contained equal energy, the ratio would be 1.0 (Fig. 14-10). Normal spectral ratios were calculated for 19 normal subjects with recordings from O_2-C_z/O_1-C_z and O_2-C_4/O_1-C_3 (international nomenclature). Spectral ratios were less or equal to 2.0 in all normal subjects.

CLINICAL APPLICATIONS

Visual disturbances can now be objectively studied with neurophysiologic methods (Halliday, 1975; Asselman, 1975; Lowitzsch, Kuhnt, Sakmann, et al., 1976; Celesia and Daly, 1977a, 1977b; Diamond, 1977; Bodis-Wollner, Hendley, Mylin, et al., 1979). Abnormalities in visual evoked responses indicate dysfunction somewhere along the visual pathways. Different disease processes affecting the same region will produce similar disturbances. Three abnormality profiles have emerged, permitting differentiation among eye proper, optic nerve, and retrochiasmatic pathway involvement (Celesia, 1978).

Diseases of the vitreous, lens, anterior chamber, or cornea produce TVEP amplitude-attenuation without, in most instances, affecting TVEP latencies. These lesions, however, are best diagnosed by clinical examination. Diseases of the retina and optic nerve may result in pattern-reversal TVEPs of low amplitude and delayed latency. In most cases, the differentiation can be made by identification of retinal lesions on fundoscopic examination. The simultaneous determination of retinal and cortical CFPD is useful in these cases. CFPD is decreased both at the retinal and cortical level in retinal disease; it is normal at the retinal level (retinal CFPD), but abnormal at the cortical level (cortical CFPD) in diseases affecting the optic nerve (Fig. 14-11). In more difficult cases, the differential diagnosis between retinal and optic nerve involvement may require the utilization of ERG with contact-lens electrodes (Armington, 1974). The amplitude distribution of TVEPs to full-field and half-field pattern stimulation in retinal and optic nerve disease is normal. Amplitude distribution to half-field stimulation needs to be studied in every patient, to exclude delayed TVEP caused by retrochiasmatic lesions. Halliday (1978) and Kuroiwa and Celesia (1981) have reported delayed TVEPs in patients with retrochiasmatic lesions, however, in each case, an abnormal amplitude distribution in response to stimulation of the affected half-field was demonstrated. Bilateral retrochiasmatic lesions have also been reported to result in attenuated and delayed TVEPs (Ashworth, Maloney, and Towsend, 1978).

Only when ocular pathology is excluded and a normal amplitude distribution to half-field stimulation is demonstrated can a delay in latency of the pattern TVEP indicate optic nerve pathology. Delayed or absent TVEPs have now been reported in optic and retrobulbar neuritis, optic atrophy, ischemic optic neuropathy, and compression of the optic nerve. A TVEP is considered to have a delayed latency when the peak latency for wave N_1 and P_1 falls outside the boundary of normality (mean ± 2½ sd, according to age), or when

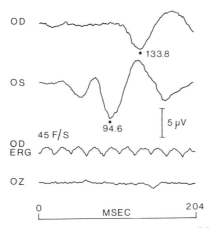

Figure 14-11. Visual evoked potentials in a 36-year-old woman with diagnosis of suspected multiple sclerosis. Visual acuity was 20/30 for both eyes. Goldmann perimetry and fundoscopic examination was normal. Note the greatly delayed TVEP in response to monocular stimulation of the right eye (OD). The normal steady-state visual evoked potentials at the retinal level (ERG) to flash stimulation (frequency, 45 flashes/sec) contrast with the absence of cortical responses (OZ-to reference), indicating dysfunction of the right optic nerve and normal retinal function.

the peak latency difference for both waves N_1 and P_1 between the stimulation of the right and left eye is greater than 6 msec. Celesia (1978) studied 74 MS patients and found delayed or absent TVEPs in 55 (74 percent) (Fig. 14-12). Every patient with a central or paracentral scotoma had an abnormal TVEP. Of 856 MS patients, 356 (65 percent) have been reported to have abnormal TVEPs (Celesia, 1982). More important is the great sensitivity of the test, and its ability to show abnormal pattern-evoked responses in early optic nerve lesions when other clinical signs of visual impairment are absent.

Celesia (1978) demonstrated delayed TVEPs in 16 (55 percent) of 29 MS patients who were without signs or symptoms of visual dysfunction (Fig. 14-12). Delays were also found in six out of seven MS patients who had normal visual acuity, visual fields, and no subjective visual complaints, but who had a history of optic neuritis. Similarly, Halliday and co-workers (1972, 1973) found delayed TVEPs in 12 of 14 patients with normal optic discs and no history of optic neuritis. Asselman, Chadwick and Marsden (1975) reported delayed VEPs in 28 percent of eyes assessed as normal by other criteria.

Not only are TVEPs useful in determining subclinical and/or early lesions of the optic nerves, but they can also be used to monitor early compression of the optic nerve and chiasma by sellar and parasellar tumors. TVEPs can also be utilized to quantify the effects of surgery and/or irradiation. Halliday, Halliday, Kriss, et al. (1976) showed marked improvement of VEP in the postoperative recordings of nine parasellar neoplasms; improvement was associated with improved visual function. Craniopharyngiomas and pituitary tumors compressing the chiasma resulted in abnormal VERs in both eyes in 9 of 10 patients.

CFPD was studied in MS patients (Fig. 14-12), and was abnormal in 44 percent of the cases. When compared to TVEP, CFPD was a less-sensitive in-

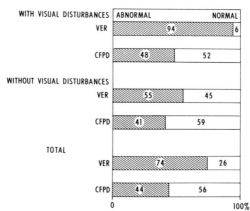

Figure 14-12. Visual evoked potential's profile in 74 multiple sclerosis patients. The results of pattern stimulation (VER) and critical frequency of photic driving (CFPD) are separately tabulated. (See text for further details.)

dicator of optic nerve pathology, but the two tests were not mutually exclusive. CFPD was the sole abnormality in 2 of the 74 patients in the study (Celesia, 1978). Similarly, Regan, Milner, and Heron (1976) identified a distinct group of MS patients having a defect to medium-frequency flicker independently of the delay in pattern-reversal VEPs. The utilization of more than one test can enhance the reliability and the yield of the procedure(s).

Considerable controversy exists regarding the effects of retrochiasmatic lesions on TVEP amplitude (Halliday, 1975; Asselman, et al., 1975; Barrett, et al., 1976; Halliday, 1978; Starr, Sohmer, and Celesia, 1978; Holder, 1978). Halliday's group, using full- and half-field pattern stimulation, was able to demonstrate clear asymmetrics of amplitude distribution in hemianopic patients, findings that were confirmed by Kuroiwa and Celesia (1981). In a study of 14 hemianopic patients, the following amplitude distribution abnormalities were noted: (1) absent TVEPs to stimulation of the affected half-field with normal amplitude distribution to stimulation of the normal half-field; (2) reversal of normal amplitude asymmetry during stimulation of the affected half-field; that is to say, higher amplitude TVEPs at occipital regions contra-

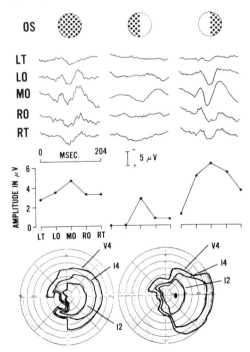

Figure 14-13. TVEP amplitude distribution in a hemianopic patient. Computerized axial tomography scan demonstrated an infarct localized to the right occipital lobe. Note normal TVEPs in response to full-field stimulation, but almost absent responses to stimulation of the affected left field. (Nomenclature as in Fig. 14-9.)

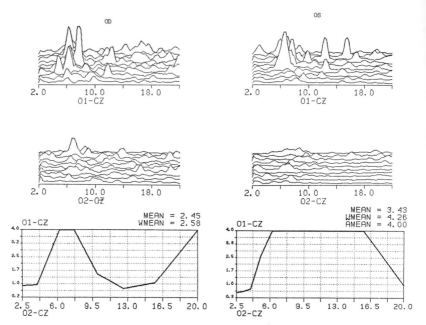

Figure 14-14. VESA in a patient with left hemianopsia. Note depressed visual evoked spectrum array over the right occipital region, both with monocular stimulation of the right (OD) and left (OS) eye. Note also the high peaks of the ratio plots and high numerical values of the ratios (all above 2).

lateral to the field stimulated, in contrast to the normal findings of higher amplitude ipsilateral to the half-field stimulated; and (3) lateral occipital ratio above 1.36. One or two of these abnormalities were present in 12 patients (Fig. 14-13).

    Another promising method for the detection of the hemianopic fields is the visual evoked spectrum array (VESA). Celesia, Soni, and Rhode, (1978) have shown the following abnormalities in four hemianopic patients (Fig. 14-14): (1) small spectral amplitude over the occipital region contralateral to the affected field, (2) visual evoked spectral ratio plot with high peaks and valleys, and (3) spectral ratio above 2.5. The major strength of VESA is its ability to be carried out in uncooperative patients. Visual stimulation at each frequency lasts 8 seconds; the test is complete in less than 2 minutes.

    As promising as these tests appear for the objective determination of retrochiasmatic lesions, a note of caution is in order. While either TVEP amplitude distribution or VESA are reliable, neither test has yet proved as sensitive as the visual-field perimetry. Further testing of these methods is needed. Nevertheless, the addition of visual (and somatosensory) potentials to the neurologic, diagnostic battery deserves consideration by both the otologist and audiologist.

Michael M. Merzenich
John N. Gardi
Michael C. Vivion

15 Animals

The use of noninvasively recorded averaged auditory evoked responses
(AERs) in animals over the past two decades has paralleled the significant increase in experimental and clinical use of these responses in humans. It is our
objective in this chapter to describe some of the basic features of AERs recorded from commonly studied animal species, and to outline, by example,
ways in which they have been, or are expected to be, of practical use in the
experimental laboratory.

In describing basic features of auditory AERs in animals, it is perhaps instructive to review the terminology adopted to identify classes of auditory
evoked responses (see Chapter 6). Transient responses recorded within 10
msec following the onset of the eliciting stimulus (either a click or a short-
onset tone burst) have been labeled as brain-stem evoked responses (BSERs)
or auditory brain-stem responses (ABRs). These names were chosen because
it has been shown that these responses arise from within or in close proximity
to various auditory brain-stem nuclei and tracts (Buchwald and Huang, 1975;
Goldenberg and Derbyshire, 1975; Achor and Starr, 1980b; Gardi, Merzenich,
and McKean, 1979; Gardi and Berlin, 1981). Sustained responses, elicited
by each cycle of a low-frequency tone burst or continuous tone, mimic signal
frequency and, therefore, have been termed frequency-following responses
(FFRs) or frequency-following potentials (FFPs), although they are also predominantly products of brain-stem auditory nuclei and/or tracts (see Gardi,
Merzenich, and McKean, 1979). Responses which occur within 10 to 80
msec of stimulus onset have usually been designated as middle-latency re-

391

sponses (MLRs) to distinguish them from the early responses, and those which occur still later. Although their sources have not been defined with certainty (Shinoda, et al., 1979; Gardi and Bledsoe, 1979; Buchwald, et al., 1981, Chapter 7), it is probable that at least initial portions of MLRs originate from brain-stem nuclei.

Thus, no systematic terminology has been applied to these various non-invasively recorded AERs. We prefer terminology that is less committal to neural origin (ABR or BSER), to phenomenology (FFR or FFP), or to time of occurrence (MLR), because all of these responses arise, at least in part, from brain-stem or mid-brain nuclei and/or fiber tracts, and they all overlap in time. Established nomenclature is difficult to change, however, and for the remainder of this chapter, we will employ the following nomenclature: auditory brain stem responses (ABRs)—transient responses generated by clicks or rapid-onset tonal stimuli that have peak latencies within the first 10 msec following stimulus presentation; frequency following responses (FFRs)—sustained responses that mimic signal frequency and are generated by tone bursts and continuous tones; and middle latency responses (MLRs)—responses that have peak latencies between 10 and 80 msec and are elicited by clicks or tone bursts.

SCALP-RECORDING TECHNIQUES

Techniques used to noninvasively record auditory evoked responses from animals are in most respects the same as those used for recording ABRs in humans. That is, at least three electrodes (a differential pair and a ground) are attached to appropriate locations on the animal's head. Electrical signals detected by the electrodes are led to the inputs of a conventional biological differential amplifier having appropriate gain, low internal noise, high common-mode rejection, and wide bandwidth characteristics. Amplified signals are appropriately filtered (see Table 12-1); filter characteristics are dependent upon which class of auditory AER is to be recorded. Repeatedly acquired signals are led to an analog-to-digital converter (either a hard-wired signal averager or a programmable computer system), where they are sampled at an appropriate rate and converted to a series of digital values (the exact number of values depends on the latency of the response and its spectral content). Finally, numbers (representing amplitude values) are stored in a memory device, in which the derived digital values are averaged together to yield an auditory evoked response. For a succinct description of these techniques, see Chapters 2 and 8.

There are some notable practical differences in the techniques commonly used to record animal auditory AERs. Conventional earphone headsets, routinely used in human AER testing, are obviously inappropriate for animal use. Therefore, when recording auditory AERs from animals, sound stimuli are either presented free-field or, more often, through a closed ear-tube system. The latter method offers two important advantages: (1) the ear tubes can be inserted in the external auditory canal with high reliability of placement so that test and retest differences in absolute stimulation levels are minimal; and (2) the ear tubes can be fitted with probe-microphone inserts so that the stimulus intensity levels at or very near the tympanic membrane can be measured and monitored during AER recordings and precisely specified in terms of spectrum.

A second difference in recording techniques for animals is the type of electrodes used. Cup-shaped or flat disc electrodes typically used in recording human AERs can also be used with animals, but, in fact, are seldom employed. This is because a more stable recording can be achieved with the use of needle electrodes, or with the use of chronically implanted, mechanically stabilized electrodes (e.g., we commonly use small stainless steel screws, connected via insulated wires to a percutaneous plug, to insure invariant recording conditions over very long periods).

A third difference is in subject state. Human AER recordings typically are taken with the subject or patient either awake or in natural sleep (i.e., for adults, infants, and young children) or under sedation (i.e., for difficult-to-test patients). As a rule, general anesthesia is administered only when the patient cannot be successfully tested in any other state. In such cases, care is still taken to anesthetize the patient for as brief a period as possible (typically, 2 hours or less). Animal AER recordings are almost never made with the animal awake or in natural sleep. Exceptions are when the animal can be safely restrained in a device that immobilizes its head and reduces other body movements, or when electrodes are chronically implanted in the animal and a remote amplification system (e.g., a telemetry system) is used to record the brain's electrical activity. More often, animals are sedated or anesthetized during testing (usually the latter). Recording animal AERs under anesthesia offers several distinct advantages. Artifacts due to movement or muscle activity are minimized. More importantly, when an animal is maintained under anesthesia for long periods, complex and highly resolved parametric sequences of stimulation can be presented and resultant AERs recorded.

A final difference in recording animal AERs relates to the nature of the evoked response itself (i.e., the signal) and of the other ongoing electrical activity of the brain (i.e., the noise), which is also detected by the recording electrodes. In laboratory animals, the smaller absolute head size and concomitant smaller brain size (together with proportionally lesser amounts of bone, muscle, sinew, and skin) result in a more favorable situation for recording the responses elicited by auditory stimuli (even though the generators of responses are also smaller). Thus, in general, evoked responses detected at the scalp in non-primate laboratory animals tend to have large absolute magnitudes as compared to humans, and there is a more favorable signal-to-noise ratio in the signal detected from an animal's scalp as compared to that detected from the human scalp. Practically, these two differences mean that the overall amount of gain required in the biological amplifier system may be less, and that the amount of averaging (the number of stimuli presented/AER) required to extract a clear response is less than that typically required for recording from human subjects.

BASIC FEATURES

The same major nuclear subdivisions can be identified within the auditory nervous system in all or nearly all mammals (Merzenich, Roth, and Anderson, et al., 1977). With few exceptions, all mammals have a cochlear nuclear (CN) complex, a superior olivary complex (SOC), a nucleus of the lateral lemniscus (LL), and central, pericentral, and external nuclei of the inferior colliculus (IC); all have the same major definable subdivisions. Hence, it is hardly surprising that a similar (i.e., resembling human) repertoire of "early" AERs have been recorded in experimental mammals.

On the other hand, several factors insure that AERs are species-specific in detail: (1) The auditory nervous system is relatively volatile in its detailed appearance in mammalian phylogeny, i.e., there are species-specific differences in detail (e.g., size of nuclei and component divisions, orientation of nuclei and fiber tracts, physical characteristics of component neurons) between auditory nuclei in all studied mammals (Merzenich, Roth, and Anderson, et al., 1977). (2) Component divisions of the auditory nervous system are scaled in size as a function of the animal's size, as are neurons and their axons (hence, conduction velocity and conduction path length). (3) There are great differences in the degree of encephalization along several lines of descent in mammals. For example, the neocortex is differentially expanded (e.g., the brain stem) in primates (especially in humans), pinnipeds, and cetaceans. The cerebellum is also differentially greatly expanded in many species, including humans. (4) There are obvious species-specific differences in bone, muscle, skin, and sinew.

Thus, while similar ABRs and FFRs can be recorded in all mammalian species, it is not surprising that their detail—the detailed post-stimulus time of occurrence and the proportional and absolute amplitudes of response components—vary in species-specific ways.

AUDITORY BRAIN-STEM EVOKED RESPONSES

ABRs to clicks were initially recorded from the scalp and shown to be distinguishable from N_1 responses by Jewett in the cat (1970). They were subsequently recorded in humans (Jewett and Williston, 1971; Moore, 1971). ABRs have now been extensively recorded in guinea pigs (Dobie and Berlin,

1979b; Gardi and Berlin, 1981), mice (Henry and Chole, 1979a, 1979b), rats (Schorn, Lennon, and Bickford, 1976), cats (Buchwald and Huang, 1975; Achor and Starr, 1977; Gardi, Merzenich, and McKean, 1979; Gardi and Merzenich, 1979), monkeys (Allen and Starr, 1978), dolphins (Ridgway, et al., 1981), as well as in other species (Corwin, Bullock, and Schweitzer, in press).

Under optimal and corresponding recording conditions (healthy adolescent animals, clean external-ear canals, clear middle-ear cavities, proper ear-tube placement, identical electrode configuration), all mammals studied exhibit a series of four or five waves. At the same time, species-specific differences in waveform morphology are readily apparent. Several examples are illustrated in Figure 15-1 (mouse, rat, guinea pig, cat, human). Among evident differences in recorded responses, observe that: (1) the first two waves of the BSER recorded from the mouse are of relatively greater magnitude than later waves; (2) in responses recorded from the rat and guinea pig, waves II and III are relatively prominent; (3) in the rat, the peak of the third wave is usually observed to fall on the downward slope of the second wave, whereas, in the guinea pig, the second peak usually occurs on the upward

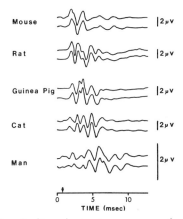

Figure 15-1. Auditory brain-stem response from five mammalian species (N = 512 for animals; 2048 for human subjects) evoked by 10 kHz, 1 msec stimuli (instaneous rise-fall times) presented at 15/sec. For animals, stimuli were presented at 80 dB pe SPL. In human subjects, stimuli were presented at a 60 dB sensation level (which, in dB SPL, was near the same level as used for the animal recordings). Stimulus onset is at 0.6 msec on the time scale (indicated by the arrow).*

---

*Stimulation is monaural; responses are recorded from the scalp between the vertex and ipsilateral mastoid or neck, and are plotted vertex-positive upward; bandwidth of the recording system is 300-3000 Hz; recordings in animals were made under sodium pentobarbitol anesthesia; and human recordings were collected from awake subjects.

slope of the third wave; (4) the guinea pig also displays an impressive third peak, while in the cat there is a more prominent fourth wave; and (5) in humans, there is a more prominent IV-V complex, and so forth. Note, however, the relative reduction in amplitude (see calibration bars) for all waves in humans.

As indicated in Chapter 7, interpretation of the sources of such differences involve complex considerations (generator size and orientation, response characteristics of neurons within generators, conduction velocities, conduction path lengths, etc.). In fact, given the possibilities for differences in the responses across species, perhaps it is more surprising that ABRs of common laboratory animals are so similar. This is especially the case with respect to peak latency and absolute amplitude values. Although specific latency values are not given for the examples in Figure 15-1, similarities in peak positions among the waveforms recorded from different species are apparent.

Response latencies are primarily a function of two anatomic-physiologic considerations. First, a large brain results in longer nerve-conduction pathways (resulting, by itself, in slower conduction times or longer interpeak latencies). Simultaneous with this increase in head volume, however, is an increase in axon diameter (with consequent higher conduction velocities). This axon diameter increase seems to approximately offset the greater delays due to greater conduction distances. We know that cochlear travel times are longer for given frequencies in larger animals (Greenwood, 1977), but for high-frequency or click stimuli, these differences are not very significant. Synaptic delays might also be expected to vary as a function of the size of synaptic structures. Human ABRs clearly have longer interpeak latencies, presumably due to a different balance of these same factors.

Amplitude differences are also surprisingly small among these illustrated animal species, except for the human. Again, absolute amplitudes reflect both a trade-off between the sizes and orientations of generators, their component neurons, the head volume, and mass of muscle, skin, bone, and sinew. The principal reasons for the observed lower response amplitude in human ABR recordings result from greater head volume (due to the dramatic differential expansion of neocortex and cerebellum with respect to brain-stem structures) and from concomitant greater head-structure thickness. These increases in anatomic dimensions increase electrical resistance, as well as remove generators further from recording sites (recall that electrical current decreases as the inverse square of distance). In addition, relative differences in synchronicity of firing could also be an important factor in accounting for absolute amplitude values.

These differences between response recording in humans and laboratory animals are actually exaggerated by signal-to-noise problems. With an absolute amplitude which is only 20-25 percent as large as that recorded from other species, the human response is more deeply embedded in noise. Thus, responses to 1000 to 2000 stimulus presentations must be averaged to obtain adequate human records; in most animals, however, readily identifiable responses can be obtained with only 200-500 stimulus presentations.

Despite the similarities outlined above, for any given recording configuration there can be significant variation of ABR waveform shape and amplitude between individuals of the same species. Thus, responses shown in Figure 15-1 should not be taken as applicable in all instances to other members (or to other recording configurations) of those species.

Frequency-Following Responses

Although there has been less extensive recording of tone-evoked FFRs in animals, they have been intensively studied in cats and guinea pigs (Smith, Marsh, and Brown, 1975; Gardi, Merzenich, and McKean, 1979; Gardi and Merzenich, 1979; Gardi, Bledsoe, and Berlin, 1979). The FFR, like the ABR, is more easily recorded in animals than in humans, requiring less averaging for equal-amplitude responses (Fig. 15-2), permitting for significantly easier definition of response thresholds (for presumably the same reasons). FFRs are also evoked at higher stimulus frequencies in commonly studied animal species than in humans. In the cat, for example, tone-evoked FFRs are recorded to frequencies above 4 kHz (Figs. 15-2, 15-3); in humans, they are difficult to record above about 1.5 kHz (Fig. 15-2). Thresholds for FFR generation in mammals, defined as using 200 stimuli/average, are commonly in the range of 45-55 dB peak equivalent SPL. Thresholds defined as using 2000 stimuli/average are commonly of the order of 10-15 dB higher in humans. Again, a clear response is commonly recorded with 200 stimuli/

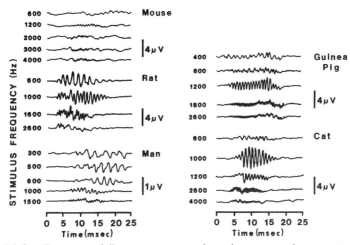

Figure 15-2. Frequency-following responses from five mammalian species (N = 512 for the animals; 2048 for human subjects) evoked by 20 msec tone bursts, (rise-fall time = 5 msec) presented at 15/sec. Stimulus intensity levels, which varied across species, were between 80 and 90 dB pe SPL. Stimulus onset is at 0.6 msec on the time scale. (See footnote on page 395.)

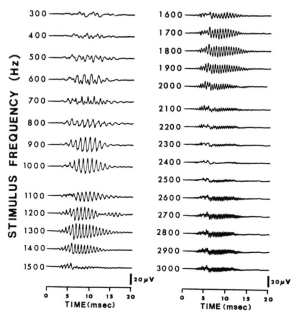

Figure 15-3. Frequency-following responses from the cat
(N = 200) evoked by 11 msec tone bursts (rise-fall time = 5
msec) presented at 20/sec and 100 dB pe SPL. Stimulus onset
is at 2 msec on the time scale. (See footnote on page 395.)

average in animals; a clear response in humans is usually generated only with
an order of magnitude greater number of stimuli/averaged response.

FFR amplitudes recorded at different frequencies in different species
must reflect differences in the animals' audiograms. Thus, in the mouse the
FFR is difficult to record at any frequency, presumably a consequence of the
mouse's high-frequency-shifted hearing range. In all other studied species (including humans), responses are of larger amplitude. As illustrated in Figure
15-3, cat FFRs generated at different frequencies are unequal in amplitude
and onset latencies. The sources of these amplitude and onset-latency fluctuations will be discussed in detail later in this chapter.

Middle-Latency Responses

Middle-latency responses (MLRs) have not been widely investigated in
animals. That is, most studies of MLRs have been conducted in humans
(Mendel, 1980). Nearly all MLR studies in animals have been directed toward
defining neural generator(s) (Buchwald and Brown, 1977; Gardi and Bledsoe, 1979; Kaga, Hink, and Shinoda, et al., 1979; Shinoda, et al., 1979;
Ichikawa, et al., 1979; Buchwald, et al., 1981). Typical middle-latency
responses recorded under pentobarbital anesthesia from some commonly
studied mammals are shown in Figure 15-4. There is a reduction or complete
absence of latter portions of the MLR in these anesthetized animals, whereas

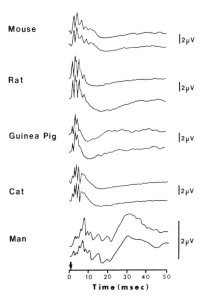

Figure 15-4. Middle-latency responses from five mammalian species (N = 512 for animals; 2048 for human subjects) evoked by 10 kHz, 1 msec stimuli (instantaneous rise-fall times) presented at 15/sec. For the animals, stimuli were presented at 80 dB pe SPL; for humans, at 60 dB SL. Bandwidth of the recording system is 10-3000 Hz. (See footnote on page 395.)

in humans, the responses are robust and easily identifiable when recorded under alert or resting conditions. When other anesthetics are used in cats and guinea pigs (e.g., urethane, chlorolose, or ketamine), more "human-like" MLRs are recorded.

Unlike the auditory brain-stem, the auditory forebrain varies considerably in different studied mammals (Merzenich, Roth, and Anderson, et al., 1977). Auditory cortical fields differ in number, orientation, and internal order across different species, with different degrees of encephalization along different lines of parallel phylogenic descent. Thus, there are almost certainly non-corresponding (non-homologous) auditory cortical fields in different advanced species (e.g., in cats as compared with monkeys) at the end of these parallel lines of mammalian evolution.

AER Uses in Animals

There have been four principal practical uses of noninvasive recording of AERs in animals. First, animal studies have been directed toward understanding the neural genesis of human evoked responses. Advantages of undertaking such studies in animals (in parallel with human observations) include (1) invasive techniques can be employed with noninvasive recording of AERs. For example, one can study the relation of discharges of neurons in auditory nuclei in parallel with generated evoked responses. One can also study AERs in parallel with evoked responses recorded intranuclearly, or one can observe the consequences of ablating or of sectioning auditory tissue in relation to the presence or absence of AER activity recorded from the scalp. (2) Virtually all of these responses are much easier to record in animals. (3) Animals are easily anesthetized over several hours, allowing extensive parametric experiments.

Second, animal studies have been directed toward defining the origins and nature of the cochlear excitation which underlies these evoked responses. Definition of the underlying cochlear origins of specific evoked responses is central to their interpretation and practical use in audiology. One decided advantage of animal studies is the availability of information about distributed neural and/or microphonic responses in several species, especially guinea pigs, cats, and squirrel monkeys. Another advantage lies, again, with the use of invasive procedures, e.g., introduction of prescribed and histologically confirmed lesions to define cochlear origins.

Third, scalp-recorded evoked responses have been employed in numerous experiments to monitor the status of the cochlear or auditory nervous system, if a change in status is likely, i.e., either detrimental or integral to the experiment (Cody, Robertson, and Bredberg, et al., 1980). The recording of N_1 potentials as well as scalp-recorded auditory evoked responses is now being extensively employed so as to monitor animal status. The technique is used to determine hearing status, similar to its use in uncooperative human subjects. Such applications in animals are, again, easier to perform and interpret, because of greater response amplitude with far less averaging, and because of less limiting conditions for idealization of chronic recording conditions.

Finally, AERs have been employed to relate evoked responses to auditory nerve array excitation patterns generated by simple stimuli to allow for quantitative application of these noninvasive recording techniques in basic auditory physiologic investigations. Several such studies have been conducted; as the data increases, a crucial link between quantitative neurophysiologic data recorded in animals and human psychophysic data should be provided. The salient feature here is that FFRs and ABRs can be translated in detail as to auditory nerve coding in animals and therefore can be recorded with identical stimuli in animals and humans.

These and other practical applications (Hamernik, Henderson, and Coling, et al., 1981) of the recording of these noninvasively recorded responses can be expected to significantly increase. It is useful, then, to briefly describe some AER uses in animals.

Definition of the Neural Origins of Auditory Evoked Responses

ABRs.   One important application of ABR recording in animals has been in studies directed toward defining their neural origins (see Chapter 7). Thus, ABRs have been recorded: (1) prior to and following surgical ablation of auditory nuclei (cochlear nucleus, superior olivary complex, nucleus of the lateral lemniscus, and nuclei of the inferior colliculus); (2) prior to and following generation of electrolytic lesions in auditory nuclei or pathways (Buchwald and Huang, 1975; Goldenberg and Derbyshire, 1975); (3) prior to and following reversible cooling of auditory nuclei or pathways (Smith, Marsh, and Brown, 1975); (4) simultaneous with recorded intranuclear evoked responses (Jewett, 1970; Lev and Sohmer, 1972); and (5) while defining phase reversals, through long penetrations crossing auditory nuclei (Jewett, 1970).

A representative ablation study (Gardi, Merzenich, and McKean, 1979) designed to determine ABR neural genesis is illustrated in Figure 15-5. In this study, ABRs were recorded prior to and following total bilateral collicular ablation (Fig. 15-5A), and prior to and following aspiration of the cochlear nuclei (Fig. 15-5B). Such invasive studies provide the strongest evidence that

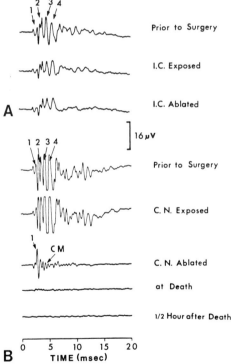

Figure 15-5. Auditory brain-stem responses from the cat (N = 100), evoked by 0.1 msec click stimuli presented at 10/ sec and 70 dB pe SPL. Stimulus onset is at 2 msec on the time scale. A. Responses were recorded before and after bilateral aspiration of the inferior colliculi (IC). B. Responses from a second cat before and after aspiration of the cochlear nuclei (CN) (the cochlear blood supply was spared); at death; and after death. (See footnote on page 395.) (Redrawn from Gardi, Merzenich, and McKean, 1979.)

successive peaks in the ABR originate predominantly from successive levels of the auditory nervous system. Specifically, almost all evidence (Buchwald and Huang, 1975; Goldenberg and Derbyshire, 1975; Huang and Buchwald, 1977; Achor and Starr, 1980b; Gardi, Merzenich and McKean, 1979; Gardi and Berlin, 1981; Gardi and Bledsoe, 1981) derived from such animal studies is consistent with the following: (1) Successive waves arise from the spiral ganglion and/or auditory nerve, cochlear nuclei, superior olivary complex, lateral lemniscus nuclei, and inferior colliculus. (2) The first wave, without doubt, corresponds to N_1. (3) There is little contribution to later waves from earlier sources. (For example, with destruction of the auditory striae, there is absolutely no response following the second wave, and hence little significant contribution from the cochlear nuclei to any later component, unless such contributions require descending connection to the cochlear nucleus.) (4) Amplitudes of successive waves follow the first or any other wave in a more or less mimicking fashion. A measure of the amplitude of the entire 6-7 msec of the ABR, for example, parallels the rate of growth of the first response (or N_1). (5) Relative amplitudes of the waves depend on the placement of the recording electrodes.

What is the neuronal source of these responses within brain-stem nuclei? In investigating neural genesis, great advantages exist in animal studies in that all basic physiology—nearly all direct understanding of auditory nerve coding and neural processes in these component divisions of the auditory system— has been derived in studies conducted in experimental animals. Several investigators (Jewett, 1970; Lev and Sohmer, 1972) have demonstrated that ABR waves are coincident with intranuclear evoked responses generated by synchronous neural responses to stimulus onset transients. Animal studies generally support the conclusion that ABR component waves arise from synchronous onset-linked neural discharges and, probably more importantly, from synchronous, powerful, post-synaptic potentials intranuclearly generated via highly coincident neural responses to stimulus transients in each of a successive, ascending series of auditory nuclei. (See Chapter 7 for a more complete description of possible central neural generators.)

FFRs. Studies of tone-evoked FFR genesis in animals have employed similar techniques used to determine neural origins of ABR activity. For example, invasive procedures, local cooling, and simultaneous intranuclear recording have also been used in attempts to define FFR neural origins (Smith, Marsh, and Brown, 1975; Gardi, Merzenich, and McKean, 1979). Experiments in cats (Gardi, Merzenich, and McKean, 1979) (Fig. 15-6) have revealed that cat FFRs originate from several sources. The principal contribution (approximately 50-60 percent) arises from the cochlear nuclear complex. There is a significant smaller contribution (20-25 percent) from at least one other brain-stem source (perhaps one or more of the component nuclei of the superior olivary complex). Further, at higher stimulus levels, there is a

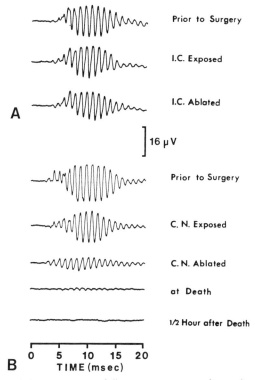

Prior to Surgery

I.C. Exposed

I.C. Ablated

A

] 16 μV

Prior to Surgery

C. N. Exposed

C. N. Ablated

at Death

1/2 Hour after Death

```
   0    5    10   15   20
B       TIME (msec)
```

Figure 15-6. Frequency-following responses from the cat (N = 200) evoked by 1 kHz, 11 msec tone burst (rise-fall time = msec) presented at 10/sec and at 100 dB pe SPL. Stimulus onset is at 2 msec on the time scale. A. Responses were recorded before and after bilateral aspiration of the inferior colliculi (IC). B. Responses from a second cat before and after aspiration of the cochlear nuclei (CN) (the cochlear blood supply was spared); at death; and after death. (See footnote on page 395.) (Redrawn from Gardi, Merzenich, and McKean, 1979.)

contribution from the cochlea itself (20-25 percent). Earlier conclusions implicated the inferior colliculus as a source of the FFR (Smith, Marsh, and Brown, 1975); it now appears that the inferior colliculus and the dorsal nucleus of the lateral lemniscus may not make very significant contributions to the FFR; other recent studies have not resolved this issue (Yamada, Marsh, and Potsic, 1980; Yamada, Kodera, and Hink, et al., 1979; Yamada, Yamane, and Kodera, 1977).

The premise that the FFR originates from multiple generators (Faingold and Caspary, 1979) is also supported by studies in cats, which reveal that the amplitude of this response varies considerably as a function of stimulus frequency (see Fig. 15-3). This variation of response amplitude is consistent with the theory of two or more generators involved in FFR production and with fixed delays existing between the generators, on the order of 1.2 msec. Fixed delays of this magnitude (conduction delays) occur between the cochlea and the ventral cochlear nucleus, between the ventral cochlear nucleus and component nuclei of the superior olivary complex, and between the superior olivary complex and the ventral nucleus of the lateral lemniscus. These delays approximately correspond to the interpeak latencies of the ABR.

As in the case of the ABR, there appears to be little mystery about the neuronal generators of the FFR. Basic physiologic studies (principally conducted in cats at the level of the cochlear nuclei see Rose, et al., 1974; Lavine, 1971; Rupert, 1970; Bledsoe, Rupert, and Moushegian, 1982; Goldberg and Brownell, 1973; at the level of the superior olivary nuclei see Brownell, 1975; Moushegian, Rupert, and Whitcomb, 1964) have demonstrated that the FFR primarily arises from component divisions of the auditory system in which there is a continuous temporal neural representation of stimulus period. As observed with recording of intranuclear evoked responses (Marsh and Worden, 1968; Worden and Marsh, 1968; Smith, Marsh, and Brown, 1975), stimulus periodicity is represented by the synchronous excitation of neurons within these contributing nuclei.

Middle-latency responses. Fewer animal studies have been directed toward determination of the neural origins of MLRs; they are, as a result, less understood. Given the differences in the auditory central nervous system in cats and primates (and differences in species susceptibility to anesthetics), perhaps later portions of the MLR may arise from non-corresponding neural generators.

Some preliminary animal results have been obtained that implicate certain auditory areas (in cats) as middle-latency response generators. Gardi and Bledsoe (1979) and Kaga, Hink, and Shinoda, et al. (1979) have shown that the second positive MLR peak (Pa) is eliminated by contralateral destruction of auditory cortex (Fig. 15-7). In fact, near-field records obtained by Kaga, Kitazumi, and Kodama, et al. (1979) showed a phase reversal in waveform polarity (for this peak) as penetrations were made through the "anterior portions of AI [AI = primary auditory cortex]" in the cat. These near-field records had similar latencies to responses obtained from the scalp that were abolished by contralateral AI damage. In a preliminary experiment, Kaga, and his colleagues (1979) attempted to define the specific area of auditory cortex responsible for the generation of the second positive peak in the scalp-recorded MLR in the cat. They concluded that lesions restricted to the "anterior boundaries of AI" in that species (actually probably principally affecting the recently described "anterior auditory field"; see Knight, 1977) most dramatically affected the second positive peak. Other recent work (Buchwald et al., 1981) suggests a very different source for the second positive peak (Pa). While recording from awake, bilaterally hemispherectomized cats, Buchwald, et al.

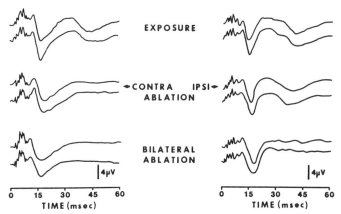

Figure 15-7. Middle-latency responses from the cat (N = 512) evoked by 6 kHz, 1 msec stimuli (instantaneous rise–fall times) presented at 15/sec and 80 dB pe SPL. Stimulus onset is at 0.6 msec on the time scale. All recordings were made between the vertex and ipsilateral mastoid. Bandwidth of the recording system was 10–3000 Hz. Responses were recorded after surgical exposure, after ablation of the contralateral primary auditory cortex in one cat (left tracings), after ablation of the ipsilateral primary auditory cortex in another cat (right tracings), and after bilateral ablation of the auditory cortices. (See footnote on page 395.) (Redrawn from Gardi and Bledsoe, 1979.)

(1981) observed no change in MLR wave Pa amplitude (see Chapter 7 for further discussion).

Lesions of the contralateral medial geniculate body abolish the initial positive peak (Po) seen in cat MLRs recorded from the scalp (Gardi and Bledsoe, 1979). Lower-level ablations, including those at the level of the inferior colliculi, do not seem to alter the prominent negative peak at 16-18 msec, while the fifth wave in the ABR (recorded with a wide band-pass) is abolished by such lesions (Buchwald and Huang, 1975). That the prominent negative peak was not abolished following these lesions, coupled with the observation that this component is resistant to anesthetic effects, suggest that this negative peak reflects slow wave activity actually arising from one or more of the brainstem nuclei caudal to the inferior colliculus.

Cochlear Excitation Sources

A principal objective of the clinical use of noninvasive recorded AERs in humans has been the determination of the status of a damaged or diseased cochlea. Related to such interpretations is an understanding of the nature of cochlear excitation that underlie these evoked responses.

Animal AERs have special importance to clinical application and interpretation of human AERs. There is an increasing quantity of information emerging from animal studies on the distributed activation of the auditory nerve array (Kim and Molnar, 1979; Evans, 1978). Since these data are derived using stimuli commonly used to record AERs in both animals and humans, it becomes possible to relate AERs in animals to their underlying origins and excitation patterns in the cochlea, and hence draw inferences about the underlying cochlear origins of human AERs.

Studies of cochlear excitation dictate absolute limits for the underlying cochlear origins of all evoked responses. That is, at relatively low stimulus levels (below 40–50 dB SPL), tonal stimulation causes place-restricted cochlear nerve excitation patterns. As stimulation exceeds 45–50 dB, cochlear nerve excitation rapidly spreads basalward. At levels of 80–100 dB SPL, all of the cochlear nerve array basal to the "best frequency" locus is being excited at or near saturation. Thus, any AER recorded using such levels of stimulation potentially (although not necessarily) reflects the status of a large proportion of the cochlea.

Another fundamental consideration must be taken into account when interpreting cochlear sources from basic neurophysiologic data. Underlying contributions of the cochlea to neural responses are weighted toward inputs that are temporally more synchronous (see Chapter 9). Even when neurons are driven at high stimulus levels by complex stimuli, sufficient to drive neurons across most of the nerve array at or near saturation, there are foci of more synchronously firing neurons for each spectral component of the complex stimulus (Sachs and Young, 1979; Kim and Molnar, 1979). These two factors, spread of excitation and distributed relative synchronicity, absolutely dictate any interpretation of cochlear sources underlying AERs.

Studies directly establishing the relationship between AERs and auditory nerve excitation as functions of cochlear position or place of excitation are still incompletely developed. Some masking studies have been conducted in animals (Gardi and Merzenich, 1979; Bledsoe and Moushegian, 1980); they offer results in support of the basic conclusion that such relationships exist. One such result is illustrated in Figure 15-8. An FFR to a low-level tonal stimulus reveals restricted cochlear excitation. When the stimulus level is increased (i.e., at stimulus levels higher than the 55 dB peSPL shown in Figure 15-8), excitation rapidly shifts toward the basal end of the cochlea (higher frequencies). At these successively higher stimulus levels, significant masking is recorded at successively higher cut-off frequencies; all masking studies have revealed similar results. Future studies should provide a quantitative basis for the use of AERs as a means for efficiently assessing distributed VIIIth nerve activation. Harris (1979) provided an elegant example of such use of electrophysiologic responses (Fig. 15-9). Using masking N_1 responses, two-tone suppression bands were derived through the use of a forward masking paradigm (Green, 1976). Tuning curves and suppression bands were demonstrated to accurately reflect distributed VIIIth nerve responses in the chinchillas studied.

AERs to Monitor Hearing Status

Noninvasively recorded AERs can be used effectively to evaluate and monitor hearing status in experimental animal preparations (Chou and Galambos, 1979). For example, we have used AERs to tonal and/or click

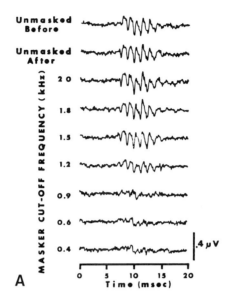

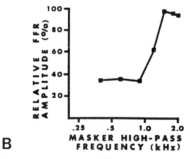

Figure 15-8. A. Frequency-following responses from the cat (N = 4096) evoked by 800 Hz, 10 msec tone bursts (rise-fall time = 5 msec) presented at 55 dB pe SPL and at 10/sec. High-pass masking noises were continuously presented at 40 dB SPL. Tonal stimulus onset is at 2 msec on the time scale. B. Percent-relative root mean square amplitude of masked FFR as a function of cut-off (−3 dB) frequency of the masker (noise). (See footnote on page 395.) (Redrawn from Gardi and Merzenich, 1979.)

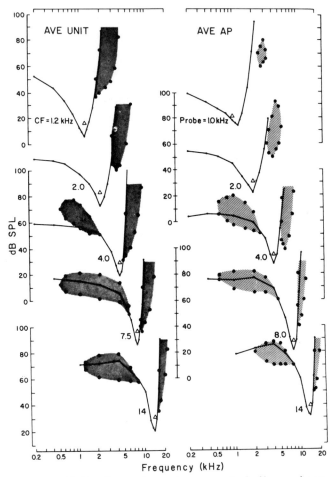

Figure 15-9. Comparison of average single-fiber and compound action potential (AP) data recorded from chinchillas. On the left are average frequency-threshold curves (solid lines) and two-tone suppression areas (shaded areas). Each threshold curve represents data from seven to eight fibers from various animals. These data were frequency-normalized to the characteristic frequency (CF), as indicated for each curve, and SPL values of the curves and the suppression areas were averaged. On the right are average AP tuning curves and suppression areas (N = 3), derived with the use of a "forward-masking" technique. (Reprinted with permission from Harris, D. Action potential suppression, tuning curves and thresholds. Comparison with single fiber data. *Hearing Research*, 1979 1:133-154.)

stimuli recorded in animals as follows: (1) To estimate hearing thresholds at a given frequency, prior to injection of the activity-dependent tracer 2-deoxy-glucose. (2) To estimate hearing thresholds prior to administration of an ototoxic drug (neomycin sulfate), and to time-track the hearing loss induced by that drug (Leake-Jones and Vivion, 1979; Osako, Tokimoto, and Matsuura, 1979). (3) To determine electrical stimulation thresholds (Dobie and Kimm, 1980) of the auditory nerve prior to and during "overstimulation" studies designed to reveal "safe" limits of electrical stimulation, i.e., to define electrical stimulation levels above which damage is induced (Spelman, Pfingst, and Miller, et al., 1980).

The advantages of using AER recording to monitor hearing status include:

1. The time course of normal (e.g., developmental) or pathologic changes in hearing status can be defined. For example, in studying a pathologic process, AER recordings provide a convenient way to stage the process (e.g., to derive specimens for histologic examination throughout the time course of the pathologic change). Thus, with such monitoring, study efficiency is greatly increased (Mikaelian, 1979). As another example, such AER monitoring techniques allow the more accurate correlation of parametric anatomic studies (e.g., in 2-deoxyglucose tracer studies, the extent of tracer transport can be related to physiologic activity evoked by stimuli applied at different defined suprathreshold sound levels).

2. Highly repeatable and reliable data about hearing status are derived, and the technique is easily applied. This advantage is illustrated in Figure 15-10, which shows typical baseline ABR thresholds obtained for successive evaluations.

3. Since the technique is noninvasive, it is virtually failsafe and can be repeatedly applied over very long periods of time.

4. Finally, reliable frequency-specific responses can be derived using low stimulus levels in animals in order to obtain cochlear place-specific information. Monitoring for this purpose is usually now achieved by recording N_1 responses using electrocochleographic techniques (Pugh, Moody, and Anderson, 1978). For most applications, however, scalp-recorded ABRs and/or FFRs would serve as well, and are much easier to obtain. Of course, N_1 responses can now be reliably recorded from the promontory at levels 10–15 dB lower than ABRs or FFRs, and require fewer stimulus repetitions to record an identifiable averaged response.

AERs as a Physiologic Measurement Tool

AER recordings are being increasingly used in the quantitative study of central auditory nervous system processes. Four examples are presented below; they indicate lines of research with great promise.

First, as described earlier, AERs have been recorded using basic psychophysical paradigms, in a first-level search to identify physiologic correlates

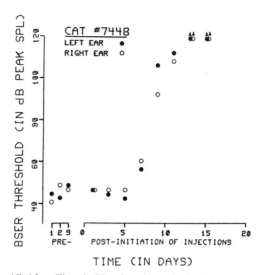

TIME (IN DAYS)

Figure 15-10. Thresholds of auditory brain-stem responses (N = 250) recorded from the cat prior to, during, and following administration of a 10-day series of intramuscular injections of neomycin sulfate (50 mg/Kg body weight). Arrowheads indicate ABR thresholds presumed greater than the maximum stimulus level. Stimuli were 0.1 msec clicks presented at 10/sec. The bandwidth of the recording system was 100-3000 Hz. (See footnote on page 395.) (Reprinted with permission from Leake-Jones, P. A., and Vivion, M. C. Cochlear pathology in cats following administration of neomycin sulfate. *SEM/1979 III.* AMF O'Hare, Ill.: SEM, Inc., 1979.)

(mechanisms) for observed psychophysical phenomena. Again, Harris' (1979) N_1 study is a significant step toward this use of AERs. His comprehensive use of the forward-masking paradigm could obviously be applied using ABR (or, possibly FFRs) to derive the same measurements of "tuning curves" and "two-tone suppression bands" in both animals and humans. Similarly, Gardi, Bledsoe, and Berlin (1979) used gap-masking paradigms to generate FFR "tuning curves" in guinea pigs (Fig. 15-11). Smith, et al., 1978, and Hall, 1979, have attempted to find a physiologic correlate of the "missing fundamental" to a series of higher, harmonically related tones in the FFR. While these attempts are fraught with interpretative problems, the potential for studies of this kind is great.

Second, noninvasively recorded AERs have been used to map excitation patterns resulting from direct electrical stimulation in studies directed toward development of cochlear prostheses. Two different excitation-mapping paradigms have been used. In one series, ABR amplitude was related to extent of cochlear nerve excitation (using a single-unit recording mapping technique) (Merzenich, et al., 1979; Merzenich and White, 1977). A very wide variety of

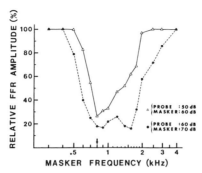

Figure 15-11. Percent relative root mean square amplitudes of frequency-following responses from the cat (N = 4096) evoked by 800 Hz, 20 msec tone bursts (rise-fall time = 5 msec) presented in a gap-masking paradigm at 20/sec. A tonal masker of 30 msec duration (rise-fall time = 5 msec) is alternated with the 800 Hz stimulus for the indicated range of frequencies (200-4000 Hz). Rise and fall portions of probe and masker stimuli overlap in time. (See footnote on page 395.) (Redrawn from Gardi, Bledsoe, and Berlin, 1979.)

nerve excitation patterns were then defined for a large variety of stimulating electrodes, simply by deriving ABR intensity functions. In a second and somewhat parallel series, one stimulating electrode pair served as a "probe" for a second electrode pair, or "test," for which excitation of the nerve array was being mapped (White, et al., 1980). By presenting just-suprathreshold stimuli to the probe within the absolute refractory period for stimulation of the test electrode, spread of excitation of the test electrode across the nerve array could be determined. This determination was made by comparing the ABRs recorded for stimulation of the probe electrode alone with those recorded for stimulation of the two electrodes. These applications of AER techniques are now being used in patients with cochlear implant prostheses.

Third, "binaural difference AERs" have now been recorded in animals and humans (Dobie and Berlin, 1979b; Dobie and Norton, 1980; Gardi and Berlin, 1981; Hosford, Fullerton, and Levine, 1979). Such responses are the numerical difference between the sum of the two responses obtained when each ear is individually stimulated, and the response obtained when both ears are simultaneously stimulated. Many binaural difference response studies will be conducted in humans, as well as in animals, because the technique offers a fundamental means for studying interactions (monaural as well as binaural) in the auditory CNS (see Chapter 10).

Fourth, recent studies (Williston, Jewett, and Martin, 1981; Gardi, Martin, and Jewett, 1980) have employed simultaneous recording of ABR and FFR activity from three orthogonally placed electrode pairs in cats, to define, at a first level, the spatial representation of given auditory stimuli within all levels of the auditory brain stem. Such studies may provide a means of studying spatial aspects of information processing within central auditory nuclei in animals and humans. Although it remains to be demonstrated, the potential clinical use of such information is enormous.

DISCUSSION

In the future, we can expect to see AERs used as techniques for studying spatial and temporal coding of auditory information in humans, just as we are beginning to obtain results of the same experiments in animals, in which we have a neurophysiologic understanding of distributed auditory nerve array excitation, and of response features of central auditory nuclei. In other words, what lies ahead is a noninvasive means of investigating the information-handling mechanisms of the central auditory nervous system in humans, through the practical use of AERs in animals.

References

Abeles, M., and Goldstein, M. H. Functional architecture in cat primary auditory cortex: Columnar organization and organization according to depth. *Journal of Neurophysiology*, 1970, *33*:172-187.

Abeles, M., and Goldstein, M. H. Responses of single units in the primary auditory cortex of the cat to tones and to tone pairs. *Brain Research*, 1972, *42*:337-352.

Achor, L. J., and Starr, A. Auditory brain stem responses in the cat. I. Intracranial and extracranial recordings. *Electroencephalography and Clinical Neurophysiology*, 1980a, *48*:154-173

Achor, L. J., and Starr, A. Auditory brain stem responses in the cat. II. Effects of lesions. *Electroencephalography and Clinical Neurophysiology*, 1980b, *48*: 174-190

Adams, G. L., Boies, L. R., and Paparella, M. M. *Fundamentals of Otolaryngology (4th ed.)*. Philadelphia: W. B. Saunders, 1978.

Adams, J. C. Morphology and physiology in the ventral nucleus of the lateral lemniscus. *Neuroscience Abstracts*, 1978, *4*:3.

Adams, J. C. Ascending projections to the inferior colliculus. *Journal of Comparative Neurology*, 1979, *183*:519-538.

Adams, J. C., and Warr, W. B. Origins of axons in the cat's acoustic striae determined by injection of horseradish peroxidase into severed tracts. *Journal of Comparative Neurology*, 1976, *170*:107-122.

Adams, R. M., and Roeser, R. The ultimate hearing test: Evoked response audiometry. *Journal of School Health*, 1979, *49*(9):536.

Adrian, E. D. The activity of the nervous system of the caterpillar. *Journal of Physiology* (London), 1930, *30*:34-36.

Adrian, E. D. The microphonic action of the cochlea in relation to theories of hearing. In *Report of a discussion of audition*. London: Physical Society of London, 1931.

413

Adrian, E. D. *The mechanism of nervous action.* Philadelphia: University of Pennsylvania Press, 1932.

Adrian, E. D., and Buytendijk, F. J. J. Potential changes in the isolated brain stem of the goldfish. *Journal of Physiology* (London), 1931, *71*:121-135.

Adrian, E. D., and Matthews, B. H. C. The Berger rhythm: Potential changes from the occipital lobe of man. *Brain*, 1934, *57*:355-385.

Adrian, E. D., and Yamagiwa, K. The origin of the Berger rhythm. *Brain*, 1935, *35*: 322-351.

Ahmed, I. Brain stem auditory evoked potentials in transtentorial herniation. *Clinical Electroencephalography*, 1980, *11*(1):34-37.

Aitkin, L. M. Medial geniculate body of the cat: Responses to tonal stimuli of neurons in medial division. *Journal of Neurophysiology*, 1973, *36*:275-283.

Aitkin, L. M., Anderson, D. J., and Brugge, J. F. Tonotopic organization and discharge characteristics of single neurons in nuceli of the lateral lemniscus of the cat. *Journal of Neurophysiology*, 1970, *33*:421-440.

Aitkin, L. M., and Boyd, J. Acoustic input to the lateral pontine nuclei. *Hearing Research*, 1978, *1*:67-77.

Aitkin, L. M., Dickhaus, H., and Schult, W., et al. External nucleus of inferior colliculus: Auditory and spinal somatosensory afferents and their interactions. *Journal of Neurophysiology*, 1978, *41*:837-847.

Aitkin, L. M., and Dunlop, C. W. Interplay of excitation and inhibition in the cat medial geniculate body. *Journal of Neurophysiology*, 1968, *31*:44-61.

Aitkin, L. M., Dunlop, C. W., and Webster, W. R. Click-evoked response patterns of single units in the medial geniculate body of the cat. *Journal of Neurophysiology*, 1966, *29*:109-123.

Aitkin, L. M., and Webster, W. R. Medial geniculate body of the cat: Organization and responses to tonal stimuli of neurons in ventral division. *Journal of Neurophysiology*, 1972, *35*:365-380.

Aitkin, L. M., Webster, W. R., and Veale, J. L., et al. Inferior colliculus. Comparison of response properties of neurons in central, pericentral, and external nuclei of adult cat. *Journal of Neurophysiology*, 1975, *38*:1196-1207.

Akiyama, Y. Schulte, F. J., and Schulz, M., et al. Acoustically evoked responses in premature and full term newborn infants. *Electroencephalography and Clinical Neurophysiology*, 1969, *26*:371-380.

Allen, A. R., and Starr, A. Auditory brain stem potentials in monkey (M. mulatta) and man. *Electroencephalography and Clinical Neurophysiology*, 1978, *45*:53-63.

Amadeo, M., and Shagass, C. Brief latency click-evoked potentials during waking and sleep in man. *Psychophysiology*, 1973, *10*:244-250.

Amassian, V. E., Waller, H. J., and Macy, J. Neural mechanisms of primary somatosensory evoked potential. *Annals of the New York Academy of Science*, 1964, *112*:5-32.

Amit, Y. Prognostic and diagnostic values of auditory nerve and brain stem responses in comatose patients. (Unpublished M.D. thesis, in Hebrew, 1978.)

Ananthanarayan, A. K., and Gerken, G. M. Masking and enhancement: A contrast of processes in the auditory brainstem response. Unpublished manuscript.

Andreev, A. M., Arapova, A. A., and Gersuni, S. V. On electrical potentials in the human cochlea. *Journal of Physiology* (London), U.S.S.R., 1939, *26*:205-212.

Anthony, P. F., Durrett, R., and Pulec, J. L., et al. A new parameter in brain stem evoked response: Component wave areas. *Laryngoscope*, 1979, *10*:1569-1578.

Antinoro, F., Skinner, P. H., and Jones, J. J. Relation between sound intensity and amplitude of the auditory evoked response at different stimulus frequencies. *Journal of the Acoustical Society of America*, 1969, *46*:1433-1436.

Antoli-Candela, F., and Kiang, N. Y.-S. Unit activity underlying the N_1 potential. In R. F. Naunton and C. Fernandez (Eds.), *Evoked electrical activity in the auditory nervous system*. New York: Academic Press, 1978.

Antonelli, A., Cazzavillan, A., and Gaini, R., et al. Some effects of the stimulus repetition rate of N_1 and N_2 in transtympanic and surface recordings. *Scandinavian Audiology*, 1981, *10*:13-19.

Anziska, B., and Cracco, R. Q. Short latency somatosensory evoked potentials in brain dead patients. *Archives of Neurology*, 1980a, *37*:222-225.

Anziska, B. J., and Cracco, R. Q. Short latency somatosensory evoked potentials in patients with focal neurological disease. *Electroencephalography and Clinical Neurophysiology*, 1980b, *49*:227-239.

Anziska, B., Cracco, R. Q., and Cook, A. W., et al. Somatosensory far field potentials: Studies in normal subjects and patients with multiple sclerosis. *Electroencephalography and Clinical Neurophysiology*, 1978, *45*:602-610.

Appleby, S. The slow vertex maximal sound evoked response in infants. In Davis, H. (Ed.). The young deaf child. Identification and management. *Acta Oto-Laryngologica* (Suppl) (Stockholm), 1973, *206*:146-152.

Aran, J. M. The electro-cochleogram. Recent results in children and in some pathological cases. *Archives für Klinische und experimentalles ohres Nases und Kehlkopf Heilkunde* (Munich), 1971, *198*:128-141.

Aran, J. M. Clinical measures of VIIIth nerve functions. *Advances in Oto-Rhino-Laryngology*, 1973, *20*:374-394.

Aran, J. M. Contributions of electrocochleography to diagnosis in infancy. An eight year survey. In S. E. Gerber, and G. T. Mencher (Eds.), *Early diagnosis of hearing loss*. New York: Grune & Stratton, 1978.

Aran, J. M., and Charlet de Sauvage, R. Clinical value of cochlear microphonic recordings. In R. J. Ruben, C. Elberling, and G. Salomon (Eds.), *Electrocochleography*. Baltimore: University Park Press, 1976.

Aran, J. M., and Delaunay, J. Étude électrophysiologique de l'audition humaine. *Revue d'Acoustique*, 1971, *14*:91-94.

Aran, J. M., and Negrévergne, M. Clinical study of some particular pathological patterns of eighth nerve responses in the human being. *Audiology*, 1973, *12*:488-503.

Aran, J. M., Pelerin, J., and Lenoir, J., et al. Aspects théoretiques et pratiques des enregistrements électrocochléographiques selon la méthode établie à Bordeaux. *Revue de Laryngologie Otologie Rhinologie* (Suppl) (Bordeaux), 1971, *92*:601-644.

Aran, J. M., and Portmann, M. L'électro cochléogramme. *Journal Francais D Oto-Rhino-Laryngologie, Audiophonologie, Chirurgie, Maxillo-Faciale*, 1972, *21*:211-221.

Aran, J. M., Portmann, M., and Portmann, C., et al. Electrochochleography in adults and children. Electrophysiological study of the peripheral receptor. *Audiology*, 1972, *11*:77-89.

Arden, G. B., Bodis-Wollner, I., and Halliday, A. M., et al. Methodology of pattern visual stimulation. In J. E. Desmedt (Ed.), *Visual evoked potentials in man: New developments.* Oxford University Press, 1977, pp. 3-15.

Arlinger, S. D., and Kylen, P. Bone-conducted stimulation in electrocochleography. *Acta Oto-Laryngologica* (Stockholm), 1977, *84*:377-384.

Armington, T. C. *The electroretinogram.* New York: Academic Press, 1974.

Ashworth, B., Maloney, A. F. J., and Towsend, H. R. A. Delayed visual evoked potentials with bilateral disease of the posterior visual pathway. *Journal of Neurology, Neurosurgery and Psychiatry*, 1978, *41*:449-451.

Asselman, P., Chadwick, D. W., and Marsden, C. D. Visual evoked responses in the diagnosis and management of patients suspected of multiple sclerosis. *Brain*, 1975, *98*:201-282.

Barnet, A. B., and Goodwin, R. S. Averaged evoked electroencephalographic response to clicks in the human newborn. *Electroencephalography and Clinical Neurophysiology*, 1965, *18*:441-450.

Barnet, A. B., Ohlrich, E. S., and Weiss, I. P., et al. Auditory evoked potentials during sleep in normal children from 10 days to 3 years of age. *Electroencephalography and Clinical Neurophysiology*, 1975, *39*:29-41.

Barrance, V., Mino, D., and Salamon, H. Treatment of relapsing polychondritis with Dapsone. *Archives of Dermatology*, 1976, *112*:1286-1288.

Barrett, G., Blumhardt, L., and Halliday, A. M., et al. A paradox in the lateralization of the visual evoked response. *Nature*, 1976, *261*:253-255.

Bartley, S. H. Action potentials of the optic cortex under the influence of strychnine. *American Journal of Physiology*, 1933, *103*:203-212.

Bartley, S. H., and Newman, E. B. Recording action currents. *Transactions of the Kansas Academy of Science*, 1930a, *33*:78-81.

Bartley, S. H., and Newman, E. B. Recording cerebral action currents. *Science*, 1930b, *71*:587.

Baschek, V., and Steinert, W. The indication for brain stem evoked response and the effect of click rate and stimulus intensity on the latencies of the auditory evoked potentials. *Laryngologie, Rhinologie, Otologie* (Stuttgart), 1980, *59*:690-697.

Bauch, C. D., Rose, D. E., and Harner, S. G. Brainstem responses to tone pip and click stimuli. *Ear and Hearing*, 1980, *1*:181-184.

Beagley, H. A., and Butler, J. Avoidance of masking difficulties using electrocochleography. Case report. *British Journal of Audiology*, 1981, *15*:11-12.

Beagley, H. A., and Kellogg, S. E. A comparison of evoked response and subjective auditory thresholds. *International Audiology*, 1969, *8*:345-353.

Beagley, H. A., and Knight, J. J. Changes in auditory evoked response with intensity. *Journal of Laryngology and Otology*, 1967, *81*:861-873.

Beagley, H. A., Legouix, J. P., and Teas, D. C., et al. Electrocochleographic changes in acoustic neuroma. Some experimental findings. *Clinical Otolaryngology*, 1977, *2*:213-219.

Beagley, H. A., and Sheldrake, J. B. Differences in brain stem response latency with age and sex. *British Journal of Audiology*, 1978, *12*:69-77.

von Békésy, G. Shearing microphonics produced by vibrations near the inner and outer hair cells. *Journal of the Acoustical Society of America*, 1953, *25*:786-790.

von Békésy, G. *Experiments in hearing.* Translated by E. G. Wever. New York: McGraw-Hill, 1960.

Benevento, L. A., Coleman, P. D., and Loe, P. R. Responses of single cells in cat inferior colliculus to binaural click stimuli. Combinations of intensity levels, time differences, and intensity differences. Brain Research, 1970, 17:387-405.
Bergamini, L., Bergamasco, B., and Fra, I., et al. Somatosensory evoked cortical potentials in subjects with peripheral nervous lesions. Electromyography, 1965, 5:121-130.
Berger, H. Uber das Elektrenkephalogramm des Menschen. Archiv für Psychiatrie und Nervenkrankheiten, 1929, 87:527-570.
Bergholtz, L. M., Arlinger, S. D., and Kylen, P., et al. Electrocochleography used as a clinical hearing test in difficult-to-test children. Acta Oto-Laryngologica (Stockholm), 1977, 84:385-392.
Bergholtz, L. M., Hooper, R. E., and Mehta, D. C. Electrocochleographic response patterns in a group of patients mainly with presbycusis. Scandinavian Audiology, 1977, 6:3-11.
Bergman, M., and Matathias, O. Personal communication, 1979.
Berlin, C. I. Electrophysiological indices of auditory function. In F. N. Martin (Ed.), Pediatric Audiology, Englewood Cliffs, N.J.: Prentice-Hall, Inc., 1978.
Berlin, C. I. Temporal and dichotic factors in central auditory testing. In J. Katz (Ed.), Handbook of clinical audiology. Baltimore: Williams & Wilkins, 1972.
Berlin, C. I. Central deafness: Fact or fiction? Birth Defects, 1980, 17:47-57.
Berlin, C. I., Cullen, J. K., and Ellis, M. S., et al. Clinical application of recording human VIIIth nerve action potentials from the tympanic membrane. Transactions of the American Academy of Ophthalmology and Otolaryngology, 1974, 78: 401-410.
Berlin, C. I., Cullen, J. K., and Gondra, M. I., et al. Clinical experience with electrocochleography. Special application in bone conduction. In G. E. Shambaugh, and J. J. Shea (Eds.), Middle ear microsurgery and fluctuant hearing loss. Huntsville, Alabama: the Strode Publishing Company, 1977.
Berlin, C. I., and Dobie, R. A. Electrophysiologic measures of auditory function via electrocochleography and brainstem-evoked responses. In W. F. Rintelman (Ed.), Hearing Assessment, Baltimore: University Park Press, 1979.
Berlin, C. I., and Gardi, J. N. Clinical application of auditory electrophysiology. In R. D. Brown and E. A. Daigneault (Eds.), The Pharmacology of Hearing: Experimental and Clinical Basis, New York: John Wiley and Sons, 1981.
Berlin, C. I., Gondra, M. I., and Casey, D. A., et al. Bone-conduction electrocochleography: Clinical applications, Laryngoscope, 1978, 5:756-763.
Bernard, P. A., Péchére, J. C., and Hebert, R. Altered objective audiometry in aminoglycoside-treated human neonates. Archives of Oto-Rhino-Laryngology, 1980, 228(3):205-210.
Berry, H., Briant, T. D., and Winchester, B. T. Electrophysiologic assessment of the lower portion of the auditory pathway in the human subject. Journal of Otolaryngology, 1976, 5:3-11.
Bhargava, V. K., Salamy, A., and McKean, C. M. Effect of cholinergic drugs on the auditory evoked responses from brain-stem (FFP) and auditory cortex (CER). Neuroscience, 1978, 3:821-826.
Bickford, R. G. Physiological and clinical studies of microflexes. Recent Contributions to Neurophysiology. EEG Suppl. Elsevier, 1972, 31:93-108.
Bickford, R. G., Fleming, N. I., and Billinger, T. W. Compression of EEG data by

isometric power spectral plots. *Electroencephalography and Clinical Neurophysiology*, 1971, *31*:631-635.

Bickford, R. G., Jacobson, J., and Cody, D. Nature of averaged evoked potential to sound and other stimuli in man. *Annals of the New York Academy of Science*, 1964, *112*:204-223.

Bishop, G. H., and Clare, M. Sequence of events in optic cortex response to volleys of impulses in the radiation. *Journal of Neurophysiology*, 1953, *16*:490-498.

Bledsoe, S. C., and Moushegian, G. The 500 Hz frequency-following potential in kangaroo rat. An evaluation with noise masking. *Electroencephalography and Clinical Neurophysiology*, 1980, *48*:654-663.

Bledsoe, S. C., Rupert, A. L., and Moushegian, G. Response characteristics of cochlear nucleus neurons to 500 Hz tones and noise: Findings relating to frequency-following potentials. *Journal of Neurophysiology*, 1982, *47*:113-127

Blegvad, B. Binaural summation of surface recorded electrocochleographic responses. Normal hearing subjects. *Scandinavian Audiology*, 1975, *4*:233-238.

Bloom, W., and Fawcett, D. W. *A Textbook of Histology* (8th ed), Philadelphia: W. B. Saunders, 1962.

Bloom, W., Fawcett, D. W. *A textbook of histology, 10th ed*. Philadelphia: W. B. Saunders, 1975.

Blumhardt, L. D., Barrett, G., and Halliday, A. M. The asymmetrical visual evoked potential to pattern reversal in one half field and its significance for the analysis of visual field defects. *British Journal of Ophthalmology*, 1977, *61*:454-461.

Bobbin, R. P., May, J. G., and Lemoine, R. L. Effects of pentobarbital and ketamine on brain stem auditory potentials. *Archives of Otolaryngology*, 1979, *105*: 467-470.

Bochenek, W., and Bochenek, Z. Postauricular (12 msec latency) responses to acoustic stimuli in patients with peripheral, facial nerve palsy. *Acta Oto-Laryngologica* (Stockholm), 1976, *81*:264-269.

Bochenek, Z., Fialkowska, D., and Bochenek, W., et al. Four-year experience with electric response audiometry. *Audiology*, 1974, *13*:403-407.

Bodis-Wollner, I., Hendley, C. D., and Mylin, L. H., et al. Visual evoked potentials and the visuogram in multiple sclerosis. *Annals of Neurology*, 1979, *5*:40-47.

de Boer, E., and Bouwmeester, J. Critical bands and sensorineural hearing loss. *Audiology*, 1974, *13*:236-259.

Bonding, P. Critical bandwidth in loudness summation in sensorineural hearing loss. *British Journal of Audiology*, 1979a, *13*:23-30.

Bonding, P. Critical bandwidth in patients with acoustic neuroma. *Scandinavian Audiology*, 1979b, *8*:15-22.

Bonding, P. Critical bandwidth in presbycusis. *Scandinavian Audiology*, 1979c, *8*:43-50.

Booth, J. B. Ménière's disease: The selection and assessment of patients for surgery using electrocochleography. *Annals of the Royal College of Surgeons of England*, 1980, *62*(6):415-425.

Bordley, J. E., Ruben, R. J., and Lieberman, A. T. Human cochlear potentials. *Laryngoscope*, 1964, *74*:463-479.

Bossy, J. Atlas of Neuroanatomy and Special Sense Organs. Philadelphia: W. B. Saunders, 1970, p. 267.

Boston, J. R., and Ainslie, P. J. Effects of analog and digital filtering on brain stem auditory evoked potentials. *Electroencephalography and Clinical Neurophysiology*, 1980, *48*:361-364.

Botte, M. D., Bujas, R., and Chocholle, R. Comparison between the growth of the averaged electroencephalic response and direct loudness estimations. *Journal of the Acoustical Society of America*, 1975, *58*:208-213.

Boudreau, J. C. Neural volleying: Upper frequency limits detectable in the auditory system. *Nature*, 1965a, *208*:1237-1238.

Boudreau, J. D. Stimulus correlates of wave activity in the superior-olivary complex of the cat. *Journal of the Acoustical Society of America*, 1965b, *37*:779-785.

Bourk, T. R. *Electrical responses of neural units in the anteroventral cochlear nucleus of the cat.* Doctoral dissertation, Massachusetts Institute of Technology, Cambridge, 1976.

Bourk, T. R. Phase-locking in AVCN units of cat. *Journal of the Acoustical Society of America*, 1977, *61*:S59.

Brackmann, D. E. Electric response audiometry in a clinical practice. *Laryngoscope*, 1977, *87*:1-33.

Brackmann, D. E., and Selters, W. A. Electrocochleography in Ménière's disease and acoustic neuromas. In R. J. Ruben, E. Elberling, and G. Salomon (Eds.), *Electrocochleography*. Baltimore: University Park Press, 1976.

Brackmann, D. E., and Selters, W. A. Electric response audiometry. Clinical applications. *Otolaryngologic Clinics of North America*, 1978, *11*:7-18.

Brama, I., and Sohmer, H. Auditory nerve and brain-stem responses to sound stimuli at various frequencies. *Audiology*, 1977, *16*:402-408.

Brawer, J. R., Morest, D. K., and Kane, E. C. The neuronal architecture of the cochlear nucleus of the cat. *Journal of Comparative Neurology*, 1974, *155*:251-300.

Brinkmann, R. D., and Ebner, A. Clinical value of the brain stem evoked response in coma. *Electroencephalography and Clinical Neurophysiology*, 1977, *43*:525.

Brinkmann, R. D., and Scherg, M. Human auditory on- and off-potentials of the brain stem. Influence of stimulus envelope characteristics. *Scandinavian Audiology*, 1979, *8*:27-32.

Brinkmann, W. F. B., and Tolk, J. Aural microphonics in man. *Practica Otorhinolaryngologica* (Basel), 1961/62, *23*:325.

Broughton, R., Maier-Ewert, M., and Abe, M. Evoked visual somatosensory and retinal potentials in photosensitive epilepsy. *Electroencephalography and Clinical Neurophysiology*, 1969, *27*:373-386.

Brownell, W. E. Organization of the cat trapezoid body and the discharge characteristics of its fibers. *Brain Research*, 1975, *94*:413-433.

Brugge, J. F., Anderson, D. J., and Aitkin, L. M. Responses of neurons in the dorsal nucelus of the lateral lemniscus of cat to binaural tonal stimulation. *Journal of Neurophysiology*, 1970, *33*:441-458.

Brugge, J. D., Dubrovsk, N. A., and Aitkin, L. M., et al. Sensitivity of single neurons in auditory cortex of cat to binaural tonal stimulation. Effects of varying interaural time and intensity. *Journal of Neurophysiology*, 1969, *32*:1005-1024.

Brugge, J. F., and Merzenich, M. M. Responses of neurons in auditory cortex of the macaque monkey to monaural and binaural stimulation. *Journal of Neurophysiology*, 1973, *36*:1138-1158.

Brush, S. G. Should the history of science by rated x? *Science*, 1974, *183*:1164-1172.

Buchwald, J. S., and Brown, K. A. The role of acoustic inflow in the development of adaptive behavior. *Annals of the New York Academy of Sciences*, 1977, *290*:270-284.

Buchwald, J. S., and Hinman, C. Unpublished observations, 1980.

Buchwald, J. S., Hinman, C., and Norman, R. J., et al. Middle- and long-latency auditory evoked responses recorded from the vertex of normal and chronically-lesioned cats. *Brain Research*, 1981, *205*:91-109.

Buchwald, J. S., and Huang, C. M. Far-field acoustic response: Origins in the cat. *Science*, 1975, *189*:382-384.

Bullock, T. H., Grinnell, A. D., and Ikezone, E., et al. Electrophysiological studies of central auditory mechanisms in cetaceans. *Zeitschrift für vergleichende Physiologie*, 1968, *59*:117-156.

Butler, R. A. The effect of changes in stimulus frequency and intensity in habituation of the human vertex potential. *Journal of the Acoustical Society of America*, 1968, *44*:945-950.

Caccia, M. R., Ubcali, E., and Andreussi, L. Spinal evoked responses recorded from the epidural space in normal and diseased humans. *Journal of Neurology, Neurosurgery and Psychiatry*, 1976, *39*:962-972.

Callaway, E. *Brain electrical potentials and individual psychological differences*. New York: Grune & Stratton, 1975.

Callaway, E., and Halliday, R. A. Evoked potential variability. Effects of age, amplitude, and methods of measurement. *Electroencephalography and Clinical Neurophysiology*, 1973, *34*:125-133.

Calmes, R. L., and Cracco, R. Q. Comparison of somatosensory and somatomotor evoked responses to median nerve and digital nerve stimulation. *Electroencephalography and Clinical Neurophysiology*, 1971, *31*:547-562.

Campbell, F. W., Atkinson, J., and Francis, M. R., et al. Estimation of auditory thresholds using evoked potentials: A clinical screening test. In J. E. Desmedt (Ed.), *Progress in clinical neurophysiology, Vol. 2. Auditory evoked potentials in man. Psychopharmacology Correlates of EPs*. Basel: Karger, 1977.

Campbell, K. B., Picton, T. W., and Wolfe, R. G., et al. Auditory potentials. Proceedings of the First International Workshop and Symposium on Evoked Potentials, Milan, 1981, *I*:21-31.

Cann, J., and Knott, J.: Polarity of acoustic click stimuli for eliciting brain-stem auditory evoked responses: A proposed standard. *American Journal of Electroencephalography and Technology*, 1979, *19*:125-132.

Caton, R. The electric currents of the brain. *British Medical Journal*, 1875, *2*:278.

Celesia, G. G. Organization of auditory cortical areas in man. *Brain*, 1976, *99*:403-414.

Celesia, G. G. Visual evoked potentials in neurological disorders. *American Journal of Electroencephalography and Technology*, 1978, *18*:47-59.

Celesia, G. G. Steady state and transient visual evoked potentials in clinical practice. *Annals of New York Academy of Science*, 1982, *388*:290-305.

Celesia, G. G., and Daly, R. F. Visual electroencephalographic computer analysis (VECA). *Neurology*, 1977a, *27*:637-641.

Celesia, G. G., and Daly, R. F. Effects of aging on visual evoked responses. *Archives of Neurology*, 1977b, *34*:403-407.

Celesia, G. G., and Puletti, F. Auditory cortical areas of man. *Neurology*, 1969, *19*: 211-220.

Celesia, G. G., and Puletti, F. Auditory input to the human cortex during states of drowsiness and surgical anesthesia. *Electroencephalography and Clinical Neurophysiology*, 1971, *31*:603–609.

Celesia, G. G., Soni, V. K., and Rhode, W. S. Visual evoked spectrum array and interhemispheric variations. *Archives of Neurology*, 1978, *35*:678–682.

Chandler, J. R. Malignant external otitis: Further considerations. *Annals of Otology, Rhinology and Laryngology*, 1977, *86*:417–428.

Charachon, R., and Dumas, G. Value of early auditory evoked potentials in nontraumatic diseases of the brain stem. *Journal Francais Oto-Rhino-Laryngologie, Audiophonologie, Chirurgie Maxillo-Faciale*, 1980, *29*(9):569–588.

Charachon, R., Dumas, G., and Richard, J. Electrocochleography and measurement of brain stem auditory potentials in the diagnosis of deafness in children. *Revue de Laryngologie Otologie Rhinologie* (Bordeaux), 1979, *100*(11-12): 645–655.

Chesney, G. L., Michie, P., and Donchin, E. Selective attention and a slow, negative component of the human event-related potential. *Psychophysiology*, 1980, 17:291–242.

Chiappa, K. H., Choi, S. K., and Young, R. R. Short latency somatosensory evoked potentials following median nerve stimulation in patients with neurological lesions. In *Clinical uses of cerebral, brain-stem and spinal somatosensory evoked potentials*, 1980, 264–281.

Chiappa, K. H., and Gladstone, K. J. The limits of normal variations in waves I through VII of the human brain stem auditory response. *Neurology*, 1978, *28*:402.

Chiappa, K. H., Gladstone, K. J., and Young, R. R. Brain stem auditory evoked responses. Studies of wave form variations in 50 normal human subjects. *Archives of Neurology*, 1979, *36*:81–87.

Chiappa, K. H., Harrison, J. L., and Brooks, E. B., et al. Brainstem auditory evoked responses in 200 patients with multiple sclerosis. *Annals of Neurology*, 1980, 7:135–143.

Chisin, R., Perlman, M., and Sohmer, H. Cochlear and brainstem responses in hearing loss following neonatal hyperbilirubinemia. *Annals of Otology, Rhinology and Laryngology*, 1979, *88*:352–356.

Chou, C. K., and Galambos, R. Middle-ear structures contribute little to auditory perception of microwaves. *Journal of Microwave Power*, 1979, *14*(4):321–326.

Chu, N. S., Squires, K. C., and Starr, A. Auditory brainstem potentials in chronic alcohol intoxication and alcohol withdrawal. *Archives of Neurology*, 1978, *35*:596–602.

Ciganek, L. Visual evoked responses. In W. S. van Leeuwen, F. M. Lopes da Silva, and A. Kamp (Eds.), *Evoked responses*. In A. Remond (Ed.), *Handbook of electroencephalography and clinical neurophysiology*. Amsterdam: Elsevier, 1975.

Clark, G. M., and Dunlop, C. W. Field potentials in the cat medial superior olivary nucleus. *Experimental Neurology*, 1968, *20*:31–42.

Clemis, J. D., and McGee, T. Brainstem electric response audiometry in the differential diagnosis of acoustic tumors. *Laryngoscope*, 1979, *84*:31–42.

Clemis, J. D., and Mitchell, C. Electrocochleography and brainstem responses used in the diagnosis of acoustic tumors. *Journal of Otolaryngology*, 1977, 6:447–459.

Coats, A. On electrocochleographic electrode design. *Journal of the Acoustical Society of America*, 1974, *56*:708-711.

Coats, A. Evaluation of "click pips" as impulsive, yet frequency-specific stimuli for possible use in electrocochleography—A preliminary report. In R. Ruben, C. Elberling, and G. Salomon (Eds.), *Electrocochleography*. Baltimore: University Park Press, 1976.

Coats, A. C. Human auditory nerve action potentials and brain-stem evoked responses. Latency-intensity functions in detection of cochlear and retrocochlear abnormality. *Archives of Otolaryngology*, 1978, *104*:709-717.

Coats, A. C. Ménière's disease and the summating potential. II. Vestibular test results. *Archives of Otolaryngology*, 1981a, *107*:263-270.

Coats, A. C. The summating potential and Ménière's disease. I. Summating potential amplitude in Ménière and non-Ménière ears. *Archives of Otolaryngology*, 1981b, *107*:199-208.

Coats, A. C., and Dickey, J. R. Nonsurgical recording of human auditory nerve action potentials and cochlear microphonics. *Annals of Otology, Rhinology and Laryngology*, 1970, *79*:844-852.

Coats, A. C., and Dickey, J. R. Postmasking recovery of human click action potentials and click loudness. *Journal of the Acoustical Society of America*, 1972, *52*:1607-1612.

Coats, A. C., and Martin, J. L. Human auditory nerve action potentials and brainstem evoked responses. *Archives of Otolaryngology*, 1977, *103*:605-622.

Coats, A. C., Martin, J. L., and Kidder, H. Normal short-latency electrophysiological filtered click responses recorded from vertex and external auditory meatus. *Journal of the Acoustical Society of America*, 1979, *65*:747-758.

Cobb, W. A., and Dawson, G. D. The latency and form in man of the occipital potentials evoked by bright flashes. *Journal of Physiology* (London), 1960, *158*:108-121.

Cobb, W. A., Morton, M. B., and Ettlinger, G. Cerebral potentials evoked by pattern reversal and their suppression in visual rivalry. *Nature*, 1967, *216*:1123-1125.

Cody, A. R., Robertson, D., and Bredberg, G., et al. Electrophysiological and morphological changes in the guinea pig cochlea following mechanical trauma to the organ of Corti. *Acta Oto-Laryngologica* (Stockholm), 1980, *89*(5-6):440-452.

Cohen, D., and Sohmer, H. Comparison of earlobe and promontorium recording sites in electrocochleography. *Audiology*, 1977, *16*:462-478.

Cohen, M. M., and Rapin, I. Evoked potential audiometry in neurologically impaired children. In R. F. Naunton, and C. Fernandez (Eds.), *Evoked electrical activity in the auditory nervous system*. New York: Academic Press, 1978.

Corwin, J. T., Bullock, T. H., and Schweitzer, J. The auditory brain-stem response in five vertebrate classes. *Journal Comparative and Physiological Psychology*, in press.

Cox, C., Hack, M., and Metz, D. Brainstem-evoked response audiometry: Normative data from the preterm infant. *Audiology*, 1981, *20*(1):53-64.

Cracco, J. B., Bosch, V. V., and Cracco, R. Q. Cerebral and spinal somatosensory evoked potentials in children with CNS degenerative disease, *Electroencephalography and Clinical Neurophysiology*, 1980, *49*:437-445.

Cracco, J. B., and Cracco, R. Q. Somatosensory spinal and cerebral evoked potentials in children with occult spinal dysraphism. *Neurology*, 1979, *29*:543.

Cracco, J. B., Cracco, R. Q., and Graziani, L. J. The spinal evoked response in infants with myelodysplasia. *Neurology*, 1974, *4*:359-360.

Cracco, J. B., Cracco, R. Q., and Graziani, L. J. The spinal evoked response in infants and children. *Neurology*, 1975, *25*:31-36.

Cracco, J. B., Cracco, R. Q., and Stolove, R. Spinal evoked potential in man. A maturational study. *Electroencephalography and Clinical Neurophysiology*, 1979, *46*:58-64.

Cracco, R. Q. Traveling waves of the human scalp-recorded somatosensory evoked response. Effects of differences in recording technique and sleep on somatosensory and somatomotor responses. *Electroencephalography and Clinical Neurophysiology*, 1972, *33*:557-566.

Cracco, R. Q. Spinal evoked response: Peripheral nerve stimulation in man. *Electroencephalography and Clinical Neurophysiology*, 1973, *35*:379-386.

Cracco, R. Q. Evoked potentials in patients with neurological disorders. In H. Begleiter (Ed.), *Evoked brain potentials and behavior*. New York: Plenum Press, 1979.

Cracco, R. Q., and Cracco, J. B. Somatosensory evoked potential in man: Far field potentials. *Electroencephalography and Clinical Neurophysiology*, 1976, *41*:460-466.

Cracco, R. Q., and Cracco, J. B. Visual evoked potential in man: Early oscillatory potentials. *Electroencephalography and Clinical Neurophysiology*, 1978, *45*: 731-739.

Cracco, R. Q., Cracco, J. B., and Anziska, B. J. Somatosensory evoked potentials in man: Cerebral, subcortical, spinal, and peripheral nerve potentials. *American Journal of Electroencephalography and Technology*, 1979, *19*:59-81.

Cracco, R. Q., Cracco, J. B., and Sarnowski, R., et al. Spinal evoked potentials. In J. E. Desmedt (Ed.), *Progress in clinical neurophysiology, Vol. 7. Clinical uses of cerebral brain-stem and spinal somatosensory evoked potentials*. Basel: Karger, 1980.

Cracco, R. Q., and Evans, B. Spinal evoked potential in the cat. Effects of asphyxia, strychnine, cord section, and compression. *Electroencephalography and Clinical Neurophysiology*, 1978, *44*:187-201.

Crowell, D. H., Pang-Ching, G., and Anderson, R. E., et al. Auditory screening of high risk infants with brainstem evoked responses and impedance audiometry. *Hawaii Medical Journal*, 1980, *39*(11):277-282.

Corwley, D. E., Davis, H., and Beagley, H. A. Survey of the clinical use of electrocochleography. *Annals of Otology, Rhinology and Laryngology*, 1975, *84*: 297-307.

Cullen, J. K., Berlin, C. I., and Gondra, M. I., et al. Electrocochleography in children: A retrospective study. *Archives of Otolaryngology*, 1976, *102*:482-486.

Cullen, J. K., Ellis, M., and Berlin, C. I., et al. Human acoustic nerve action potential recordings from the tympanic membrane without anesthesia. *Acta Oto-Laryngologica* (Stockholm), 1972, *74*:15-22.

Dallos, P. *The auditory periphery. Biophysics and physiology*. New York: Academic Press, 1973.

Dallos, P. Cochlear electrophysiology. In R. F. Naunton, and C. Fernandez (Eds.), *Evoked electrical activity in the auditory nervous system*. New York: Academic Press, 1978.

Dallos, P., and Cheatham, M. A. Compound action potential (AP) tuning curves. *Journal of the Acoustical Society of America*, 1976, *59*:591-597.

Daly, D. M., Roeser, R. J., and Moushegian, G. The frequency-following response in subjects with profound unilateral hearing loss. *Electroencephalography and Clinical Neurophysiology*, 1976, *40*:132-142.

David, S., and Sohmer, H. Experiments on cats to determine the nature of the auditory evoked response in man. *Israel Journal of Medical Sciences*, 1972, *8*:571.

Davis, H. (Ed.). *Hearing and Deafness: A Guide for Layman*. New York: Murray Hill Books, 1947.

Davis, H. Enhancement of evoked cortical potentials in humans related to a task requiring a decision. *Science*, 1964, *145*:182-183.

Davis, H. Brain-stem and other responses in electric response audiometry. *Annal of Otology, Rhinology and Laryngology*, 1976a, *85*:3-14.

Davis, H. Principles of electric response audiometry. *Annals of Otology, Rhinology and Laryngology* (Suppl), 1976b, *28*:1-96.

Davis, H. United States-Japan seminar on auditory responses from the brainstem. *Laryngoscope*, 1979, *39*:1336-1339.

Davis, H., and Hirsh, S. K. The audiometric utility of brain stem response to low-frequency sounds. *Audiology*, 1976, *15*:181-195.

Davis, H., and Hirsh, S. K. A slow brainstem response for low-frequency audiometry. *Audiology*, 1979, *18*:445-461.

Davis, H., Hirsh, S. K., and Shelnutt, J. J., et al. Further evaluation of evoked response audiometry (ERA). *Journal of Speech and Hearing Research*, 1967, *10*:717-732.

Davis, H., Hirsch, S. K., and Shelnutt, J. J., et al. Validation of clinical ERA at Central Institute for the Deaf. *Revue de Laryngologie Otologie Rhinology* (Bordeaux), 1974, *95*:475-480.

Davis, H., Mast, T., and Yoshie, N., et al. The slow response of the human cortex to auditory stimuli: Recovery process. *Electroencephalography and Clinical Neurophysiology*, 1966, *21*:105-113.

Davis, H., and Onishi, S. Maturation of auditory evoked potentials. *International Audiology*, 1969, *8*:24-33.

Davis, H., Osterhammel, R. A., and Weir, C. C., et al. Slow vertex potentials: Interactions among auditory, tactile, electric, and visual stimuli. *Electroencephalography and Clinical Neurophysiology*, 1972, *33*:537-545.

Davis, H., and Saul, L. J. Action currents in the auditory tracts of the midbrain of the cat. *Science*, 1931, *74*:205-206.

Davis, H., and Zerlin, S. Acoustic relations of the human vertex potential. *Journal of the Acoustical Society of America*, 1966, *39*:109-116.

Dawson, G. D. Auto-correlation and automatic integration. *Electroencephalography and Clinical Neurophysiology* (Suppl), 1954a, *4*:26-37.

Dawson, G. D. A summation technique for the detection of small evoked potentials. *Electroencephalography and Clinical Neurophysiology*, 1954b, *6*:65-84.

Derbyshire, A. J., and Davis, H. The action potentials of the auditory nerve. *American Journal of Physiology* (London), 1935, *113*:476-504.

Desmedt, J. E., Brunko, E., and Debecker, J., et al. The system bandpass required to avoid distortion of early components when averaging somatosensory evoked potentials. *Electroencephalography and Clinical Neurophysiology*, 1974, *37*: 407-410.

Desmedt, J. E., Brunko, E., and Debecker, J. Maturation of the somatosensory evoked potentials in normal infants and children, with special reference to the early N_1 component. *Electroencephalography and Clinical Neurophysiology*, 1976, *40*:43-58.

Desmedt, J. E., Noel, P., and Debecker, J., et al. Maturation of afferent conduction velocity as studied by sensory nerve potentials and cerebral evoked potentials. In J. E. Desmedt (Ed.), *New developments in electromyography and clinical neurophysiology. Vol. 2*. Basel: Karger, 1973.

Despland, P. A., and Galambos, R. The auditory brainstem response (ABR) is a useful diagnostic tool in the intensive care nursery. *Pediatric Research*, 1980, *14*(2): 154-158.

von Deuster, C., and Seiler, C. F. Brainstem auditory evoked response (BER) in paedaudiological diagnosis (author's translation). *Laryngologie, Rhinologie, Otologie* (Stuttgart), 1979, *58*(1):43-47.

Diamond, A. L. Latency of the steady state visual evoked potential. *Electroencephalography and Clinical Neurophysiology*, 1977, *42*:125-127.

Diamiani, J. M., and Levine, H. L. Relapsing polychondritis—report of ten cases. *Laryngoscope*, 1979, *89*:929-946.

Dimitrijevic, M. R., Larsson, L. E., and Lehmkuhl, D., et al. Evoked spinal cord and nerve root potentials in humans using a non-invasive recording technique. *Electroencephalography and Clinical Neurophysiology*, 1978, *45*:331-340.

Dobie, R. A., and Berlin, C. I. Influence of otitis media on hearing and development. *Annals of Otology, Rhinology and Laryngology* (Suppl. 60), 1979a, *88*:48-53.

Dobie, R. A., and Berlin, C. I. Binaural interaction in brainstem evoked response. *Archives of Otolaryngology*, 1979b, *105*:391-398.

Dobie, R. A., and Kimm, J. Brainstem responses to electrical stimulation of cochlea. *Archives of Otolaryngology*, 1980, *106*(9):573-577.

Dobie, R. A., and Norton, S. J. Binaural interaction in human auditory evoked potentials. *Electroencephalography and Clinical Neurophysiology*, 1980, *49*:303-313.

Don, M., Allen, A. R., and Starr, A. Effect of click rate on the latency of auditory brain stem responses in humans. *Annals of Otology, Rhinology and Laryngology*, 1977, *86*:186-196.

Don, M., and Eggermont, J. J. Analysis of the click-evoked brainstem potentials in man using high-pass noise masking. *Journal of the Acoustical Society of America*, 1978, *63*:1084-1092.

Don, M., Eggermont, J. J., and Brackmann, D. E. Reconstruction of the audiogram using brain-stem responses and high-pass noise masking. *Annals of Otology, Rhinology and Laryngology* (Suppl 57), 1979, *88*:1-20.

Donchin, E. Event-related brain potentials: A tool in the study of human information processing. In H. Begleiter (Ed.), *Evoked brain potentials and behavior*. New York: Plenum Press, 1979.

Donchin, E., Callaway, E., and Cooper, R., et al. Publication criteria for studies of evoked potentials (EP) in man. In J. E. Desmedt (Ed.), *Progress in clinical neurophysiology. Vol. 1. Attention, voluntary contraction, and event-related cerebral potentials*. Basel: Karger, 1977.

426   References

Donchin, E., Kubovy, M., and Kutas, M., et al. Graded changes in evoked response (P300) amplitude as a function of cognitive activity. *Perception and Psychophysics*, 1973, *14*:319-324.

Donchin, E., Ritter, W., and McCallum, W. C. Cognitive psychophysiology: The endogenous components of the ERP. In E. Callway, P. Tueting, and S. H. Koslow (Eds.), *Event-related brain potentials in man*. New York: Academic Press, 1978.

Dorfman, L. J. Indirect estimation of spinal cord conduction velocity in man. *Electroencephalography and Clinical Neurophysiology*, 1977, *42*:26-34.

Dorfman, L. J., and Bosley, T. M. Age related changes in peripheral and central nerve conduction in man. *Neurology*, 1979, *29*:38-44.

Dorfman, L. J., Bosley, T. M., and Cummins, K. L. Electrophysiological localization of central somatosensory lesions in patients with multiple sclerosis. *Electroencephalography and Clinical Neurophysiology*, 1978, *44*:742-753.

Douek, E., Gibson, W., and Humphries, K. The crossed acoustic response. *Journal of Laryngology and Otology*, 1973, *87*:711-726.

Dublin, W. B. Neurologic lesions of erythroblastosis fetalis in relation to nuclear deafness. *American Journal of Clinical Pathology*, 1951, *21*:935-939.

du Bois-Reymond, E. *Untersuchungen über thierische Elektricitat. Vol. I*. Berlin: Reimer, 1848.

Duncan-Johnson, C. C., and Donchin, E. On quantifying surprise: The variation in event-related potentials with subjective probability. *Psychophysiology*, 1977, *14*:456-467.

Duncan-Johnson, C. C., and Donchin, E. The time constant in P300 recording. *Psychophysiology*, 1979, *16*:53-55.

Dunlop, C. W., Itzkowic, D. J., and Aitkin, L. M. Tone-burst response patterns of single units in the cat medial geniculate body. *Brain Research*, 1969, *16*: 149-164.

Durrant, J. D. Anatomic and physiologic correlates of the effects of noise on hearing. In D. M. Lipscomb (Ed.). *Noise and Audiology*. Baltimore: University Park Press, pp. 109-141, 1978.

Durrant, J. D., Gabriel, S., and Walter, M. Psychophysical tuning functions for brief stimuli: Preliminary report. *American Journal of Otolaryngology*, 1981, *2*:108-113.

Durrant, J. D., and Lovrinic, J. H. *Bases of hearing science*. Baltimore: Williams & Wilkins, 1977.

Dustman, R. E., Schenkenberg, T., and Beck, E. C. The development of the evoked response in a diagnostic and evaluative procedure. In R. Karrer (Ed.), *Developmental psychophysiology of mental retardation*. Springfield: C. C. Thomas, 1976.

Dustman, R. E., Snyder, E. W., and Callner, D. A., et al. The evoked response as a measure of cerebral dysfunction. In H. Begleiter (Ed.), *Evoked brain potentials and behavior*. New York: Plenum Press, pp. 321-363, 1979.

von Economo, C. *The cytoarchitectonics of the human cerebral cortex*. (S. Parker translator.) London: H. Milford Univ. Press, 1929.

Edwards, R., Buchwald, J., and Tanguay, P., et al. Sources of variability in brainstem potential measures over time. *Electroencephalography and Clinical Neurophysiology*, 1982, *53*:125-132.

Eggermont, J. J. Electrocochleography. In W. D. Keidel, and W. D. Neff (Eds.), *Handbook of sensory physiology, Vol. V/3. Auditory system. Clinical and special topics.* Heidelberg: Springer-Verlag, 1976a.

Eggermont, J. J. Analysis of compound action potential responses to tone bursts in the human and guinea pig cochlea. *Journal of the Acoustical Society of America*, 1976b, *60*:1132-1139.

Eggermont, J. J. Summating potentials in electrocochleography: Relation to hearing disorders. In R. J. Ruben, C. Elberling, and G. Salomon (Eds.), *Electrocochleography*. Baltimore: University Park Press, 1976c.

Eggermont, J. J. Unpublished results, 1977.

Eggermont, J. J. Detection of acoustic neurinoma on basis of brainstem electrical responses. *Electroencephalography and Clinical Neurophysiology*, 1977a, *43*:582.

Eggermont, J. J. Compound action potential tuning curves in normal and pathological human ears. *Journal of the Acoustical Society of America*, 1977b, *62*:1247-1251.

Eggermont, J. J. Electrocohleography and recruitment. *Annals of Otology, Rhinology and Laryngology*, 1977c, *86*:138-149.

Eggermont, J. J. Stimulus-response relations for promontory recorded compound action potentials in normal and recruiting ears. In R. F. Naunton, and C. Fernandez (Eds.), *Evoked electrical activity in the auditory nervous system.* New York: Academic Press, 1978.

Eggermont, J. J. Summating potentials in Ménière's disease. *Archives of Oto-Rhino-Laryngology*, 1979a, *222*:63-75.

Eggermont, J. J. Narrow-band AP latencies in normal and recruiting human ears. *Journal of the Acoustical Society of America*, 1979b, *65*:463-470.

Eggermont, J. J., and Don, M. Analysis of the click-evoked brainstem potentials in humans using high-pass noise masking. II. Effect of click intensity. *Journal of the Acoustical Society of America*, 1980, *68*:1671-1675.

Eggermont, J. J., Don, M., and Brackmann, D. E. Electrocochleography and auditory brainstem electric responses in patients with pontine angle tumors. *Annals of Otology, Rhinology and Laryngology* (Suppl), 1980, *89*:Suppl. 75, 1-19.

Eggermont, J. J., and Odenthal, D. W. Action potentials and summating potentials in the normal human cochlea. In J. J. Eggermont, D. W. Odenthal, and P. H. Schmidt, et al. (Eds.), *Electrocochleography. Basic principles and clinical application.* Acta Oto-Laryngology (Suppl) (Stockholm), 1974a, *316*:39-61.

Eggermont, J. J., and Odenthal, D. W. Electrophysiological investigation of the human cochlea: Recruitment, masking, and adaptation. *Audiology*, 1974b, *13*:1-22.

Eggermont, J. J., and Odenthal, D. W. Frequency selective masking in electrocochleography. *Revue de Laryngologie Otologie Rhinologie* (Bordeaux), 1974c, *95*: 489-496.

Eggermont, J. J., and Odenthal, D. W. Methods in electrocochleography. In J. J. Eggermont, D. W. Odenthal, and P. H. Schmidt, et al. (Eds.) *Electrocochleography. Basic principles and clinical application. Acta Oto-Laryngologica* (Suppl) (Stockholm), 1974d, *316*:17-24.

Eggermont, J. J., and Odenthal, D. W. Potentialities of clinical electrocochleography. *Clinical Otolaryngology*, 1977, *2*:275-286.

Eggermont, J. J., Odenthal, D. W., and Schmidt, P. H., et al. (Eds.). Electrococh-leography: Basic principles and clinical application. *Acta Oto-Laryngologica* (Suppl) (Stockholm), 1974, *316*:1-84.

Eisen, A., Steward, J., and Nudleman, K., et al. Short latency somatosensory responses in multiple sclerosis. *Neurology*, 1979, *29*:827-834.

Eisenberg, R. B. Auditory behavior in the human neonate. I. Methodologic problems and the logical design of research procedures. *Journal of Auditory Research*, 1965, *5*:159-177.

Elberling, C. Transitions in cochlear action potentials recorded from the ear canal in man. *Scandinavian Audiology*, 1973, *2*:151-159.

Elberling, C. Action potentials along the cochlear partition recorded from the ear canal in man. *Scandinavian Audiology*, 1974, *3*:13-19.

Elberling, C. Stimulation of cochlear action potentials recorded from the ear canal in man. In R. J. Ruben, C. Elberling, and G. Salomon (Eds.), *Electrocochleography*. Baltimore: University Park Press, 1976a.

Elberling, C. Action potentials recorded from the promontory and the surface, com-pared with recordings from the ear canal in man. *Scandinavian Audiology*, 1976b, *5*:69-78.

Elberling, C. High-frequency evoked action potentials recorded from the ear canal of man. *Scandinavian Audiology*, 1976c, *5*:157-164.

Elberling, C. Compound impulse response for the brain stem derived through com-binations of cochlear and brain stem recordings. *Scandinavian Audiology*, 1978, *7*:147-157.

Elberling, C. Auditory electrophysiology: Spectral analysis of cochlear and brainstem evoked potentials. *Scandinavian Audiology*, 1979a, *8*:57-64.

Elberling, C. Auditory electrophysiology. The use of templates and cross correlation functions in the analysis of brain stem potentials. *Scandinavian Audiology*, 1979b, *8*:187-190.

Elberling, C., Bak, C., and Kofoed, B., et al. Magnetic auditory responses from the human brain. A preliminary report. *Scandinavian Audiology*, 1980, *9*(3): 185-190.

Elberling, C., and Salomon. Personal communication, 1979.

Elberling, C., and Salomon, G. Cochlear microphonics recorded from the ear canal in man. *Acta Oto-Laryngologica* (Stockholm), 1973, *75*:489-495.

Elberling, C., and Salomon, G. Action potentials from pathological ears compared to potentials generated by a computer model. In R. J. Ruben, C. Elberling, and G. Salomon (Eds.), *Electrocochleography*. Baltimore: University Park Press, 1976.

Ellingson, R. J., Danahy, T., and Nelson, B., et al. Variability of auditory evoked potentials in human newborns. *Electroencephalography and Clinical Neurology*, 1974, *36*:155-162.

Elverland, H. H. Ascending and intrinsic projections of the superior olivary complex in the cat. *Experimental Brain Research*, 1978, *32*:117-134.

Emmett, J. R., and Shea, J. J. Recent advances in pediatric otology. *Southern Medical Journal*, 1980, *73*(1):36-9; 42.

Engel, R. Early waves of the electroencephalic auditory response in neonates. *Neuro-paediatrie*, 1971, *3*:147-154.

Engler, L. L., Spielholz, N. I., and Bernhard, W. N., et al. Somatosensory evoked potentials during Harrington instrumentation for scolioses. *Journal of Bone and Joint Surgery* (London), 1978, *60*:528-532.

Ertekin, C. Studies in the human evoked electrospinogram. I. The origin of the segmental evoked potentials. *Acta Neurologica Scandinavica*, 1976a, *53*:2-30.

Ertekin, C. Studies in the human evoked electrospinogram. II. The conduction velocity along the dorsal funiculus. *Acta Neurologica Scandinavica*, 1976b, *53*:21-38.

Erulkar, S. D., Rose, J. E., and Davies, P. W. Single unit activity in the auditory cortex of the cat. *Johns Hopkins Hospital Bulletin*, 1956, *99*:55-86.

Evans, E. F. The sharpening of cochlear frequency selectivity in the normal and abnormal cochlea. *Audiology*, 1975, *14*:419-442.

Evans, E. F. Place and time coding of frequency in the peripheral auditory system: Some physiological pros and cons. *Audiology*, 1978, *17*:369-420.

Evans, E. F., and Nelson, P. G. The responses of single neurons in the cochlear nucleus of the cat as a function of their location and the anesthetic state. *Experimental Brain Research*, 1973, *17*:402-427.

Evans, E. F., and Whitfield, I. C. Classification of unit responses in the auditory cortex of the unanesthetized and unrestrained cat. *Journal of Physiology* (London), 1964, *171*:476-493.

Evans, T. R., and Deatherage, B. H. The effect of frequency on the auditory evoked response. *Psychonomic Science*, 1969, *15*:95-96.

Fabiani, M., Sohmer, H., and Tait, C., et al. A functional measure of brain activity: Brainstem transmission time. *Electroencephalography and Clinical Neurophysiology*, 1979, *47*:483-491.

Fahn, M. Correlation between auditory nerve and brainstem recordings and the location of pathology as defined in clinical examination. (Unpublished M.D. thesis, in Hebrew, 1979.)

Faingold, C. L., and Caspary, D. M. Frequency-following responses in primary auditory and reticular formation structures. *Electroencephalography and Clinical Neurophysiology*, 1979, *47*:12-20.

Feinmesser, M., and Sohmer, H. Contribution of cochlear, brainstem and cortical responses to differential diagnosis and lesion localization in hearing loss. In, S. K. Hirsh, I. J. Hirsh, and D. H. Eldredge, et al. (Eds.), *Hearing and Davis: Essays Honoring Hallowell Davis*. St. Louis, Missouri: Washington University Press, 1976.

Feldman, M. H., Cracco, R. Q., and Farmer, P., et al. Spinal evoked potential in the monkey. *Annals of Neurology*, 1980, *7*:238-244.

Fialkowska, D., Janozewski, G., and Sulkowski, W., et al. Acoustic nerve adaptation in chronic acoustic trauma. *Medycyna Pracy* (Lodz), 1980, *31*:355-362.

Ferraro, J. A., and Minckler, J. The human lateral lemniscus and its nuclei. The human auditory pathways: A quantitative study. *Brain and Language*, 1977, *4*: 277-294.

Ferriss, G. S., Davis, G. D., and Dorsen, M., et al. Maturation of the evoked response to auditory stimuli in human infants. *Electroencephalography and Clinical Neurophysiology*, 1967, *23*:83.

Finck, A., Ronis, M. L., and Rosenberg, P. E. Some relationships between audiometry and cochlear microphonics in man. *Journal of Speech and Hearing Research*, 1969, *12*:156-160.

Finitzo-Hieber, T., Hecox, K., and Cone, B. Brainstem auditory evoked potentials in patients with congenital atresia. *Laryngoscope*, 1979, *89*:1151-1158.

Firth, H. Habituation during sleep. *Psychophysiology*, 1973, *10*:43-51.

Fischer, M. H. Elektrobiologische erscheinungen an der hirnrinde. *Pfluegers Archiv. European Journal of Physiology*, 1932, *230*:161-178.

Flach, M., and Seidel, P. Mikrophon-potentiale (MP) des menschlichen Ohres. *Archiven für Klinische und experimentelles Ohres Nases und Kehlkopf Heilkunde* (Munich), 1968, *190*:229.

Fletcher, H., and Munson, W. A. Loudness, its definition, measurement and calculation. *Journal of the Acoustical Society of America*, 1933, *5*:82-108.

Flock, Å., Jorgensen, M., and Russell, I. The physiology of individual hair cells and their synapses. In A. R. Møller (Ed.), *Basic mechanisms in hearing*. New York: Academic Press, 1973.

Ford, J. M., and Pfefferbaum, A. The utility of ERPs in determining age-related changes in CNJ and cognitive functions. In L. Poon (Ed.), *Aging in the 1980s: Selected contemporary issues in the phsychology of aging*. Washington, D. C.: American Psychology Association, 1980.

Ford, J. M., Roth, W. T., and Dirks, S. J., et al. Evoked potential correlates of signal recognition between and within modalities. *Science*, 1973, *181*:465-466.

Ford, J. M., Roth, W. T., and Kopell, B. S. Attention effect on auditory evoked potentials to infrequent events. *Biological Psychology*, 1976, *4*:65-77.

Ford, J. M., Roth, W. T., and Mohs, R. C., et al. Event-related potentials recorded from young and old adults during a memory retrieval task. *Electroencephalography and Clinical Neurophysiology*, 1979, *47*:450-459.

Fria, T. J., The auditory brain stem response: Background and clinical applications. *Monographs in Contemporary Audiology*, 1980, *2*:1-44.

Fria, T. J., and Sabo, D. L. Auditory brainstem responses in children with otitis media with effusion. *Annals of Otology, Rhinology and Laryngology* (Suppl), 1980, *68*(2):200-206.

Fromm, B., Nylen, C. O., and Zotterman, Y. Studies in the mechanism of the Wever-Bray effect. *Acta Oto-Laryngologica* (Stockholm), 1934/35, *22*:477-486.

Fruhstrofer, H. Habituation and dishabituation of the human vertex response. *Electroencephalography and Clinical Neurophysiology*, 1971, *30*:306-312.

Fruhstrofer, H., and Bergstrom, R. M. Human vigilance and auditory evoked responses. *Electroencephalography and Clinical Neurophysiology*, 1969, *27*: 346-355.

Fruhstrofer, H., Soveri, P., and Jarvilehto, T. Short-term habituation of the auditory evoked response in man. *Electroencephalography and Clinical Neurophysiology*, 1970, *28*:153-161.

Fujikawa, S. M., and Weber, B. A. Effects of increased stimulus rate on brainstem electric response (BER) audiometry as a function of age. *Journal of the American Audiology Society*, 1977, *3*:147-150.

Fujita, M., Hosoki, M., and Miyazaki, M. Brainstem auditory evoked responses in spinocerebellar degeneration and Wilson disease. *Annals of Neurology*, 1981, *9*:42-47.

Fullerton, B. C., and Hosford, H. L., Effects of midline brain stem lesions on the short-latency auditory evoked responses. *Neuroscience Abstract*, 1979, *5*:20.

Funasaka, S., and Abe, H. Cochlear and fast electrical responses to frequency modulated tones: A frequency specific stimulus. *Auris, Nasus, Larynx*, 1979, 6:59-69.

Furukawa, T., and Ishii, Y. Neurophysiological studies on hearing in goldfish. *Journal of Neurophysiology*, 1967, 30:1377-1403.

Gabor, D. Acoustical quanta and the theory of hearing. *Nature*, 1947, 159:591-594.

Gabriel, S. Dependence of Psychophysical Tuning Curves on Probe Bandwidth: Relation to Critical Bandwidth, unpublished Ph.D. dissertation, Temple University, Philadelphia, Pennsylvania, 1981.

Gacek, R. R., and Rasmussen, G. L. Fiber analysis of the statoacoustic nerve of the guinea pig, cat and monkey. *Anatomical Record*, 1961, 139:455-463.

Galambos, R. Microelectrode studies on medial geniculate body of cat. III. Response to pure tones. *Journal of Neurophysiology*, 1952, 15:381-400.

Galambos, R. The BER in the ICU. In R. F. Naunton and C. Fernandez (Eds.), *Evoked electrical activity in the auditory nervous system*. New York: Academic Press, 1978.

Galambos, R. (Ed.). U.S.-Japan seminar on auditory responses from the brain stem. Honolulu, Hawaii, unpublished abstracts, 1979.

Galambos, R., and Despland, P. A. The auditory brainstem response (ABR) evaluates risk factors for hearing loss in the newborn. *Pediatric Research*, 1980, 14(2):159-163.

Galambos, R., and Hecox, K. Clinical applications of the human brainstem evoked potentials to auditory stimuli. In J. E. Desmedt (Ed.), *Progress in clinical neurophysiology. Vol. 2. Auditory evoked potentials in man: Psychopharmacology correlates of evoked potentials*. Basel: Karger, 1977.

Galambos, R., and Hecox, K. Clinical application of the auditory brainstem response. In J. M. Page (Ed.), *Otolaryngologic Clinics of North America*, 1978, 11:709-722.

Galambos, R., Makeig, S., and Talmachoff, P. A 40-Hz auditory potential recorded from the human scalp. *Proceedings of the National Academy of Sciences of the United States of America*, 1981, 78:2643-2647.

Galambos, R., Rose, J. E., and Bromiley, R. G., et al. Microelectrode studies of medial geniculate body of cat. II. Response to clicks. *Journal of Neurophysiology*, 1952, 15:359-380.

Galvani, L. De viribus electricitatis in motu musculari. *Commentarius de bonomens: Scientarium et artium instituto atque academia commentarii*, 1791, 7:363-418.

Gardi, J. N., and Berlin, C. I. A preliminary report on the origin(s) of the binaural-interaction component of the brainstem evoked response (BSER) in the guinea pig. *Society for Neuroscience*, 1979, 5(61):20.

Gardi, J. N., and Berlin, C. I. A preliminary report on the origin(s) of the Binaural-interaction components of the buinea pig ABR: Possible origins. *Archives of Otolaryngology*, 1981, 107:164-168.

Gardi, J. N., and Bledsoe, S. C. Elucidation of the origins of the middle components of the auditory evoked response (AER) in the cat using a serial ablation technique. Sixth Biennial Symposium of the International Electric Response Audiometry Group. Santa Barbara, California, 1979.

Gardi, J. N., and Bledsoe, S. C. The use of kainic acid for studying the origins of scalp-recorded auditory brain-stem responses in the guinea pig. *Neuroscience Letters*, 1981, 26:143-149.

Gardi, J. N., Bledsoe, S. C., and Berlin, C. I. Frequency following potential (FFP) tone-on-tone masking studies in cats and guinea pigs. Abstracts of the Second Midwinter Research Meeting, Association for Research in Otolaryngology; St. Petersburg, Florida, 1979.

Gardi, J. N., Martin, W. H., and Jewett, D. L. Planar-curve analysis of auditory brain stem responses: Preliminary observations. *Journal Acoustical Society America* (Abstract), 1980, *68*:S19.

Gardi, J. N., and Mendel, M. I. Evoked brainstem potentials. In S. E. Gerber (Ed.), *Audiometry in infancy*. New York: Grune & Stratton, 1978.

Gardi, J. N., and Merzenich, M. M. The effect of high-pass noise on the scalp-recorded frequency following response (FFR) in humans and cats. *Journal of the Acoustical Society of America*, 1979, *65*:1491-1500.

Gardi, J. N., Merzenich, M. M., and McKean, C. Origins of the scalp-recorded frequency following response in the cat. *Audiology*, 1979, *18*:353-381.

Gardi, J. N., Salamy, A., and Mendelson, T. Scalp-recorded frequency-following responses in neonates. *Audiology*, 1979, *18*(6):494-506.

Gavilan, C., and Sanjuan, J. Microphonic potential picked up from the human tympanic membrane. *Annals of Otology, Rhinology and Laryngology*, 1964, *73*:101-109.

Geisler, C. D. Average responses to clicks in man recorded by scalp electrodes. *Research Laboratory of Electronics, Massachusetts Institute of Technology*, Technical Report No. 380, 1960.

Geisler, C. D., Frishkopf, L. S., and Rosenblith, W. A. Extracranial responses to acoustic clicks in man. *Science*, 1958, *128*:1210-1211.

Geniec, P., and Morest, D. K. The neuronal architecture of the human posterior colliculus. A study with the Golgi method. *Acta Oto-Laryngologica* (Suppl) (Stockholm), 1971, *295*:1-33.

Gerard, J. Nuclear jaundice and deafness. *Journal of Laryngology and Otology*, 1964, *66*:39-46.

Gerard, R. W., Marshall, W. H., and Saul, L. G. Cerebral action potentials. *Proceedings of the Society for Experimental Biology and Medicine*, 1933, *30*:1123-1125.

Gerken, G. M., Moushegian, G., and Stillman, R. D., et al. Human frequency-following responses to monaural and binaural stimuli. *Electroencephalography and Clinical Neurophysiology*, 1975, *38*:379-386.

Gerull, G., Giesen, M., and Mrowinski, D. Quantitative Assuagen der Hirnstammaudiometrie bei Mittelohr- , Kochlearen und Retrokochlearen Horschaden. *Laryngologie, Rhinologie, Otologie* (Stuttgart), 1979, *57*:54-62.

Gerull, G. M., Giesen, D., and Mrowinski, N., et al. Properties of an early AER of 6-10 msec latency. *Revue de Laryngologie Otologie Rhinologie* (Bordeaux), 1974, *95*:560-

Gescheider, G. A. *Psychophysics: Method and theory*. Hillsdale, New Jersey: Lawrence Erlbaum Associates, 1976.

Giblin, D. R. Somatosensory evoked potentials in healthy subjects and in patients with lesions of the nervous system. *Annals of the New York Academy of Sciences*, 1964, *112*:93-142.

Gibson, W. P. R., and Beagley, H. A. Electrocochleography in the diagnosis of acoustic neuroma. *Journal of Laryngology and Otology*, 1976a, *90*:127-139.

Gibson, W. P. R., and Beagley, H. A. Transtympanic electrocochleography in the investigation of retrolabyrinthine disorders. *Revue de Laryngologie Otologie Rhinologie* (Suppl) (Bordeaux), 1976b, *97*:507.

Gilliat, R. W., Melville, I. P., and Velate, A. S., et al. A study of normal nerve action potential using an averaging technique (barrier grid storage tube). *Journal of Neurology, Neurosurgery and Psychiatry*, 1965, *28*:191-200.

Glaser, E. M., Suter, C. M., and Dashieff, R., et al. The human frequency-following response: Its behavior during continuous tone burst stimulation. *Electroencephalography and Clinical Neurophysiology*, 1976, *40*:25-32.

Glassock, M. E., Jackson, C. G., and Josey, A. F., et al. Brainstem evoked response audiometry in a clinical practice. *Laryngoscope*, 1979, *89*:1021-1035.

Goblick, T. J., and Pfeffer, R. R. Time-domain measurements of cochlear nonlinearities using combination click stimuli. *Journal of the Acoustical Society of America*, 1969, *46*:924-938.

Godfrey, D. A., Kiang, N. Y.-S., and Norris, B. E. Single-unit activity in the posteroventral cochlear nucleus of the cat. *Journal of Comparative Neurology*, 1975a, *162*:247-268.

Godfrey, D. A., Kiang, N. Y.-S., and Norris, B. E. Single unit activity in the dorsal cochlear nucleus of the cat. *Journal of Comparative Neurology*, 1975b, *162*:269-284.

Goff, W. The scalp distribution of auditory evoked potentials. In R. F. Naunton and C. Fernandez (Eds.), *Evoked electrical activity in the auditory nervous system*. New York: Academic Press, 1978.

Goff, W. R. The scalp distribution of auditory evoked potentials. *Audiology*, 1979, *18*:505-524.

Goff, W. R., Allison, T., and Lyons, W., et al. Origins of short latency auditory evoked response components in man. In J. E. Desmedt (Ed.), *Progress in clinical neurophysiology. Vol. 2. Auditory evoked potentials in man. Pharmacology correlates of evoked potentials*. Basel: Karger, 1977.

Goff, W. R., Allison, T., and Vaughan, H. G. The functional neuroanatomy of event-related potentials. In E. Callaway, P. Tueting, and S. H. Koslow (Eds.), *Event-related brain potentials in man*. New York: Academic Press, 1978.

Goff, G. D., Matsumiya, Y., and Allison, T., et al. The scalp topography of human somatosensory and and auditory evoked potentials. *Electroencephalography and Clinical Neurophysiology*, 1977, *42*:57-76.

Goff, W. R., Rosner, B. S., and Allison, T. Distribution of cerebral somatosensory evoked responses in normal man. *Electroencephalography and Clinical Neurophysiology*, 1962, *14*:697-713.

Goff, W. R., Williamson, P. O., and VanGilder, J. C., et al. Neural origins of long latency evoked cortical potentials recorded from the depth and cortical surfaces of the brain in man. In J. E. Desmedt (Ed.), *Progress in clinical neurophysiology, Vol. 2. Clinical area of cerebral, brain stem and spinal evoked potentials, Vol. 2*. Basel: Karger, 1980.

Goldberg, J. M., Adrian, H. O., and Smith, F. D. Responses of neurons of the superior olivary complex of the cat to acoustic stimulation of long duration. *Journal of Neurophysiology*, 1964, *27*:706-749.

Goldberg, J. M., and Brown, P. B. Functional organization of the dog superior olivary complex: An anatomical and electrophysiological study. *Journal of Neurophysiology*, 1968, *31*:639-656.

Goldberg, J. M., and Brown, P. B. Response of binaural neurons of dog superior olivary complex to dichotic tonal stimuli: Some physiological mechanisms of sound localization. *Journal of Neurophysiology*, 1969, *32*:613-635.

Goldberg, J. M., and Brownell, W. E. Discharge characteristics of neurons in anteroventral and dorsal cochlear nuclei of cat. *Brain Research*, 1973, *64*:35-54.

Goldberg, J. M., and Moore, R. Y. Ascending projections of the lateral lemniscus in the cat and monkey. *Journal of Comparative Neurology*, 1967, *129*:143-156.

Goldenberg, R. A., and Derbyshire, A. J. Average evoked potentials in cats with lesions of auditory pathway. *Journal of Speech and Hearing Research*, 1975, *18*:420-429.

Goldie, W. D., Chiappa, K. H., and Young, R. R., et al. Brainstem auditory and short-latency somatosensory evoked responses in brain death. *Neurology*, 1981, *31*(3):248-256.

Goldman, Z., Sohmer, H., and Godfrey, C., et al. Auditory nerve, brain stem and cortical response correlates of learning capacity. *Physiology and Behavior*, 1981, *26*:637-645.

Goldstein, B. A. Early identification of hearing-impaired infants: Public law 94-142 falls short. *International Journal of Pediatric Otorhinolaryngology*, 1979, *1*(3):181-191.

Goldstein, J. L. Is the power law simply related to the driven spike response rate from the whole auditory nerve? In H. R. Moskowitz, B. Scharf, and J. C. Stevens (Eds.), *Sensation and measurement*. Dordrecht: D. Reidel Publishing Cie, 1974.

Goldstein, J. L., Baer, T., and Kiang, N. Y.-S. A theoretical treatment of latency, group delay and tuning characteristics for auditory nerve responses to clicks and tones. In M. B. Sachs, (Ed.), *The physiology of the auditory system*. Baltimore: National Educational Consultants, Inc., 1971.

Goldstein, M. H., Hall, J. L., and Butterfield, B. O. Single-unit activity in the primary auditory cortex of unanesthetized cats. *Journal of the Acoustical Society of America*, 1968, *43*:444-455.

Goldstein, R., and McRandle, C. C. Middle components of the averaged electroencephalic response to clicks in neonates. In S. K. Hirsh, D. H. Eldredge, and I. J. Hirsh, et al. (Eds.), *Hearing and Davis: Essays honoring Hallowell Davis*. St. Louis: Washington University Press, 1976.

Goldstein, R., Rodman, L. B., and Karlovish, R. S. Effects of stimulus rate and number on the early components of the averaged electroencephalic response. *Journal of Speech and Hearing Research*, 1972, *15*:559-566.

Goodin, D. S., Squires, K. C., and Henderson, B. H., et al. An early event-related cortical potential. *Psychophysiology*, 1978a, *15*:360-365.

Goodin, D. S., Squires, K. C., and Henderson, B. H., et al. Age-related variations in evoked potentials to auditory stimuli in normal human subjects. *Electroencephalography and Clinical Neurophysiology*, 1978b, *44*:447-458.

Goodin, D. S., Squires, K. C., and Starr, A. Long latency event-related components of the auditory evoked potential in dementia. *Brain*, 1978, *101*:635-648.

Graham, C. H., Bartlett, N. R., and Brown, J. L., et al. *Vision and visual perception*. New York: Wiley & Sons, Inc., 1965.

Green, D. M. *An introduction to hearing*. Hillsdale, New Jersey: Lawrence Erlbaum Assoc., 1976.

Greenberg, R. P., Becker, D. P., and Miller, J. D., et al. Evaluation of brain function in severe head trauma with multimodality evoked potentials. *Journal of Neuro-surgery*, 1977a, *47*:150-162.

Greenberg, R. P., Becker, D. P., and Miller, J. D., et al. Evaluation of brain function in severe human head trauma with multimodality evoked potentials. II. Localization of brain dysfunction and correlation with posttraumatic neurological conditions. *Journal of Neurosurgery*, 1977b, *47*:163-177.

Greenwood, D. D. Empirical travel time functions on the basilar membrane. In E. F. Evans and J. P. Wilson (Eds.), *Psychophysics and physiology of hearing*. London: Academic Press, 1977.

Gros, J. C. The ear in skull trauma. *Southern Medical Journal*, 1967, *60*:705-708.

Guild, S. R., Crowe, S. J., and Bunch, C. C., et al. Correlations of differences in the density of innervation of the organ of Corti with differences in acuity of hearing. *Acta Oto-Laryngologica* (Stockholm), 1931, *15*:269-308.

Guinan, J. J., Guinan, S. S., and Norris, B. E. Single auditory units in the superior olivary complex. I. Responses to sounds and classifications based on physiological properties. *International Journal of Neuroscience*, 1972, *4*:101-120.

Guinan, J. J., Norris, B. E., and Guinan, S. S. Single auditory units in the superior olivary complex. II. Locations of unit categories and tonotopic organization. *International Journal of Neuroscience*, 1972, *4*:147-166.

Guinan, J. J., and Peake, W. T. Middle-ear characteristics of anesthetized cats. *Journal of the Acoustical Society of America*, 1967, *41*:1237-1261.

Gutnick, H. N., and Goldstein, R. Effect of contralateral noise on the middle components of the averaged electroencephalic response. *Journal of Speech and Hearing Research*, 1978, *21*:613-625.

Halgren, E., Squires, N. K., and Wilson, C. L., et al. Endogenous potentials generated in the human hippocampal formation and amygdala by infrequent effects. *Science*, 1980, *210*:803-805.

Hall, J. G. On the neuropathological changes in the central nervous system following neonatal asphyxia. *Acta Oto-Laryngologica* (Suppl) (Stockholm), 1964, *188*: 331-338.

Hall, J. L., and Goldstein, M. H. Representation of binaural stimuli by single units in primary auditory cortex of unanesthetized cats. *Journal of the Acoustical Society of America*, 1968, *43*:456-461.

Hall, J. W. Auditory brainstem frequency following responses to waveform envelope periodicity. *Science*, 1979, *205*:1297-1299.

Halliday, A. M. The incidence of large cerebral evoked responses in myoclonic epilepsy. *Electroencephalography and Clinical Neurophysiology*, 1965, *19*:102.

Halliday, A. M. The effect of lesions of the visual pathways and cerebrum on the visual evoked response. In W. S. Van Leeuwen, F. M. Lopes da Silva, and A. Kamp (Eds.), *Evoked responses. 8:A.* In A. Remond (Ed.), *Handbook of electroencephalography and clinical neurophysiology*. Amsterdam: Elsevier, 1975.

Halliday, A. M. Commentary: Evoked potentials in neurological disorders. In E. Callaway, P. Tueting, and S. H. Koslow (Eds.), *Event-related brain potentials in man*. New York: Academic Press, 1978.

Halliday, A. M., Barrett, G., and Halliday, E., et al. The topography of the pattern-evoked potential. In J. E. Desmedt (Ed.), *Visual evoked potentials in man: New developments*. Oxford: Clarendon Press, 1977.

Halliday, A. M., and Halliday, E. Cortical evoked potentials in patients with benign essential myoclonus and progressive myoclonic epilepsy. *Electroencephalography and Clinical Neurophysiology*, 1970, *29*:106.

Halliday, A. M., Halliday, E., Kriss, A., et al. The pattern-evoked potentials in compression of the anterior visual pathways. *Brain*, 1976, *99*:357-374.

Halliday, A. M., McDonald, W. I., and Mushin, J. Delayed visual evoked responses in optic neuritis. *Lancet*, 1972. *1*:982-985.

Halliday, A. M., McDonald, W. I., and Mushin, J. The visual evoked response in the diagnosis of multiple sclerosis. *British Medical Journal*, 1973, *4*:661-664.

Halliday, A. M., and Michael, E. F. Changes is pattern-evoked responses in man associated with the vertical and horizontal meridians of the visual field. *Journal of Physiology* (London), 1970, *208*:499-513.

Halliday, A. M., and Wakefield, G. S. Cerebral evoked potentials in patients with dissociated sensory loss. *Journal of Neurology, Neurosurgery and Psychiatry*, 1963, *26*:211-219.

Hamernik, R. P., Henderson, D., and Coling, D., et al. Influence of vibration on asymptotic threshold shift produced by impulse noise. *Audiology*, 1981, *20*(3): 259-269.

Hansen, J. C., and Hillyard, S. A. Endogenous brain potentials associated with selective auditory attention. *Electroencephalography and Clinical Neurophysiology*, 1980, *49*:277-290.

Hanson, D. G., and Ulverstad, R. F. (Eds.), Otitis media and child development: Speech, language and education. *Annals of Otology, Rhinology and Laryngology*, 1979, *88*:(Suppl 60).

Harder, H., Kylén, P., and Arlinger, S. D., et al. Preoperative bone-conducted electrocochleography in otosclerosis. *Archives of Otolaryngology*, 1980, *106*(12): 757-762.

Harker, L. A., Hosick, E. C., and Voots, R. J., et al. Influence of succinylcholine on middle component auditory evoked potentials. *Archives of Otolaryngology*, 1977, *103*:133-137.

Harkins, S. W., McEvoy, T. M., and Scott, M. L. Effects of interstimulus interval on latency of the brainstem auditory evoked potential. *International Journal of Neuroscience*, 1979, *10*:7-14.

Harris, D. Action potential suppression, tuning curves and thresholds: Comparison with single fiber data. *Hearing Research*, 1979, *1*:133-154.

Harrison, J. M., and Irving, R. Ascending connections of the anterior ventral cochlear nucleus in the rat. *Journal of Comparative Neurology*, 1966, *126*:51-64.

Harter, M. R., and White, C. T. Evoked cortical responses to checkerboard patterns: Effects of check-size and function of visual acuity. *Electroencephalography and Clinical Neurophysiology*, 1969, *28*:48-54.

Hashimoto, I., Ishiyama, Y., and Mizutani, H. Monitoring brainstem function during posterior fossa surgery with brainstem auditory evoked potentials. In C. Barber (Ed.), *Evoked Potentials*, Lancaster: MTP Press, 1980.

Hashimoto, I., Ishiyama, Y., and Tozuka, G. Bilaterally recorded brainstem auditory responses. Their asymmetric abnormalities and lesions of the brainstem. *Archives of Neurology*, 1979, *36*:161-167.

Hashimoto, I., Ishiyama, Y., Yoshimoto, T., et al. Brain-stem auditory evoked potentials recorded directly from human brain-stem and thalamus. *Brain*, 1981, *104*: 841-859.

Hassler, R. Anatomy of the thalamus. In G. Schaltenbrand, and P. Bailey (Eds.), *Introduction to stereotaxis with an atlas of the human brain*. Vol. 1. New York: Grune & Stratton, 1959.

Hawes, M. D., and Greenberg, H. J. Slow brain stem responses (SN10) to tone pips in normally hearing newborns and adults. *Audiology*, 1981, *20*(2):113-122.

Hayes, D. Effect of degree of hearing loss on diagnostic audiometric tests. *American Journal of Otology*, 1980, *2*(2):91-96.

Hayes, D., and Jerger, J. The effect of degree of hearing loss on diagnostic test strategy: Report of a case. *Archives of Otolarngology*, 1980, *106*(5):266-268.

Hay, I. S., and Davis, H. Slow cortical evoked potential: Interactions of auditory, vibrotactile and shock stimuli. *Audiology*, 1971, *10*:9-17.

Hecox, K. Electrophysiological correlates of human auditory development. In L. B. Cohen, and P. Salapatek (Eds.), *Infant perception: From sensation to cognition*. Vol. 11. New York: Academic Press, 1975.

Hecox, K., and Galambos, R. Brainstem auditory evoked responses in human infants and adults. *Archives of Otolaryngology*, 1974, *99*:30-33.

Hecox, K., Squires, N., and Galambos, R. The effect of stimulus duration and rise-fall time on the human brainstem auditory evoked response. *Journal of the Acoustical Society of America*, 1976, *60*:1187-1192.

Hellekson, C., Allen, A., and Greeley, H., et al. Comparison of interwave latencies of brain-stem auditory evoked responses in narcoleptics, primary insomniacs and normal controls. *Electroencephalography and Clinical Neurophysiology*, 1979, *47*:742-744.

Hellman, R. P. Dependence of loudness growth on skirts of excitation patterns. *Journal of the Acoustical Society of America*, 1978, *63*:1114-1119.

Hellman, W. S., and Hellman, R. P. Relation of the loudness function to the intensity characteristic of the ear. *Journal of the Acoustical Society of America*, 1975, *57*:188-192.

Henderson, D. Behavioral and human evoked response thresholds as a function of frequency. *Journal of Speech and Hearing Research*, 1972, *15*:390-394.

Hennerici, M., Weznel, D., and Freund, H. J. The comparison of small-size rectangle and checkerboard stimulation for the evaluation of delayed visual evoked responses in patients suspected of multiple sclerosis. *Brain*, 1977, *100*:119-136.

Henry, K. R. Auditory nerve and brain stem volume-conducted potentials evoked by pure-tone pips in the CBA/J laboratory mouse. *Audiology*, 1979a, *18*:93-108.

Henry, K. R. Auditory brainstem volume conducted responses. Origins in the laboratory mouse. *Journal of American Auditory Society*, 1979b, *4*:173-178.

Henry, K. R., and Chole, R. A. Cochlear electrical activity in the C57BL/6 laboratory mouse: Volume conducted vertex and round window responses. *Acta Oto-Laryngologica* (Stockholm), 1979, *87*:61-68.

Henry, K. R., and Lepkowski, C. Evoked potential correlates of genetic progressive hearing loss: Age-related changes from the ear to inferior colliculus of C57BL/6 and CBA/J mice. *Acta Oto-Laryngologica* (Stockholm), 1978, *86*:366-374.

Heron, J. R., Regan, D., and Milner, B. A. Delay in visual perception in unilateral optic atrophy after retrobulbar neuritis. *Brain*, 1974, *97*:69.

Hicks, G. E. Auditory brainstem response. Sensory assessment by bone conduction masking. *Archives of Otolaryngology*, 1980, *106*(7):392-395.

Hillyard, S. A. The CNV and human behavior. *Electroencephalography and Clinical*

Neurophysiology (Suppl), 1973, *33*:161-171.

Hillyard, S. A., Hink, R. F., and Schwent, V. L., et al. Electrical signs of selective attention in the human brain. *Science*, 1973, *182*:177-180.

Hillyard, S. A., and Picton, T. W. Event-related brain potentials and selective information processing in man. In J. E. Desmedt (Ed.), *Progress in clinical neurophysiology. Vol. 6. Cognitive components in cerebral event-related potentials and selective attention*. Basel: Karger, 1979.

Hillyard, S. A., Picton, T. W., and Regan, D. Sensation, perception and attention: Analysis using ERPs. In E. Callaway, P. Tueting, and S. H. Koslow (Eds.), *Event-related brain potentials in man*. New York: Academic Press, 1978.

Hillyard, S. A., Squires, K. C., and Bauer, J. W., et al. Evoked potential correlates of auditory signal detection. *Science*, 1971, *172*:1357-1360.

Hind, J., Anderson, D., and Brugge, J., et al. Coding of information pertaining to paired low-frequency tones in single auditory nerve fibers of the squirrel monkey. *Journal of Neurophysiology*, 1967, *30*:794-816.

Hind, J. E., Goldberg, J. M., and Greenwood, D. D., et al. Some discharge characteristics of single neurons in the inferior colliculus of the cat. II. Timing of the discharges and observations on binaural stimulation. *Journal of Neurophysiology*, 1963, *26*:321-341.

Hink, R. F., Fenton, W. H., and Pfefferbaum, A., et al. The distribution of attention across auditory input channels: An assessment using the human evoked potential. *Psychophysiology*, 1978, *15*:466-473.

Hink, R. F., and Hillyard, S. A. Auditory evoked potentials during selective listening to dichotic speech messages. *Perception and Psychophysics*, 1976, *20*:236-242.

Hink, R. F., Van Voorhis, S., and Hillyard, S. A. The division of attention and the auditory evoked potential. *Neuropsychologia*, 1977, *15*:597-605.

Hinman, C. L., Buchwald, J. S., and Brown, K. A., et al. Origins and significance of middle latency auditory evoked response in cat. *Anatomical Record*, 1978, *190*:423.

Holder, G. E. The effects of chiasmal compression on the pattern visual evoked potential. *Electroencephalography and Clinical Neurophysiology*, 1978, *45*:278-280.

Hood, D. C. Central effects on the human peripheral auditory system. Unpublished Ph.D. dissertation, Northwestern University, Chicago, 1971.

Hood, D. C. Evoked cortical response audiometry. In L. J. Bradford (Ed.), *Physiological measures of the audio-vestibular system*. New York: Academic Press, 1975.

Hosford, H. L., Fullerton, B. C., and Levine, R. A. Binaural interaction in human and cat brain stem evoked responses. *Journal of the Acoustical Society of America*, 1979, *65*(1):s86.

Hosick, E. C., and Mendel, M. I. Effects of secobarbitol on the late components of the auditory evoked potentials. *Revue de Laryngologie Otologie Rhinologie* (Bordeaux), 1975, *96*:185-191.

Houtgast, T. Psychophysical evidence for lateral inhibition in hearing. *Journal of the Acoustical Society of America*, 1972, *51*:1885-1894.

Howe, J. R., and Miller, C. A. Midbrain deafness following head injury. *Neurology*, 1975, *25*:286-289.

Howes, W. L. Loudness function derived from data on electrical discharge rates in auditory nerve fibers. *Acoustica*, 1974, *30*:247-259.

Hrbek, A., Hrbkova, M., and Lenard, H. Somatosensory, auditory, and visual evoked response in newborn infants during sleep and wakefulness. *Electroencephalography and Clinical Neurophysiology*, 1969, *26*:597-603.

Huang, C. M. A comparative study of the brain stem auditory response in mammals. *Brain Research*, 1980, *184*:215-219.

Huang, C. M., and Buchwald, J. S. Interpretation of the vertex short latency acoustic response: A study of single neurons in the brainstem. *Brain Research*, 1977, *137*:291-303.

Huang, C. M., and Buchwald, J. S. Factors that affect the amplitudes and latencies of the vertex short latency acoustic responses in the cat. *Electroencephalography and Clinical Neurophysiology*, 1978, *44*:179-186.

Huis in't Veld, F., Osterhammel, P., and Terkildsen, K. The frequency selectivity of the 500 Hz frequency following response. *Scandinavian Audiology*, 1977, *6*:35-42.

Hume, A. L., and Cant, B. R. Conduction time in central somatosensory pathways in man. *Electroencephalography and Clinical Neurophysiology*, 1978, *45*: 361-375.

Hume, A. L., Cant, B. R., and Shaw, N. A. Central somatosensory conduction time in comatose patients. *Annals of Neurology*, 1979, *5*:379-384.

Humphrey, D. R. Re-analysis of the antidromic cortical response. II. On the contribution of cell discharge and PSPs to the evoked potentials. *Electroencephalography and Clinical Neurophysiology*, 1968, *25*:421-442.

Hyde, M. L., Stephens, S. D. G., and Thornton, A. R. D. Stimulus repetition rate and the early brainstem responses. *British Journal of Audiology*, 1976, *10*:41-50.

Ichikawa, G., Kawamura, S., and Uchida, T., et al. Nature of auditory evoked middle latency response. U.S.-Japan Seminar on Auditory Responses from the Brainstem. Honolulu, Hawaii, 1979.

Imig, T. J., and Adrian, H. O. Binaural columns in the primary field (AI) of cat auditory cortex. *Brain Research*, 1977, *138*:241-257.

Irving, R., and Harrison, J. M. The superior olivary complex and audition: A comparative study. *Journal of Comparative Neurology*, 1967, *130*:77-86.

Isreal, J. B., Chesney, G. L., and Wickens, C. D., et al. P300 and tracking difficulty: Evidence for multiple resources in dual-task performance. *Psychophysiology*, 1980, *17*:259-273.

Isreal, J. B., Wickens, C. D., and Chesney, G. L., et al. The event-related brain potential as an index of display-monitoring workload. *Human Factors*, 1980, *22*:211-224.

Jacobson, J. T., Novotny, G. M., and Elliott, S. Clinical considerations in the interpretation of auditory brainstem response audiometry. *Journal of Otolaryngology*, 1980, *9*(6):493-504.

Jasper, H. H., and Carmichael, L. Electrical potentials from the intact human brain. *Science*, 1935, *81*:51-53.

Jarvilehto, T., Hari, R., and Sams, M. Effect of stimulus repetition on negative sustained potentials elicited by auditory and visual stimuli in the human EEG. *Biological Psychology*, 1978, *7*:1-12.

Jerger, J., and Hall, J. Effects of age and sex on the auditory brainstem response. *Archives of Otolaryngology*, 1980, *106*:382-391.

Jerger, J., Hayes, D., and Jordan, C. Clinical experience with auditory brainstem response audiometry in pediatric assessment. *Ear and Hearing*, 1980, *1*(1): 19-25.

Jerger, J., Neeley, J. G., and Jerger, S. Speech, impedance and auditory brainstem response audiometry in brainstem tumors. *Archives of Otolaryngology*, 1980, *106*:218-223.

Jewett, D. L. Averaged volume-conducted potentials to auditory stimuli in the cat. *Physiologist*, 1969, *12*:262.

Jewett, D. L. Volume-conducted potentials in response to auditory stimuli as detected by averaging in the cat. *Electroencephalography and Clinical Neurophysiology*, 1970, *28*:609-618.

Jewett, D. L., and Romano, M. N. Neonatal development of auditory system potentials from the scalp of rat and cat. *Brain Research*, 1972, *36*:101-115.

Jewett, D. L., Romano, M. N., and Williston, J. S. Human auditory evoked potentials: Possible brain-stem components detected on the scalp. *Science*, 1970, *167*:1517-1518.

Jewett, D. L., and Williston, J. S. Auditory-evoked far fields averaged from scalp of humans. *Brain*, 1971, *94*:681-696.

Johnson, D. H. The response of single auditory-nerve fibers in the cat to single tones: Synchrony and average discharge rate. Unpublished Ph.D. Thesis, Massachusetts Institute of Technology, Cambridge, Mass., 1974.

Johnson, R., and Donchin, E. P300 and stimulus categorization: Two plus one is not so different from one plus one. *Psychophysiology*, 1980, *17*:167-178.

Johnston, B. M., and Boyle, A. J. T. Basilar membrane vibration examined with the Mössbauer technique. *Science*, 1967, *158*:389-390.

Jones, S. J. Short-latency potentials recorded from the neck and scalp following median nerve stimulation in man. *Electroencephalography and Clinical Neurophysiology*, 1977, *43*:853-863.

Jones, T. A., Stockard, J. J., and Rossiter, V. S., et al. Application of cryogenic technique in the evaluation of afferent pathways and coma mechanisms. Proceedings San Diego Biomedical Symposium, 1976, *15*:249-255.

Josey, A. F., Jackson, C. G., and Glasscock, M. E. Brainstem evoked response audiometry in confirmed eighth nerve tumors. *American Journal of Otolaryngology*, 1980, *1*(4):285-290.

Kaga, K., Hink, R. F., and Shinoda, Y., et al. Origin of a middle latency component in cats. Sixth Biennial Symposium of the International Electric Response Audiometry Study Group, Santa Barbara, California, 1979.

Kaga, K., Kitazumi, E., and Kodama, K. Auditory brain stem responses of kernicterus infants. *International Journal of Pediatric Otorhinolaryngology*, 1979, *1*(3): 255-264.

Kaga, K., and Tanaka, Y. Auditory brainstem response and behavioral audiometry. *Archives of Otolaryngology*, 1980, *106*:564-566.

Kane, E. S. Descending inputs to the cat dorsal cochlear nucleus: An electron microscopic study. *Journal of Neurocytology*, 1977, *6*:583-605.

Kazaki, A., Shiota, R., and Terada, C., et al. Clinical studies on the somatosensory evoked response in neurosurgical patients. *Electroencephalography and Clinical Neurophysiology*, 1971, *31*:184-191.

Keating, L. W., and Ruhm, H. B. Some observations on the effects of attention to stimuli on the amplitude of the acoustically evoked response. *Audiology*, 1971, *10*:177-184.

Keidel, W. D. D. C. potentials in the auditory evoked response in man. *Acta Oto-Laryngologica* (Stockholm), 1971, *71*:242-248.

Kemp, E. H., Coppée, G. E., and Robinson, E. H. Electric responses of the brain stem to unilateral auditory stimulation. *American Journal of Physiology*, 1937, *120*:304-315.

Kemp, E. H., and Robinson, E. H. Electric responses of the brain stem to bilateral auditory stimulation. *American Journal of Physiology*, 1937, *120*:316-322.

Khechinashvili, S. N., and Kevanishvili, Z. S. Experiences in computer audiometry (ECoG and ERA). *Audiology*, 1974, *13*:391-402.

Khechinashvili, S. N., Kevanishvili, Z. S., and Kajaia, O. A. Amplitude and latency studies of the averaged auditory evoked response to tones of different intensities. *Acta Oto-Laryngologica* (Suppl) (Stockholm), 1973, *76*:395-401.

Khechinashvili, S. N., Kevanishvili, Z. S., and Khachijdze, O. A., et al. Electrocochleographical studies in humans. *British Journal of Audiology*, 1974, *8*:6-13.

Kiang, N. Y.-S. The use of computers in studies of auditory neurophysiology. *Transactions of the American Academy of Ophthalmology and Otolaryngology*, 1961, *65*:735-747.

Kiang, N. Y.-S., Liberman, M. C., and Baer, T. Tuning curves of auditory-nerve fibers. *Journal of the Acoustical Society of America*, 1977, *61*:27A.

Kiang, N. Y.-S., Liberman, M. C., and Levine, R. A. Auditory nerve activity in cats exposed to ototoxic drugs and high-intensity sounds. *Annals of Otology, Rhinology and Laryngology*, 1976, *75*:752-768.

Kiang, N. Y.-S., and Moxon, E. C. Tails of tuning curves of auditory-nerve fibers. *Journal of the Acoustical Society of America*, 1974, *55*:620-630.

Kiang, N. Y.-S., Moxon, E. C., and Kahn, A. R. The relationship of gross cochlear potentials recorded from the cochlea to single unit activity in the auditory nerve. In R. J. Ruben, C. Elberling, and G. Salomon (Eds.), *Electrocochleography*. Baltimore: University Park Press, 1976.

Kiang, N. Y.-S., Moxon, E. C., and Levine, R. A. Auditory nerve activity in cats with normal and abnormal cochleas. In G. E. W. Wolstenhome and J. Knight (Eds.), *Sensorineural hearing loss*. London: J. & A. Churchill, 1970.

Kiang, N. Y.-S., Pfeiffer, R. R., and Warr, W. B., et al. Stimulus coding in the cochlear nucleus. *Annals of Otology, Rhinology, and Laryngology*, 1965, *74*: 463-485.

Kiang, N. Y.-S., Watanabe, T., and Thomas, E. C., et al. *Discharge patterns of single fibers in the cat's auditory nerve*. Cambridge, Mass., The M.I.T. Press, 1965.

Kim, D. O., and Molnar, C. E. A population study of cochlear nerve fibers: Comparison of spatial distributions of average-rate and phase-locking measures of response to single tones. *Journal of Neurophysiology*, 1979, *42*:16-30.

Kimmelman, C. P., Marsh, R., and Yamane, H., et al. The effect of rise time on the latency and amplitude of the guinea pig brain stem response. *Transactions — Pennsylvania Academy of Ophthalmology and Otolaryngology*, 1979, *32*:160-165.

Kitzes, L. M., Gibson, M. M., and Rose, J. E., et al. Initial discharge latency and threshold considerations for some neurons in the cochlear nucleus complex of the cat. *Journal of Neurophysiology*, 1978, *41*:1165-1182.

Klein, A. J., and Teas, D. C. Acoustically dependent latency shifts of BSER (wave V) in man. *Journal of the Acoustical Society of America*, 1978, *63*:1887-1895.

Klinke, R. Physiology of hearing. In R. F. Schmidt (Ed.), *Fundamentals of Sensory Physiology*. Heidelberg: Springer-Verlag, 1978.

Klinke, R., Fruhstorfer, H., and Finkerzeller, P. Evoked responses as a function of external and stored information. *Electroencephalography and Clinical Neurophysiology*, 1968, *25*:119-122.

Klorman, R., Salzman, L. F., and Pass, H. L., et al. Effects of methylphenidate on hyperactive children's evoked response during passive and active attention. *Psychophysiology*, 1979, *16*:23-29.

Knight, P. L. Representation of the cochlea within the anterior auditory field (AAF) of the cat. *Brain Research*, 1977, *130*:447-467.

Knight, R. T., Hillyard, S. A., and Woods, D. L., et al. The effects of frontal and temporal-parietal lesions in the auditory evoked potential in man. *Electroencephalography and Clinical Neurophysiology*, 1980, *50*:112-124.

Kodera, K., Hink, R. F., and Yamaha, O., et al. Effects of rise time on simultaneously recorded auditory-evoked potentials from the early, middle and late ranges. *Audiology*, 1979, *18*:395-402.

Kodera, K., Yamane, H., and Yamada, O., et al. Brainstem response audiometry at speech frequencies. *Audiology*, 1977, *16*:469-479.

Koeber, K. C., Pfeiffer, R. R., and Warr, W. B., et al. Spontaneous spike discharges from single units in the cochlear nucleus after destruction of the cochlea. *Experimental Neurology*, 1966, *16*:119-130.

Kohllöffel, L. U. E. A study of basilar membrane vibrations. III. The basilar membrane frequency response in the living guinea pig. *Acoustica*, 1972, *27*:82-89.

Kohn, M., Lifshitz, K., and Litchfield, D. Averaged evoked potentials and frequency modulation. *Electroencephalography and Clinical Neurophysiology*, 1978, *45*:236-243.

Kooi, K. A., and Bagchi, B. K. Visual evoked responses in man: Normative data. *Annals of the New York Academy of Sciences*, 1964, *112*:254-269.

Kooi, K. A., Tipton, A. C., and Marshall, R. E. Polarities and field configurations of the vertex components of the human auditory evoked response: A reinterpretation. *Electroencephalography and Clinical Neurophysiology*, 1971, *31*: 166-169.

Kornmuller, A. E. Architektonische lokalisation bioelektrischer erscheinungen auf grosshirnrinde. I. Mitteilung: Unterschungen am kanichen bei augenbelichtung. *Journal für Psychologie und Neurologie*, 1932, *44*:447-459.

Krejci F. Utersuchungen zur frage der biolektorischen fundtion—sprufung der schnecke. *Monatsschrift f. Ohrenheilkunde Und Laryngo-Rhinologie*, 1949, *83*:224-230.

Krejci, F., and Bornschein, H. Untersuchungen uber die topische abhanglgkeit des electrocochleogramma. *Mschr Onrenheilk*, 1950, *84*:1-10.

Kritchesky, M., and Wiederholt, W. C. Short latency somatosensory evoked potentials. *Archives of Neurology*, 1978, *35*:706-711.

Krogh, H. J., Blegvad, B., and Stephens, S. D. G. Harmonics in frequency-following responses. *Scandinavian Audiology*, 1977, *6*:157-162.

Krough, H. J., Khan, M. A., and Fosuig, L., et al. N1 to P2 component of the auditory evoked potential during alcohol intoxication and interaction of pyrithioxine in healthy adults. *Electroencephalography and Clinical Neurophysiology*, 1977, *44*:1-7.

Kruidenier, C. FFR and BER; in models of the auditory system and related signal processing techniques (M. Hoke and E. de Boen , eds.). Scandinavian Audiology (Suppl), 1979, 9:179-187.

Krumholz, A., Goldstein, P., and Felix, J., et al. Maturation of the brainstem-evoked potential in premature infants. Neurology, 1978, 28:347.

Kupperman, G. L., and Mendel, M. I. Threshold of the early components of the averaged electroencephalic response determined with tone pips and clicks during drug-induced sleep. Audiology, 1974, 13:379-390.

Kuroiwa, Y., and Celesia, G. G. Visual evoked potentials with hemifield pattern stimulation. Their use in the diagnosis of retrochiasmatic lesions. Archives of Neurology, 1981, 38:86-90.

Kylen, P., Arlinger, S. D., and Bergholtz, L. M. Preoperative temporary threshold-shift in ear surgery. Acta Oto-Laryngologica (Stockholm), 1977, 84:393-401.

Lacquaniti, F., Benna, P., and Gilli, M., et al. Brainstem auditory evoked potentials and blink reflex in quiescent multiple sclerosis. Electroencephalography and Clinical Neurophysiology, 1979, 47:607-610.

Laget, P., Mamo, H., and Houdart, H. De l'interet des potentiels évoques més-thésiques dans l'étude des lesions due lobe parietal de l'homme. Etude préliminaire. Neuro-Chirurgie, 1967, 13:841-853.

Lakritz, T. Recording of auditory nerve and brainstem responses in thyroid disorders. (Unpublished M.D. thesis, in Hebrew, 1979.)

Lane, R. H., Kupperman, G. L., and Goldstein, R. Early components of the averaged electroencephalic response in relation to rise-decay time and duration of pure tones. Journal of Speech and Hearing Research, 1971, 14:408-415.

Lavine, R. A. Phase locking in response of single neurons in cochlear nuclear complex of the cat to low frequency tonal stimuli. Journal Neurophysiology, 1971, 34:467-483.

Leake-Jones, P. A., and Vivion, M. C. Cochlear pathology in cats following administration of neomycin sulfate. Scanning Electron Microscopy/1979/AMF O'Hare, Ill.: SEM, Inc., 1979.

Legoiux, J-P., and Pierson, A. Investigations on the sources of whole-nerve action potentials recorded from various places in the guinea pig cochlea. Journal of the Acoustical Society of America, 1974, 56:1222-1225.

Lehnhardt, E., and Battmer, R. D. Behavior of the fast brain stem response P6 under noise influence, an "objective noise audiometry." Laryngologie, Rhinologie, Otologie (Stuttgart), 1979, 58:822-826.

Leiberman, A., Sohmer, H., and Szabo, G. Cochlear audiometry (Electro-cochleography) during neonatal period. Developmental Medicine and Child Neurology, 1973a, 15:8-13.

Leiberman, A., Sohmer, H., and Szabo, G. Standard values of amplitude and latency of cochlear audiometry (electrocochleography) responses in different age groups. Arch Klin Exp Ohren Nasen Kehlkopf, 1973b, 203:267-273.

Lempert, J., Meltzer, P. E., and Wever, E. G., et al. The cochleogram and its clinical applications. Concluding observations. Archives of Otolaryngology, 1950, 51:307-311.

Lempert, J., Wever, E. G., and Lawrence, M. The cochleogram and its clinical applications. A preliminary report. Archives of Otolaryngology, 1947, 45:61-67.

Lenard, H., von Bernuth, H., and Hutt, S. J. Acoustic evoked responses in newborn infants: The influence of pitch and complexity of the stimulus. *Electroencephalography and Clinical Neurophysiology*, 1969, *27*:121-127.

Lentz, W. E., and McCandless, G. A. Averaged electroencephalic audiometry in infants. *Journal of Speech and Hearing Disorder*, 1971, *36*:19-28.

Leshowitz, B., and Lindstrom, R. Measurement of non linearities in listeners with sensorineural hearing loss. In E. F. Evans and J. P. Wilson (Eds.), *Psychophysics and physiology of hearing*. London: Academic Press, 1977.

Lev, A., and Sohmer, H. Sources of averaged neural responses recorded in animals and human subjects during cochlear audiometry. (Electro-cochleogram). *Arch Klin Exp Ohren, Nasen Kehlkopfheilk*, 1972, *201*:79-90.

Liberman, M. C. Auditory-nerve response from cats raised in a low-noise chamber. *Journal of the Acoustical Society of America*, 1978, *63*:442-455.

Liberman, M. C., and Kiang, N. Y.-S. Acoustic trauma in cats: Cochlear pathology and auditory-nerve activity. *Acta Oto-Laryngologica* (Suppl) (Stockholm), 1978, *358*:1-63.

Liberson, W. T. Study of evoked potentials in aphasics. *American Journal of Physical Medicine*, 1965, *5*:135-142.

Liberson, W. T., Gratzur, M., and Zales, A., et al. Comparison of conduction velocity of motor and sensory fibers determined by different methods. *Archives of Physical Medicine Rehabilitation* (Chicago), 1966, *47*:17-23.

Lifshitz, K., Susswein, S., and Lee, K. Auditory evoked potentials and psychopathology. In H. Begleiter (Ed.), *Evoked brain potentials and behavior*. New York: Plenum Press, 1979.

Lindsley, D. Average evoked potentials—Achievements, failures and prospects. In E. Donchin and D. Lindsley (Eds.), *Average evoked potentials: Methods, results, and evaluations*. Washington, D. C.: National Aeronautics and Space Administration, 1969.

Loiselle, D. L., Stamm, J. S., and Maitinsky, S., et al. Evoked potential and behavioral signs of attentive dysfunction in hyperactive boys. *Psychophysiology*, 1980, *17*:193-201.

Lolas, F., Hoeppner, T. J., and Morrell, F. The BAER profile: A method for reporting electrophysiologic brain-stem examinations in clinical practice. *Neurology*, 1979, *29*(2):242-244.

Love, J. A., and Scott, J. W. Some response characteristics of cells of the magnocellular division of the medial geniculate body. *Canadian Journal of Physiology and Pharmacology*, 1969, *47*:881-888.

Lowell, S., and Paparella, M. M. Presbycusis: What is it? *Laryngoscope*, 1977, *87*:1710-1717.

Lowitzsch, K., Kuhnt, U., and Sakmann, Ch., et al. Visual pattern evoked responses and blink reflexes in assessment of MS diagnosis. *Journal of Neurology*, 1976, *213*:17-32.

MacKay, A. R., Hosobuchi, Y., and Williston, J. S. Brain stem auditory evoked response and brain-stem compression. *Neurosurgery*, 1980, *6*(6):632-638.

MacKay, D. M., Evans, E. F., and Hammond, P., et al. Evoked brain potentials as indicators of sensory information processing. *Neurosciences Research Program Bulletin*, 1969, *9*:181-276.

Madell, J. R., and Goldstein, R. Relation between loudness and the amplitude of the early components of the averaged electroencephalic response. *Journal of Speech and Hearing Research*, 1972, *15*:134-141.

Magladery, J. W., Porter, W. E., and Park, A. M., et al. Electrophysiological studies of nerve and reflex activity in normal man. IV. The two neuron reflex and identification of certain action potentials from spinal roots and cord. *Bulletin of Johns Hopkins Hospital*, 1951, *88*:499-519.

Mair, I. W. S., Elverland, H. H., and Laukli, E. Bilateral recording of early auditory evoked responses in the cat. *Hearing Research*, 1978, *1*:11-23.

Mair, I. W., Søhoel, P., and Elverland, H. H. Brain stem electrical response audiometry and middle ear effusion. *Scandinavian Audiology*, 1979, *8*(4):227-231.

Marsh, J. T., Brown, J. S., and Smith, J. C. Differential brainstem pathways for the conduction of auditory frequency-following responses. *Electroencephalography and Clinical Neurophysiology*, 1974, *36*:415-424.

Marsh, J. T., Brown, W., and Smith, J. Far-field recorded frequency-following responses: Correlates of low pitch auditory perception in humans. *Electroencephalography and Clinical Neurophysiology*, 1975, *38*:113-119.

Marsh, J. T., Smith, J. C., and Worden, F. G. Receptor and neural responses in auditory masking of low frequency tones. *Electroencephalography and Clinical Neurophysiology*, 1972, *32*:63-74.

Marsh, J. T., and Worden, F. G. Sound evoked frequency-following responses in the central auditory pathway. *Laryngoscope*, 1968, *78*:1149-1163.

Martin, J. L., and Coats, A. C. Short-latency auditory evoked responses recorded from nasopharynx. *Brain Research*, 1973, *60*:496-502.

Martin, M. E., and Moore, E. J. Scalp distribution of early (0 to 10 msec) auditory evoked responses. *Archives of Otolaryngology*, 1978, *103*:326-328.

Mast, T. Muscular versus cerebral sources for the short latency human evoked responses to clicks. *Physiologist*, 1963, *6*:229.

Mast, T. Short latency human evoked responses to clicks. *Journal of Applied Physiology: Respiratory, Environmental and Exercise Physiology*, 1965, *20*: 725-730.

Mast, T. E. Dorsal cochlear nucleus of the chinchilla: Excitation by contralateral sound. *Brain Research*, 1973, *62*:61-70.

Mastaglia, F. L., Black, J. L., and Cala, L. A., et al. Evoked potentials, saccadic velocities and computerized tomography in diagnosis of multiple sclerosis. *British Medical Journal*, 1977, *1*:1315-1317.

Matsunaga, E. The dimorphism in human normal cerumen. *Annals of Human Genetics*, 1962, *25*:273-286.

McCallum, W. C. and Curry, S. H. The form and distribution of auditory evoked potentials and CNVs when stimuli and responses are lateralized. In H. H. Kornhuber and L. Deecke (Eds.), *Progress in brain research. Vol. 54. Motivation, motor and sensory processes of the brain: Electrical potentials, behavior and clinical use.* Amsterdam: Elsevier, 1980, 767-775.

McCandless, G. A. Clinical application of evoked response audiometry. *Journal of Speech and Hearing Research, 1967, 10*:468-478.

McCandless, G. A., and Best, L. Summed evoked response using pure-tone stimuli. *Journal of Speech and Hearing Research*, 1966, *9*:256-262.

McCandless, G. A., and Lentz, W. E. Amplitude and latency characteristics of the auditory evoked response at low sensation levels. *Journal of Auditory Research*, 1968, *8*:273-282.

McCandless, G. E., and Rose, D. E. Evoked cortical response to stimulus change. *Journal of Speech and Hearing Research*, 1970, *13*:624-634.

McClelland, R. J., and McCrea, R. S. Intersubject variability of the auditory-evoked brain stem potentials. *Audiology*, 1979, *18*(6):462-471.

McFarland, W. H., Vivion, M. C., and Goldstein, R. Middle components of the AER to tone-pips in normal-hearing and hearing-impaired subjects. *Journal of Speech and Hearing Research*, 1977, *20*:781-798.

McFarland, W. H., Vivion, M. C., and Wolf, K. E., et al. Reexamination of effects of stimulus rate and number on the middle components of the averaged electroencephalic response. *Audiology*, 1975, *14*:456-465.

McGee, T. J., and Clemis, J. D. The approximation of audiometric thresholds by auditory brain stem responses. *Otolaryngology and Head and Neck Surgery*, 1980, *88*(3):295-303.

McRandle, C. C., Smith, M. A., and Goldstein, R. Early averaged electroencephalic response to clicks in neonates. *Annals of Otology, Rhinology and Laryngology*, 1974, *83*:695-702.

Mendel, D., and Robinson, M. Electrocochleography in congenital hypothyroidism. *Developmental Medicine and Child Neurology*, 1978, *20*:664-667.

Mendel, M. I. Influence of stimulus level and sleep stage on the early components of the averaged electroencephalic response to clicks during all-night sleep. *Journal of Speech and Hearing Research*, 1974, *17*:5-17.

Mendel, M. I. Electroencephalic tests of hearing. In S. Gerber (Ed.), *Audiometry in infancy*. New York: Grune & Stratton, 1977.

Mendel, M. I. Evoked cochlear potentials. In S. Gerber (Ed.), *Audiometry in infancy*. New York: Grune & Stratton, 1978.

Mendel, M. I. Clinical use of primary cortical responses. *Audiology*, 1980, *19*(1): 1-15.

Mendel, M. I., Adkinson, C., and Harker, L. Middle components of the auditory evoked potentials in infants. *Annals of Otology, Rhinology and Laryngology*, 1977, *86*:293-299.

Mendel, M. I., and Goldstein, R. The effect of test conditions on the early components of the averaged electroencephalic response. *Journal of Speech and Hearing Research*, 1969a, *12*:344-350.

Mendel, M. I., and Goldstein, R. Stability of the early components of the averaged electroencephalic response. *Journal of Speech and Hearing Research*, 1969b, *12*:351-361.

Mendel, M. I., and Goldstein, R. Early components of the averaged electroencephalic response to constant level clicks during all-night sleep. *Journal of Speech and Hearing Research*, 1971, *14*:829-840.

Mendel, M. I., and Hosick, E. C. Effects of secobarbitol on the early components of the auditory evoked potentials. *Revue de Laryngologie Otologie Rhinologie* (Bordeaux), 1975, *96*:178-184.

Mendel, M. I., Hosick, E. C., and Windman, T. R., et al. Audiometric comparison of the middle and late components of the adult auditory evoked potentials awake and asleep. *Electroencephalography and Clinical Neurophysiology*, 1975, *38*:27-33.

Mendel, M. I., and Kupperman, G. L. Early components to constant level clicks during rapid eye movement sleep. *Audiology*, 1974, *13*:23-32.

Mendelson, T., Salamy, A., and Lenoir, M., et al. Brainstem evoked potential findings in children with otitis media. *Archives of Otolaryngology*, 1979, *105*:17-20.

Merzenich, M. M., and Brugge, J. F. Representation of the cochlear partition on the superior temporal plane of the macaque monkey. *Brain Research*, 1973, *50*:275-296.

Merzenich, M. M., and Kass, J. H. Principles of organization of sensory-perceptual systems in mammals. In J. M. Sprague, and A. N. Epstein (Eds.), *Progress in psychobiology and physiological psychology*. Vol. 9. New York: Academic Press, 1980.

Merzenich, M. M., Knight, P. L., and Roth, G. L. Representation of cochlea within primary auditory cortex in the cat. *Journal of Neurophysiology*, 1975, *38*:231-249.

Merzenich, M. M., and Reid, M. D. Representation of the cochlea within the inferior colliculus of the cat. *Brain Research*, 1974, *77*:397-415.

Merzenich, M. M., Roth, G. L., and Andersen, R. A., et al. Some basic features of organization of the central auditory nervous system. In E. F. Evans and J. P. Wilson (Eds.), *Psychophysics and physiology of hearing*. New York: Academic Press, 1977.

Merzenich, M. M., and White, M. W. Cochlear implant. The interface problem. In T. Hambrecht and J. Reswick (Eds.), *Functional electrical stimulation: Applications in neural prostheses*. New York: Marcel Dekker, 1977.

Merzenich, M. M., White, M., and Vivion, M. C., et al. Some considerations of multichannel electrical stimulation of the auditory nerve in the profoundly deaf: Interfacing electrode arrays with the auditory nerve array. *Acta Oto-Laryngologica* (Stockholm), 1979, *87*:196-203.

Meyerhoff, W. L. Symposium on hearing loss—The otolaryngologist's responsibility. Medical management of hearing loss. *Laryngoscope*, 1978, *88*:960-973.

Michalewski, H. J., Patterson, J. V., and Thompson, L. W., et al. A comparison of the emitted late positive potential in older and young adults. Paper presented at the meeting of the Society for Psychophysiological Research, Vancouver, 1980.

Michelson, R. P., and Vincent, W. R. Auditory evoked frequency following responses in man. *Archives of Otolaryngology*, 1975, *101*:6-10.

Mikaelian, D. O. Development and degeneration of hearing in the C57/b16 mouse: Relation of electrophysiologic responses from the round window and cochlear nucleus to cochlear anatomy and behavioral responses. *Laryngoscope*, 1979, *89*:1-15.

Milner, B. A. Evaluation of auditory function by computer techniques. *International Audiology*, 1969, *8*:361-370.

Moffat, D. A., Gibson, W. P. R., and Ramsden, R. T., et al. Transtympanic electrocochleography during glycerol dehydration. *Acta Oto-Laryngologica* (Stockholm), 1977, *85*:158-166.

Mokotoff, B., Schulman-Galambos, C., and Galambos, R. Brainstem auditory evoked potentials in children. *Archives of Otolaryngology*, 1977, *103*:38-43.

Møller, A. R. Function of the middle ear. In W. D. Keidel and W. D. Neff (Eds.),

Handbook of sensory physiology. Vol. V/1. Berlin: Springer-Verlag, 1974.

Møller, A. R., and Janetta, P. J. Evoked potentials from the inferior colliculus in man, *Electroencephalography and Clinical Neurophysiology*, 1982, *53*:612-620.

Monod, N., and Garma, L. Auditory responsivity in the human premature. *Biology of the Neonate*, 1971, *17*:292-316.

Mononen, L. J., and Seitz, M. R. An AER analysis of contralateral advantage in the transmission of auditory information. *Neurophysiology*, 1972, *15*:165-173.

Montandon, P. B. Clinical application of auditory nerve responses recorded from the ear canal. *Acta Oto-Laryngologica* (Stockholm), 1976, *81*:283-290.

Montandon, P. B., Cao, M., and Engel, R., et al. Auditory nerve and brainstem responses in the newborn and in preschool children. *Acta Otolaryngologica* (Stockholm), 1979, *87*:279-286.

Montandon, P. B., Megill, N. D., and Kahn, A. R., et al. Recording auditory-nerve potentials as an office procedure. *Annals of Otology, Rhinology and Laryngology*, 1975, *84*:2-10.

Montandon, P. B., Shepard, N. T., and Marr, E. M., et al. Auditory-nerve potentials from ear canals of patients with otologic problems. *Annals of Otology, Rhinology and Laryngology*, 1975, *84*:164-173.

Moore, E. Human cochlear microphonics and auditory nerve action potentials from surface electrodes. Unpublished Ph.D. dissertation, University of Wisconsin. Madison, Wisconsin, 1971.

Moore, E. Auditory brain stem electrical responses. Audiology: An audio journal for continuing education. New York: Grune & Stratton, 1978.

Moore, E. J., Baker, D., and McCoy, D. Follow-up services of a psychiatric population after audiometric screening: Results of pre-otologic clinic. *Eye, Ear, Nose and Throat*, 1969, *48*:585-588.

Moore, E. J., and Harris, H. Brain-stem evoked responses to bone-conducted stimuli. In preparation.

Moore, E. J., and Rose, D. E. Variability of latency and amplitude of acoustically evoked responses to pure tones of moderate to high intensities. *International Audiology*, 1969, *8*:172-181.

Moore, J. K., and Moore, R. Y. A comparative study of the superior olivary complex in the primate brain. *Folia Primatologica*, 1971, *16*:35-51.

Moore, J. K., and Osen, K. K. The cochlear nuclei in man. *American Journal of Anatomy*, 1979, *154*:393-418.

Morest, D. K. The neuronal architecture of the medial geniculate body of the cat. *Journal of Anatomy* (London), 1964, *98*:611-630.

Morest, D. K. The collateral system of the medial nucleus of the trapezoid body of the cat, its neuronal architecture and relation to the olivocochlear bundle. *Brain Research*, 1968, *9*:288-311.

Morest, D. K. Auditory neurons of the brain stem. *Advances in Oto-Rhino-Laryngology* (Basel), 1973, *20*:337-356.

Morest, D. K. Synaptic relationships of Golgi type II cells in the medial geniculate body of the cat. *Journal of Comparative Neurology*, 1975a, *162*:157-194.

Morest, D. K. Structural organization of the auditory pathways. In D. B. Tower, (Ed.), *The nervous system. Vol. 3. Human communication and its disorders.* New York: Raven Press, 1975b, pp. 19-29.

Morest, D. K., Kiang, N. Y.-S., and Kane, E. C., et al. Stimulus coding at caudal levels of the cat's auditory nervous system. II. Patterns of synaptic organization. In A. Møller (Ed.), *Basic mechanisms in hearing.* New York: Academic Press, 1973, pp. 479-509.

Morgon, A., Charachon, D., and Gerin, P. Electro-encephalographic audiometry for young children. *Archives für Klinische und Experimentelles Ohres Nases und Kehlkopf Keilkunde* (Munich), 1971, *198*:144-150.

Morgon, A., and Salle, B. A study of brain stem evoked responses in prematures. *Acta Oto-Laryngologica* (Stockholm), 1980, *89*(3-4):370-375.

Morrison, A. S., Gibson, W. P. R., and Beagley, H. A. Transtympanic electrococh-leography in the diagnosis of retrocochlear tumours. *Clinical Otolaryngology,* 1976, *1*:153

Morrison, A. W., Moffat, D. A., and O'Connor, A. F. Clinical usefulness of electro-cochleography in Ménière's disease: An analysis of dehydrating agents. *Otolaryn-gologic Clinics of North America,* 1980, *13*(4):703-731.

Mouney, D. F., Berlin, C. I., and Cullen, J. K., et al. Changes in human eighth nerve action potential as a function of stimulation rate. *Archives of Otolaryngology,* 1978, *104*:551-554.

Mouney, D. F., Cullen, J. K., and Gondra, M. I., et al. Tone burst electrocochleog-raphy in humans. *Transactions of the American Academy of Ophthalmology and Otolaryngology,* 1976, *82*:348-355.

Moushegian, G., Rupert, A., and Galambos, R. Microelectrode study of ventral coch-lear nucleus of the cat. *Journal of Neurophysiology,* 1962, *25*:515-529.

Moushegian, G., Rupert, A. L., and Stillman, R. D. Scalp-recorded early response in man to frequencies in the speech range. *Electroencephalography and Clinical Neurophysiology,* 1973, *35*:665-667.

Moushegian, G., Rupert, A. L., and Stillman, R. D. Evaluation of frequency-following potentials in man: Masking and clinical studies. *Electroencephalography and Clin-ical Neurophysiology,* 1978, *45*:711-718.

Moushegian, G., Rupert, A., and Whitcomb, M. A. Medial superior-olive-unit re-sponse patterns to monaural and binaural clicks. *Journal of the Acoustical Society of America,* 1964, *36*:196-202.

Mulroy, M. J. Altmann, D. W., and Weiss, T. F., et al. Intracellular electric responses to sound in a vertebrate cochlea. *Nature,* 1974, *249*:482-485.

Näätänen, R., Gaillard, A. W. K., and Mantysulo, S. Early selective attention effect on evoked potential reinterpreted. *Acta Psychologia,* 1978, *42*:313-329.

Näätänen, R., and Michie, P. T. Early selective-attention effects on the evoked poten-tial: A critical review and reinterpretation. *Biological Psychology,* 1979, *8*:81-136.

Nadol, J. B. Value and cost analysis of recent ear tests: Considerations in clinical appli-cation of electrocochleography in 1978. *Laryngoscope,* 1979, *89*:698-704.

Nagao, S., Roccaforte, P., and Moody, R. A. Acute intracranial hypertension and auditory brain-stem responses. *Journal of Neurosurgery,* 1979, *51*(6):846-851.

Nagao, S., Roccaforte, P., and Moody, R. A. Acute intracranial hypertension and auditory brain-stem responses. Part 3. The effects of posterior fossa mass lesions on brain-stem function. *Journal of Neurosurgery,* 1980, *52*(3):351-358.

Nagel, D. Compound action potential of the cochlear nerve evoked electrically. *Ar-chives Oto-Rhino-Laryngology,* 1974, *206*:293-298.

Namerow, N. S. Somatosensory evoked responses in multiple sclerosis patients with varying sensory loss. *Neurology*, 1968, *18*:1197-1204.

Nash, C. L., Lorig, R. A., and Schatzinger, L. A., et al. Spinal cord monitoring during operative treatment of the spine. *Clinical Orthopaedics and Related Research*, 1977, *126*:100-105.

Naunton, R. F., and Fernandez, C. *Evoked electrical activity in the auditory nervous system*. New York: Academic Press, 1978.

Naunton, R. F., and Zerlin, S. Basis and some diagnostic implications of electrocochleography. *Laryngoscope*, 1976a, *86*:475-482.

Naunton, R. F., and Zerlin, S. Human whole-nerve response to clicks of various frequency. *Audiology*, 1976b, *15*:1-9.

Naunton, R. F., and Zerlin, S. The evaluation of peripheral auditory function in infants and children. *Otolaryngologic Clinics of North America*, 1977, *10*:51-58.

Nelms, C. R., and Paparella, M. M. Early external auditory canal tumors. *Laryngoscope*, 1968, *78*:986-100.

Nelson, D. A., and Lassman, F. M. Effects of intersignal interval on the human auditory evoked response. *Journal of the Acoustical Society of America*, 1968, *44*:1529-1532.

Nishida, H., Kumagami, H., and Baba, M. Electrocochleographic study of patients with cerebral vascular lesions. *Archives of Otolaryngology*, 1981, *107*(2):74-78.

Nishida, H., Kumagami, H., and Katsunori, D. Prognostic criteria of sudden deafness as deduced by electrocochleography. *Archives of Otolaryngology*, 1976, *102*: 601-607.

van Noort, J. *The structure and connections of the inferior colliculus: An investigation of the lower auditory system*. Assen, The Netherlands: Van Gorcum, 1969.

Ochs, R. F., and Markand, O. N. Maturational changes of brainstem auditory evoked responses (BAERs) in children and the effect of increased frequency of stimulation. *Neurology*, 1978, *28*:408.

Odenthal, D. W., and Eggermont, J. J. Clinical electrocochleography. *Acta Oto-Laryngologica* (Suppl) (Stockholm), 1974, *316*:62-74.

Odenthal, D. W., and Eggermont, J. J. Electrocochleography study in Ménière's disease and pontine angle neuronoma. In R. J. Ruben, C. Elberling, and G. Salomon (Eds.), *Electrocochleography*. Baltimore: University Park Press, 1976.

Ohlrich, E. S., and Barnet, A. B. Auditory evoked responses during the first year of life. *Electroencephalography and Clinical Neurophysiology*, 1972, *32*:161-169.

Ohlrich, E. S., Barnet, A. B., and Weiss, I. P., et al. Auditory evoked potential development in early childhood: A longitudinal study. *Electroencephalography and Clinical Neurophysiology*, 1978, *44*:411-423.

Ohman, A., and Lader, M. Selective attention and "habituation" of the auditory averaged evoked response in humans. *Physiology and Behavior*, 1972, *8*:79-85.

Okita, T. Event-related potentials and selective attention to auditory stimuli varying in pitch and localization. *Biological Psychology*, 1979, *9*:271-284.

Okita, T., and Ohtani, A. The effects of active attention switching between the ears on averaged evoked potentials. *Electroencephalography and Clinical Neurophysiology*, 1977, *42*:198-204.

Okitsu, T., Kusakari, J., and Ito, K., et al. Study of a simultaneous lobe-vertex, and membrane-vertex recording technique in auditory brain-stem response. *Journal for Oto-Rhino-Laryngology and Its Related Specialties*, 1980, *42*:282-291.

Onishi, S., and Davis, H. Effects of duration and rise time of tone bursts on evoked potentials. *Journal of the Acoustical Society of America*, 1968, *44*:582-591.

Ornitz, E. M., Lee, J. C. M., and Tanguay, P. E., et al. The effect of stimulus interval on the auditory evoked response during sleep in normal children. *Electroencephalography and Clinical Neurophysiology*, 1972, *33*:159-166.

Ornitz, E. M., Ritvo, E. R., and Carr, E. M., et al. The variability of the auditory averaged evoked response during sleep and dreaming in children and adults. *Electroencephalography and Clinical Neurophysiology*, 1967a, *22*:514-524.

Ornitz, E. M., Ritvo, E. R., and Carr, E. M., et al. The effect of sleep onset on the auditory averaged evoked response. *Electroencephalography and Clinical Neurophysiology*, 1967b, *23*:335-341.

Ornitz, E. M., Tanguay, P. E., and Forsythe, A. B., et al. The recovery cycle of the averaged auditory evoked response during sleep in normal children. *Electroencephalography and Clinical Neurophysiology*, 1974, *37*:113-122.

Ornitz, E. M., Tanguay, P. E., and Lee, J. C. M., et al. The effect of stimulus interval on the auditory evoked response during sleep in autistic children. *Journal of Autism Child Schizophrenia*, 1972, *2*:140-150.

Ornitz, E. M., and Walter, D. O. The effect of sound pressure waveform on human brainstem auditory evoked responses. *Brain Research*, 1975, *92*:490-498.

Osako, S., Tokimoto, T., and Matsuura, S. Effects of kanamycin on the auditory evoked responses during postnatal development of the hearing of the rat. *Acta Oto-Laryngologica* (Stockholm), 1979, *88*(5-6):359-368.

Osen, K. K. Course and termination of the primary afferents in the cochlear nuclei of the cat. An experimental anatomical study. *Archives Italiennes de Biologie*, 1970, *108*:21-51.

Osen, K. K. Projection of the cochlear nuclei on the inferior colliculus in the cat. *Journal of Comparative Neurology*, 1972, *144*:355-372.

Osterhammel, P. A., Davis, H., and Wier, C. C., et al. Adult auditory evoked vertex potentials in sleep. *Audiology*, 1973, *12*:116-128.

Ott, H. *Noise reduction techniques in electronic systems.* New York: John Wiley & Sons, 1976.

Paparella, M. M., and Meyerhoff, W. L. Meatoplasty. *Laryngoscope*, 1978, *88*: 357-359.

Paparella, M. M., and Shumrick, D. A. *Otolaryngology. Vol. 2. (EAR)*. Philadelphia: W. B. Saunders, 1973.

Paparella, M. M., and Shumrick, D. A. *Otolaryngology. Vol. 2. (EAR).* Philadelphia: W. B. Saunders, 1980.

Parasuraman, R. Auditory evoked potentials and divided attention. *Psychophysiology*, 1978, *15*:460-465.

Parker, D. J., and Thornton, A. R. D. The validity of the derived cochlear nerve and brainstem evoked responses of the human auditory system. *Scandinavian Audiology*, 1978a, *7*:45-52.

Parker, D. J., and Thornton, A. R. D. Frequency specific components of the cochlear nerve and brainstem evoked responses of the human auditory system. *Scandinavian Audiology*, 1978b, *7*:53-60.

Parker, D. J., and Thornton, A. R. D. Cochlear travelling wave velocities calculated from the derived components of the cochlear nerve and brainstem evoked responses of the human auditory system. *Scandinavian Audiology*, 1978c, *7*:67-70.

Parker, D. J., and Thornton, A. R. D. Derived cochlear nerve and brainstem evoked responses of the human auditory system. *Scandinavian Audiology*, 1978d, 7:73-80.

Parving, A., Elberling, C., and Smith, T. Auditory electrophysiology: Findings in multiple sclerosis. *Audiology*, 1981, 20(2):123-142.

Parving, A., Salomon, G., and Elberling, C., et al. Middle components of the auditory evoked response in bilateral temporal lobe lesions. *Scandinavian Audiology*, 1980, 9:161-167.

Perkins, F. T. A study of cerebral action currents in the dog under sound stimulation. *Psychological Monograph*, 1933, 44(197):1-29.

Perl, E. R., and Whitlock, D. G. Potentials evoked in cerebral somatosensory region. *Journal of Neurophysiology*, 1955, 18:486-501.

Perlman, M. B. and Case, T. J. Electrical phenomena of the cochlea in man. *Archives of Otolaryngology*, 1941, 34:710-718.

Perot, P. L. The clinical use of somatosensory evoked potentials in spinal cord injury. *Clinical Neurosurgery*, 1973, 20:367-382.

Peters, J. F., and Mendel, M. I. Early components of the averaged electroencephalic response to monaural and binaural stimulation. *Audiology*, 1974, 13:195-204.

Pfefferbaum, A., Ford, J. M., and Roth, W. T., et al. Age differences in P3-reaction time association. *Electroencephalography and Clinical Neurophysiology*, 1980a, 49:257-265.

Pfefferbaum, A., Ford, J. M., and Roth, W. T., et al. Age-related changes in auditory event-related potentials. *Electroencephalography and Clinical Neurophysiology*, 1980b, 49:266-276.

Pfefferbaum, A., Horvath, T. B., and Roth, W. T., et al. Event-related potential changes in chronic alcoholics. *Electroencephalography and Clinical Neurophysiology*, 1979, 47:637-647.

Pfeiffer, R. R. Consideration of the acoustic stimulus. In W. D. Keidel and W. D. Neff (Eds.), *Auditory System, Anatomy and Physiology (EAR), Handbook of Physiology*, Vol. V/1, New York: Springer-Verlag, 1974, pp. 13, 15.

Pfurtscheller, G., and Aranibar, A. Event-related cortical desynchronization detected by power measurements of scalp EEG. *Electroencephalography and Clinical Neurophysiology*, 1977, 42:817-826.

Pick, G. F., Evans, E. F., and Wilson, J. P. Frequency resolution in patients with hearing loss of cochlear origin. In E. F. Evans and J. P. Wilson (Eds.), *Psychophysics and physiology of hearing*. London: Academic Press, 1977.

Picton, T. W. The strategy of evoked potential audiometry. In S. E. Gerber and G. T. Mencher (Eds.), *Early diagnosis of hearing loss*. New York: Grune & Stratton, 1978.

Picton, T. W., Campbell, K. B., and Baribeau-Braun, J., et al. The neurophysiology of human attention: A tutorial review. In J. Requin (Ed.), *Attention and performance. VII.* Hillsdale, N.J.: Lawrence Erlbaum Associates, 1978.

Picton, T. W., Goodman, W. S., and Bryce, D. P. Amplitude of evoked responses to tones of high intensity. *Acta Oto-Laryngologica* (Stockholm), 1970, 70:77-82.

Picton, T. W., and Hillyard, S. A. Human auditory evoked potentials. II. Effects of attention. *Electroencephalography and Clinical Neurophysiology*, 1974, 36:191-199.

Picton, T. W., Hillyard, S. A., and Galambos, R., et al. Human auditory attention: A central or peripheral process? *Science*, 1971, 173:351-353.

Picton, T. W., Hillyard, S. A., and Galambos, R. Habituation and attention in the auditory system. In W. D. Keidel and W. D. Neff (Eds.), *Handbook of sensory physiology. Vol. V. Auditory systems, part 3.* Heidelberg: Springer-Verlag, 1976.

Picton, T. W., Hillyard, S. H., and Krauz, H. J., et al. Human auditory evoked potentials. I. Evaluation of components. *Electroencephalography and Clinical Neurophysiology*, 1974, *36*:179-190.

Picton, T. W., Ouellette, J., and Hamel, G., et al. Brainstem evoked potentials to tonepips in notched noise. *Journal of Otolaryngology*, 1979, *8*:289-314.

Picton, T. W., and Smith, A. D. The practice of evoked potential audiometry. *Otolaryngologic Clinics of North America*, 1978, *11*:263-282.

Picton, T. W., Stapells, D. R., and Campbell, K. B. Auditory evoked potentials from the human cochlea and brainstem. *Journal of Otolaryngology*, 1981, *10* (Supp. 9):1-41.

Picton, T. W., and Stuss, D. T. The component structure of the human event-related potentials. In H. H. Kornhuber and L. Deecke (Eds.), *Progress in brain research. Vol. 54. Motivation, motor and sensory processes of the brain: Electrical potentials, behavior and clinical use.* Amsterdam: Elsevier, 1980, pp. 17-49.

Picton, T. W., Woods, D. L., and Baribeau-Braun, J., et al. Evoked potential audiometry. *Journal of Otolaryngology*, 1977, *6*:90-118.

Picton, T. W., Woods, D. L., and Proulx, G. B. Human auditory sustained potentials. I. The nature of the response. *Electroencephalography and Clinical Neurophysiology*, 1978a, *45*:186-187.

Picton, T. W., Woods, D. L., and Proulx, G. B. Human auditory sustained potentials. II. Stimulus relationships. *Electroencephalography and Clinical Neurophysiology*, 1978b, *45*:198-210.

Picton, T. W., Woods, D. L., and Stuss, D. T., et al. Methodology and meaning of human evoked potential scalp distribution studies. In D. Otto (Ed.), *Multidisciplinary perspectives in event-related brain potential research.* Washington, D.C.: U.S. Government Printing Office, 1978.

Plantz, R. G., Williston, J. S., and Jewett, D. L. Spatio-temporal distribution of auditory-evoked far field potentials in rat and cat. *Brain Research*, 1974, *68*:55-71.

Poland, R. M., Wells, D. H., and Ferlauto, J. J. Methods for detecting hearing impairment in infancy. *Pediatric Annals*, 1980, *9*(1):31-32.

Polyak, S. L. *The human ear.* Elmsford, N.Y.: Sonotone Corp., 1946.

Portmann, M., and Aran, J. M. Electro-cochleography. *Laryngoscope*, 1971a, *81*:899-910.

Portmann, M., Aran, J. M. Électro-cochléographie sur le nourrisson et le jeune enfant. *Acta Oto-Laryngologica* (Stockholm), 1971b, *71*:243-261.

Portmann, M., and Aran, J. M. Rélations entre pattern cochléographique et pathologie rétrolabyrinthique. *Acta Oto-Laryngologica* (Stockholm), 1972, *73*:190-196.

Portmann, M., Aran, J. M., and Lagourge, P. Testing for "recruitment" by electrocochleography. *Annals of Otology, Rhinology and Laryngology*, 1973, *82*: 36-43.

Portmann, M., Aran, J. M., and LeBert, G. Potentiels cochleaires obténues chez l'homme en dehors de toute intervention chirurgicale. Note préliminaire. *Revue de Laryngologie Otologie Rhinologie* (Bordeaux), 1967, *88*:157-164.

Portmann, M., Cazals, Y., and Negrevergne, M., et al. Transtympanic and surface recordings in the diagnosis of retrocochlear disorders. *Acta Oto-Laryngologica* (Stockholm), 1980, *89*(3-4):362-369.

Portmann, M., Portmann, C., and Negrevergne, M. Four years of clinical use of electrocochleography. *Revue de Laryngologie Otologie Rhinologie* (Bordeaux), 1974, *95*:537-539.

Powell, W. H., and Hatton, J. B. Projections of the inferior colliculus in the cat. *Journal of Comparative Neurology*, 1969, *136*:183-192.

Pratt, H., Amlie, R. N., and Starr, A. Short latency mechanically evoked somatosensory potentials in humans. *Electroencephalography and Clinical Neurophysiology*, 1979, 47:524-531.

Pratt, H., and Sohmer, H. Intensity and rate functions of cochlear and brainstem evoked responses to click stimuli in man. *Archives of Oto-Rhino-Laryngology*, 1976, *212*:85-93.

Pratt, H., and Sohmer, H. Correlations between psychophysical magnitude estimates and simultaneously obtained auditory nerve, brain stem and cortical responses to click stimuli in man. *Electroencephalography and Clinical Neurophysiology*, 1977, *43*:802-812.

Pratt, H., and Sohmer, H. Comparison of hearing threshold determined by auditory pathway electric responses and by behavioral responses. *Audiology*, 1978, *17*:285-292.

Pratt, H., Starr, A., and Amlie, R. N., et al. Mechanically and electrically evoked somatosensory potentials in normal humans. *Neurology*, 1979, *29*:1236-1244.

Price, L. L., Rosenblut, B., and Goldstein, R. The averaged evoked response to auditory stimulation. *Journal of Speech and Hearing Research*, 1966, *9*:361-370.

Pugh, J. E., Moody, D. B., and Anderson, D. J. Electrocochleography and experimentally-induced loudness recruitment. *Archives of Oto-Rhino-Laryngology*, 1979, *224*:241-255.

Pujol, R. Development of tone-burst responses along the auditory pathway in the cat. *Acta Oto-Laryngologica* (Stockholm), 1972, *74*:383-391.

Pulec, J. L. Ménière's disease: Etiology, natural history, and result of treatment. *Otolaryngologic Clinics of North America*, 1973, *6*:25-39.

Purpura, D. P. Nature of electrocortical potentials and synaptic organizations in cerebral and cerebellar cortex. *International Review of Neurobiology*, 1959, *1*:47-163.

Ramón y Cajal, S. R. *The acoustic nerve: Its cochlear branch or cochlear nerve*. In, *Histologie du système nerveux de l'homme et des vertébrés. Vol. I* 1899 (English translation by Information Center for Hearing, Speech and Disorders of Human Communications. Baltimore: The Johns Hopkins Medical Institutions, 1967).

Ramsden, R. T., Wilson, P., and Gibson, W. P. Immediate effects of intravenous tobramycin and gentamicin on human cochlear function. *Journal of Laryngology and Otology*, 1980, *94*(5):521-531.

Rapin, I., and Graziani, L. J. Auditory-evoked responses in normal, brain damaged, and deaf infants. *Neurology*, 1967, *17*:888-894.

Rapin, I., Schimmel, H., and Cohen, M. M. Reliability in detecting the auditory evoked response (AER) for audiometry in sleeping subjects. *Electroencephalography and Clinical Neurophysiology*, 1972, *32*:521-528.

Rapin, I., Schimmel, H., and Tourk, L. M., et al. Evoked response to clicks and tones of varying intensity in waking adults. *Electroencephalography and Clinical Neurophysiology*, 1966, *21*:335-344.

Rasmussen, A. T. Studies of the VIIIth cranial nerve of man. *Laryngoscope*, 1940, *50*:67-83.

Rasmussen, G. L. Further observations on the efferent cochlear bundle. *Journal of Comparative Neurology*, 1953, *99*:61-74.

Rasmussen, G. L. Efferent fibers of the cochlear nerve and cochlear nucleus. In G. L. Rasmussen and W. Windle (Eds.), *Neural mechanisms of the auditory and vestibular systems*. Springfield, Illinois: Charles C. Thomas, 1960.

Rasmussen, G. L. Anatomic relationships of the ascending and descending auditory systems. In W. S. Fields and B. R. Alford (Eds.), *Neurological aspects of auditory and vestibular disorders*. Springfield, Illinois: Charles C. Thomas, 1964.

Regan, D. *Evoked potentials in psychology, sensory physiology and clinical medicine*. London: Chapman and Hall, 1972.

Regan, D. Recent advances in electrical recording from the human brain. *Nature*, 1975, *253*:401-407.

Regan, D. Steady state evoked potentials: *Journal of the Optical Society of America*, 1977, *67*:1475-1489.

Regan, D., and Heron, J. R. Clinical investigation of lesions of the visual pathway: A new objective technique. *Journal of Neurology, Neurosurgery and Psychiatry*, 1969, *32*:479-483.

Regan, D., Milner, B. A., and Heron, J. R. Delayed visual perception and delayed visual potentials in the spinal form of multiple sclerosis and in retrobulbar neuritis. *Brain*, 1976, *99*:43-66.

Regan, D., and Richards, W. A. Independence of evoked potentials and apparent size. *Vision Research*, 1971, *11*:679-684.

Reneau, J. P., and Hnatiow, G. Z. *Evoked response audiometry: A topical and historical review*. Baltimore: University Park Press, 1975.

Rhode, W. S. Observation of the vibration of the basilar membrane in squirrel monkeys using the Mössbauer technique. *Journal of the Acoustical Society of America*, 1971, *49*:1218-1231.

de Ribaupierre, F., Goldstein, M. H., and Yeni-Komshian, G. Cortical coding of repetitive acoustic pulses. *Brain Research*, 1972, *48*:205-225.

Ridgeway, S. H., Bullock, T. H., and Garder, D. A., et al. Auditory brain-stem response in dolphins. *Proceedings of the National Academy Sciences*, 1981, *78*: 1943-1947.

Rietema, S. J. The clinical significance of electrocochleography. Unpublished Ph.D. thesis, Leyden University, Leyden, The Netherlands, 1979.

Ritter, W., Simson, R., and Vaughan, H. G. Association cortex potentials and reaction time in auditory discrimination. *Electroencephalography and Clinical Neurophysiology*, 1972, *33*:547-555.

Ritter, W., Simson, R., and Vaughan, H. G., et al. A brain event related to the making of a sensory discrimination. *Science*, 1979, *203*:1358-1361.

Ritter, W., and Vaughan, H. G. Averaged evoked responses in vigilance and discrimination: A reassessment. *Science*, 1969, *164*:326-328.

Ritter, W., Vaughan, H. G., and Costa, L. O. Orienting and habituation to auditory stimuli: A study of short term changes in averaged evoked responses. *Electroen-*

cephalography and Clinical Neurophysiology, 1969, *25*:550-556.

Robertson, D. Cochlear neurons: Frequency selectivity altered by perilymph removal. *Science*, 1974, *186*:153-155.

Robertson, D., and Manley, G. A. Manipulation of frequency analysis in the cochlear ganglion of the guinea pig. *Journal of Comparative Physiological Psychology*, 1974, *91*:363-375.

Robinson, D. W., and Dadson, R. S. A redetermination of the equal loudness relations for pure tones. *British Journal of Applied Physiology*, 1956, *7*:166-181.

Robinson, K., and Rudge, P. Auditory evoked responses in multiple sclerosis. *Lancet*, 1975, *i*:1164-1166.

Robinson, K., and Rudge, P. Abnormalities of the auditory evoked potentials in patients with multiple sclerosis. *Brain*, 1977, *100*:19-40.

Robinson, K., and Rudge, P. The stability of the auditory evoked potentials in normal man and patients with multiple sclerosis. *Journal of the Neurological Sciences*, 1978, *36*:147-156.

Rockel, A. J. Observations on the inferior colliculus of the adult cat, stained by the Golgi technique. *Brain Research*, 1971, *30*:407-410.

Rockel, A. J., and Jones, E. G. The neuronal organization of the inferior colliculus. I. The central nucleus. *Journal of Comparative Neurology*, 1973a, *147*:11-60.

Rockel, A. J., and Jones, E. G. The neuronal organization of the inferior colliculus. II. The pericentral nucleus. *Journal of Comparative Neurology*, 1973b, *149*:301-334.

Roeser, R. J., and Price, L. L. Effects of habituation on the auditory response. *Journal of Auditory Research*, 1969, *9*:306-313.

Roeser, R. J., Price, L. L., and Hnatiow, G. Z. Evoked response audiometry: Psychiatric patients. *Archives of Otolaryngology*, 1971, *94*:208-213.

Rohrbaugh, J. W., Syndulko, K., and Lindsley, D. B. Cortical slow waves following non-paired stimuli: Effects of task factors. *Electroencephalography and Clinical Neurophysiology*, 1978, *45*:551-567.

Rohrbaugh, J. W., Syndulko, K., and Lindsley, D. B. Cortical slow waves following non-paired stimuli: Effects of modality, intensity and rate of stimulation. *Electroencephalography and Clinical Neurophysiology*, 1979, *46*:416-427.

Romand, R., and Marty, R. Postnatal maturation of the cochlear nuclei in the cat: A neurophysiological study. *Brain Research*, 1975, *83*:225-233.

Ronis, B. J. Cochlear potentials in otosclerosis. *Laryngoscope*, 1966, *73*:212-231.

Rose, D. E., Keating, L. W., and Hedgecock, L. D., et al. A comparison of evoked response audiometry and routine clinical audiometry. *Audiology*, 1972, *11*: 238-243.

Rose, J. E. The cellular structure of the auditory region of the cat. *Journal of Comparative Neurology*, 1949, *91*:409-440.

Rose, J. E., Galambos, R., and Hughes, J. R. Microelectrode studies of the cochlear nuclei of the cat. *Johns Hopkins Hospital Bulletin*, 1959, *104*:211-251.

Rose, J. E., Greenwood, D. D., and Goldberg, J. M., et al. Some discharge characteristics of single neurons in the inferior colliculus of the cat. I. Tonotopic organization, relation of spike-counts to tone intensity and firing patterns of single elements. *Journal of Neurophysiology*, 1963, *26*:294-320.

Rose, J. E., Gross, N. B., and Geisler, C. D., et al. Some neural mechanisms in the inferior colliculus of the cat which may be relevant to localization of a sound source. *Journal of Neurophysiology*, 1966, *29*:288-314.

Rose, J. E., Hind, J. E., and Anderson, D. J., et al. Some effects of stimulus intensity on response of auditory nerve fibers in the squirrel monkey. *Journal of Neurophysiology*, 1971, *34*:685-699.

Rose, J. E., Kitzes, L. M., and Gibson, M. M., et al. Observations on phase sensitive neurons of antereoventral cochlear nucleus of the cat: Linearity of cochlear output. *Journal of Neurophysiology*, 1974, *37*:218-253.

Rosenblith, W. A., and Rosenzweig, M. R. Electrical responses to acoustic clicks: Influence of electrode location in cats. *Journal of the Acoustical Society of America*, 1951, *23*:583-588.

Rosenhamer, H. J. Observations on the electric brain-stem responses in retrocochlear hearing loss. *Scandinavian Audiology*, 1977, *6*:179-196.

Rosenhamer, H. J., Lindstrom, B., and Lundborg, T. On the use of click-evoked electric brainstem responses in audiological diagnosis. II. The influence of sex and age upon the normal response. *Scandinavian Audiology*, 1980, *9*(2):93-100.

Rosenzweig, M. R., and Sutton, D. Binaural interaction in the lateral lemniscus of cat. *Journal of Neurophysiology*, 1958, *21*:17-23.

Rossi, G., Solero, P., and Cortesina, M. F. Brainstem electric response audiometry. Value and significance of "latency" and "amplitude" in absolute sense and in relation to the auditory threshold. *Acta Oto-Laryngologica* (Suppl) (Stockholm), 1979, *364*:1-13.

Roth, G. L., Aitkin, L. M. and Anderson, R. A., et al. Some features of the spatial organization of the central nucleus of the inferior colliculus of the cat. *Journal of Comparative Neurology*, 1978, *182*:661-680.

Roth, W. T., Ford, J. M., and Pfefferbaum, A., et al. Event related potential research in psychiatry. In D. Lehman and E. Callaway (Eds.), *Human evoked potentials: Applications and problems*. New York: Plenum Press, 1979.

Roth, W. T., Krainz, J. M., and Ford, J. R., et al. Parameters of temporal recovery of the human auditory evoked potential. *Electroencephalography and Clinical Neurophysiology*, 1976, *40*:623-632.

Rothman, H. H. Effects of high frequencies and intersubject variability in the auditory evoked cortical response. *Journal of the Acoustical Society of America*, 1970, *47*:569-573.

Rothman, H. H., Davis, H., and Hay, I. S. Slow evoked cortical potentials and temporal features of stimulation. *Electroencephalography and Clinical Neurophysiology*, 1970, *29*:225-236.

Rowe, M. J. Normal variability of the brainstem auditory evoked response in young and old adults. *Electroencephalography and Clinical Neurophysiology*, 1978, *44*:459-470.

Ruben, R. J. Cochlear potentials as a diagnostic test in deafness. In A. B. Graham, (Ed.), *Sensorineural hearing processes and disorders*. Boston: Little, Brown, 1967.

Ruben, R. J., Bordley, J. E., and Lieberman, A. T. Cochlear potentials in man. *Laryngoscope*, 1961, *71*:1141-1164.

Ruben, R. J., Knickerbocker, G. G., and Sekula, J., et al. Cochlear microphonics in man. A preliminary report. *Laryngoscope*, 1959, *69*:665-671.

Ruben, R. J., Lieberman, A. T., and Bordley, J. E. Some observations on cochlear potentials and nerve action potentials in children. *Laryngoscope*, 1962, *72*: 545-554.

Ruben, R. J., Sekula, J., and Bordley, J. E., et al. Human cochlear responses to sound stimuli. *Annals of Otology, Rhinology and Laryngology*, 1960, *69*: 459-479.

Ruben, R. J., and Walker, A. E. The VIIIth nerve action potential in Ménière's disease. *Laryngoscope*, 1963, *73*:1456-1461.

Ruchkin, D., and Glaser, E. Simple digital filter for examining CNV and P300 on a single-trial basis. In D. Otto, (Ed.), *Multi-disciplinary perspective in event-related brain potential research*. Washington, D.C.: U.S. Government Printing Office, 1978.

Ruchkin, D. S., Sutton, S., and Kietsman, M. L., et al. Slow wave and P300 in signal detection. *Electroencephalography and Clinical Neurophysiology*, 1980, *50*:35-47.

Ruchkin, D. S., Sutton, S., and Stega, M. Emitted P300 and slow wave event-related potentials in guessing and detection tasks. *Electroencephalography and Clinical Neurophysiology*, 1980, *49*:1-14.

Ruhm, H. B., and Jansen, J. W. Rate of stimulus change and the evoked response. I. Signal rise-time. *Journal of Auditory Research*, 1969, *3*:211-216.

Rupert, A. L., and Moushegian, G. Neuronal responses of kangaroo rat ventral nucleus of the cochlea nucleus to low frequency tones. *Experimental Neurology*, 1970, *26*:84-102.

Russell, I. J., and Sellick, P. M. Intracellular studies of hair cells in the mammalian cochlea. *Journal of Physiology* (London), 1978, *284*:261-290.

Ryerson, S. G., and Beagley, H. A. Brainstem electric responses and electrocochleography: A comparison of threshold sensitivities in children. *British Journal of Audiology*, 1981, *15*(1):41-48.

Sabat, S. R. Selective attention, cortical evoked responses, and brain function in human subjects: A critical review and theory. *Biological Psychology*, 1978, *7*: 175-210.

Sachs, M. B., and Abbas, P. J. Rate versus level functions for auditory-nerve fibers in cats: Tone-burst stimuli. *Journal of the Acoustical Society of America*, 1974, *56*:1835-1847.

Sachs, M. B., and Young, E. D. Effects of nonlinearities on speech encoding in the auditory nerve. *Journal of the Acoustical Society of America*, 1979, *65*:102.

Sagales, T., Gimeno, V., and Vallet, M., et al. Far-field auditory brain-stem potentials in acoustic neuromas. *Electroencephalography and Clinical Neurophysiology*, 1977, *543*:515-516.

Salamy, A., and Birtley-Fenn, C. Ontogenesis of human brainstem evoked potential amplitude. *Developmental Psychobiology*, in press.

Salamy, A., and McKean, C. M. Postnatal development of human brainstem potentials during the first year of life. *Electroencephalography and Clinical Neurophysiology*, 1976, *140*:418-426.

Salamy, A., and McKean, C. M. Habituation and dishabituation of cortical and brainstem evoked potentials. *International Journal of Neuroscience*, 1977, *7*: 175-182.

Salamy, A., McKean, C., and Buda, F. Maturational changes in auditory transmission as reflected in human brainstem potentials. *Brain Research*, 1975, *96*:361-366.

Salamy, A., McKean, C. M., and Pettett, G., et al. Auditory brainstem recovery processes from birth to adulthood. *Psychophysiology*, 1978, *15*:214-220.

Salomon, G. Electric response audiometry based on rank correlation. *Audiology*, 1974, *13*:181-194.

Salomon, G. Electric response audiometry (ERA) from the vertex in paedoaudiology: Technical basis, clinical results and new developments. *Journal of Audiological Techniques*, 1976, *15*:2-27.

Salomon, G., and Barford, J. A new concept of vertex ERA and EEG analysis applying inverse filtering. *Acta Oto-Laryngologica* (Stockholm), 1977, *83*:200-210.

Salomon, G., and Elberling, C. Cochlear nerve potentials recorded from the ear canal in man. *Acta Oto-Laryngologica* (Stockholm), 1971, *71*:4-15.

Salomon, G., Elberling, C., and Tos, M. Combined use of electrocochleography and brain stem recordings in the diagnosis of acoustic neuromas. *Revue de Laryngologie Otologie Rhinologie* (Bordeaux), 1979, *100*(11-12):697-707.

Sando, I. The anatomical interrelationships of the cochlear nerve fibers. *Acta Oto-Laryngologica* (Stockholm), 1965, *59*:417-436.

Sarno, M. A., and Clemis, M. D. A workable approach to the identification of neonatal hearing impairment. *Laryngoscope*, 1980, *8*:1313-1320.

Sarnowski, R. J., Cracco, R. Q., and Vogel, H. B., et al. Spinal evoked response in the cat. *Journal of Neurosurgery*, 1975, *43*:329-336.

Saul, L. J., and Davis, H. Action currents in the central nervous system. I. Action currents of the auditory tracts. *Archives of Neurology and Psychiatry*, 1932, *28*: 1104-1116.

Sayers, B. M., Beagley, H. A., and Riha, J. Pattern analysis of auditory-evoked EEG potentials. *Audiology*, 1979, *18*:1-16.

Scheibel, M. E., and Scheibel, A. B. Neuropil organization in the superior olive of the cat. *Experimental Neurology*, 1974, *43*:339-348.

Schein, J. D., and Delk, M. T. National census of the deaf population; interview responses. Silver Spring, MD.: The Deaf Populations of the United States, National Association of the Deaf, 1974.

Schimmel, H., Rapin, I., and Cohen, M. M. Improving evoked response audiometry: Results of normative studies for machine scoring. *Audiology*, 1975, *14*:466-479.

Schlag, J. Generation of brain evoked potentials. In R. F. Thompson, and N. M. Patterson (Eds.), *Bioelectric recording techniques. Part A. Cellular processes and brain potentials*. New York: Academic Press, 1973.

Schmidt, P. H., Eggermont, J. J., and Odenthal, D. W. Study of Ménière's disease by electrocochleography. *Acta Oto-laryngologica* (Suppl) (Stockholm), 1974, *316*: 75-84.

Schorn, V. F., Lennon, V. A., and Bickford, R. G. Brainstem auditory evoked responses (BAERs) in the rat—Effect of field extension, asphyxia and autoimmune encephalomyelitis. *Society for Neuroscience Abstracts*, 1976, *2*:9.

Schuknecht, H. F. Neuroanatomical correlates of auditory sensitivity and pitch discrimination in the cat. In G. L. Rasmussen, and W. Windle (Eds.), *Neural mechanisms of the auditory and vestibular systems*. Springfield, Illinois: Charles C. Thomas, 1960.

460   References

Schulman-Galambos, C., and Galambos, R. Brainstem auditory-evoked responses in premature infants. *Journal of Speech and Hearing Research*, 1975, *18*: 456-465.

Schwent, V. L., and Hillyard, S. A. Evoked potential correlates of selective attention with multi-channel auditory inputs. *Electroencephalography and Clinical Neurophysiology*, 1975, *38*:131-138.

Schwent, V. L., Hillyard, S. A., and Galambos, R. Selective attention and the auditory vertex potential. I. Effects of stimulus delivery rate. *Electroencephalography and Clinical Neurophysiology*, 1976a, 40:604-614.

Schwent, V. L., Hillyard, S. A., and Galambos, R. Selective attention and the auditory vertex potential. II. Effects of signal intensity and masking noise. *Electroencephalography and Clinical Neurophysiology*, 1976b, 40:615-622.

Schwent, V. L., and Jewett, D. L. Far field recording of the cochlear microphonic to pure tones from the scalp of animals. *Society for Neuroscience Abstracts*, 1976, *2*:25.

Schwent, V. L., Snyder, E., and Hillyard, S. A. Auditory evoked potentials during multichannel selective listening: Role of pitch and localization cues. *Journal of Experimental Psychology: Human Perception and Performance*, 1976, *2*:313-325.

Schwent, V. L., Williston, J. S., and Jewett, D. L. The effects of ototoxicity on the auditory brain stem response and the scalp-recorded cochlear microphonic in guinea pigs. *Laryngoscope*, 1980, *90*(8): 1350-1980.

Seales, D. M., Rossiter, V. S., and Weinstein, M. E. Brainstem auditory evoked responses in patients comatose as a result of blunt head injury. *Journal of Trauma*, 1979, *19*:347-353.

Selters, W. A., and Brackmann, D. E. Acoustic tumor detection with brainstem electric response audiometry. *Archives of Otolaryngology*, 1977, *103*:181-187.

Shagass, C. *Evoked brain potentials in psychiatry*. New York: Plenum Press, 1972.

Shagass, C., Ornitz, E. M., and Sutton, S., et al. Event-related potentials and psychopathology. In E. Calloway, P. Tueting, and S. H. Koslow (Eds.), *Event-related brain potentials in man*. New York: Academic Press, 1978.

Shaia, F. T., and Albright, P. Clinical use of brainstem evoked response audiometry. *Virginia Medical Journal*, 1980, *107*(1):44-45.

Shanon, E., Gold, S., and Himmelfarb, M. Z., et al. Auditory potentials of cochlear nerve and brainstem responses in multiple sclerosis. *Archives of Otolaryngology*, 1979, *105*:505-508.

Shanon, E., Gold, S., and Himelfarb, M. Z. Auditory brain stem responses in cerebellopontine angle tumors. *Laryngoscope*, 1981, *2*:254-259.

Shaw, E. A. G. The external ear. In W. D. Keidel and W. D. Neff (Eds.), *Handbook of sensory physiology. Vol. V/1. Auditory System: Anatomy of Physiology (EAR)*. Berlin: Springer-Verlag, 1974.

Shimoji, K., Matsuki, M., and Shimizu, H. Wave form characteristics and spatial distribution of evoked spinal electrogram in man. *Journal of Neurosurgery*, 1977, *46*:304-310.

Shimoji, K., Shimizu, H., and Maruzama, Y. Origin of somatosensory evoked response recorded from the cervical skin surface. *Journal of Neurosurgery*, 1978, *48*:980-984.

Shinoda, Y., Kaga, K., and Hink, R. T. Origin of a middle latency component in cats. *U.S.-Japan seminar on auditory responses from the brain stem*. Honolulu, Hawaii: 1979.

Shipley, C., and Buchwald, J. S. Unpublished observations, 1980.

Shipley, C., Buchwald, J. S., and Norman, R., et al. Brain stem auditory evoked response development in the kitten. *Brain Research*, 1980, *182*:313-326.

Simmons, F. B. Electrical stimulation of the auditory nerve in man. *Archives of Otolaryngology*, 1966, *84*:2-54.

Simmons, F. B. Electrocochleography. *Annals of Otology, Rhinology, and Laryngology*, 1974, *83*:312-313.

Simmons, F. B. Human auditory nerve responses: A comparison of three commonly used recording sites. *Laryngoscope*, 1975, *85*:1564-1581.

Simmons, F. B. Clinical evaluation of hearing loss. In R. Ruben, C. Elberling, and G. Salomon (Eds.), *Electrocochleography*. Baltimore: University Park Press, 1976.

Simmons, F. B., Epley, J., and Lummis, R., et al. Auditory nerve: Electrical stimulation in man. *Science*, 1965, *148*:104-106.

Simmons, F. B., and Glattke, T. Electrocochleography. In L. J. Bradford (Ed.), *Physiological measures of the audio-vestibular system*. New York: Academic Press, 1975.

Simson, R., Vaughan, H. G., and Ritter, W. The scalp topography of potentials associated with missing visual or auditory stimuli. *Electroencephalography and Clinical Neurophysiology*, 1976, *40*:33-42.

Simson, R., Vaughan, H. G., and Ritter, W. The scalp topography of potentials in auditory and visual discrimination tasks. *Electroencephalography and Clinical Neurophysiology*, 1977, *42*:528-535.

Singh, C. B., and Mason, S. M. Simultaneous recording of extra tympanic electrocochleography and brainstem evoked responses in clinical practice. *Journal of Laryngology and Otology* (London), 1981, *95*(3):279-290.

Skinner, P. H., and Antinoro, F. Auditory evoked response in normal hearing adults and children before and during sedation. *Journal of Speech and Hearing Research*, 1969, *12*:394-400.

Skinner, P. H., and Antinoro, F. The effect of signal rise time and duration on the early components of the auditory evoked cortical response. *Journal of Speech and Hearing Research*, 1971, *14*:552-558.

Skinner, P. H., and Glattke, T. J. Electrophysiologic response audiometry: State of the art. *Journal of Speech and Hearing Research*, 1977, *42*:179-198.

Skinner, P. H., and Jones, H. C. Effects of signal duration and rise time on the auditory evoked potential. *Journal of Speech and Hearing Research*, 1968, *11*:301-306.

Skinner, P. H., and Shimoto, J. A comparison of the effects of sedative on the auditory evoked cortical response. *Journal of the American Audiological Society*, 1975, *1*:71-78.

Small, D. G., Matthews, W. B., and Small, M. The cervical somatosensory evoked potential in the diagnosis of multiple sclerosis. *Journal of Neurological Sciences*, 1978, *35*:211-224.

Smith, C. A. The inner ear: Its embryological development and microstructure. In D. B. Tower (Ed.), *The nervous system. Vol. 3. Human communication and its disorders.* New York: Raven Press, 1975.

Smith, D. B. D., Thompson, L. W., and Michalewski, H. J. Averaged evoked potential research in adult aging—Status and prospects. In L. Poon (Ed.), *Aging in the 1980's: Psychological issues.* Washington, D. C.: American Psychological Association, 1980.

Smith, J. C., Marsh, J. T., and Brown, W. S. Far-field recorded frequency-following responses: Evidence for the locus of brainstem sources. *Electroencephalography and Clinical Neurophysiology,* 1975, *39*:465-472.

Smith, J. C., Marsh, J. T., and Greenburg, S., et al. Human auditory frequency-following responses to a missing fundamental. *Science,* 1978, *201*:639-641.

Smith, R. L., and Zwislocki, J. J. Short-term adaptation and incremental responses of single auditory-nerve fibers. *Biological Cybernetics,* 1975, *17*:169-182.

Snyder, E., and Hillyard, S. A. Long-latency evoked potentials to irrevelevant, deviant stimuli. *Behavioral Biology,* 1976, *16*:319-331.

Snyder, E., Hillyard, S. A., and Galambos, R. Similarities and differences among the P3 waves to detected signals in three modalities. *Psychophysiology,* 1980, *17*:112-122.

Sohmer, H., and Cohen, D. Responses of the auditory pathway in several types of hearing loss. In R. Ruben, C. Elberling, and G. Salomon (Eds.), *Electrocochleography,* Baltimore: University Park Press, 1976.

Sohmer, H., Fahn, M., and Amit, Y., et al. Brain-lesion diagnosis by recording cochlear and brainstem responses to sound stimuli. *Scandinavian Journal of Rehabilitation Medicine,* 1978, *10*:11-13.

Sohmer, H., and Feinmesser, M. Cochlear action potentials recorded from the external ear in man. *Annals of Otology, Rhinology and Laryngology,* 1967, *76*: 427-435.

Sohmer, H., and Feinmesser, M. Cochlear and cortical audiometry conveniently recorded in the same subject. *Israel Journal of Medical Sciences,* 1970, *6*: 219-223.

Sohmer, H., and Feinmesser, M. Routine use of electrocochleography (cochlear audiometry) in human subjects. *Audiology,* 1973, *12*:167-173.

Sohmer, H., and Feinmesser, M. Electrocochleography in clinical-audiological diagnosis. *Archives of Oto-Rhino-Laryngology,* 1974, *206*:91-102.

Sohmer, H., Feinmesser, M., and Bauberger-Tell, L., et al. Routine use of cochlear audiometry in infants with uncertain diagnosis. *Annals of Otology, Rhinology and Laryngology,* 1972, *81*:72-75.

Sohmer, H., Feinmesser, M., and Szabo, G. Sources of electrocochleographic responses as studied in patients with brain damage. *Electroencephalography and Clinical Neurophysiology,* 1974, *37*:663-669.

Sohmer, H., Gafni, M., and Tannenbaum, M., et al. Auditory nerve brainstem response abnormalities in infants with developmental disabilities. In S. Harel (Ed.), *The Infant at Risk.* Amsterdam: Excerpta Medica, 1979, 272-276.

Sohmer, H., and Pratt, H. Electrocochleography during noise-induced temporary threshold shift. *Audiology,* 1975, *14*:130-134.

Sohmer, H., and Pratt, H. Recording of the cochlear microphonic potential with surface electrodes. *Electroencephalography and Clinical Neurophysiology*, 1976, 40:253-260.

Sohmer, H., Pratt, H., and Feinmesser, M. Electrocochleography or evoked cortical responses: Which is preferable in diagnosis of hearing loss? *Revue de Laryngologie Otologie, Rhinologie* (Bordeaux), 1974, 95:515-522.

Sohmer, H., Pratt, H., and Kinarti, R. Sources of frequency-following responses (FFR) in man. *Electroencephalography and Clinical Neurophysiology*, 1978, 44:380-388.

Sohmer, H., and Student, M. Auditory nerve and brain stem evoked responses in normal, autistic, minimal brain dysfunction and psychomotor retarded children. *Electroencephalography and Clinical Neurophysiology*, 1978, 44:380-388.

Søhoel, P., Mair, I. W., and Elverland, H. H., et al. BSER-audiometry in difficult-to-test patients. *Acta Oto-Laryngologica* (Suppl) (Stockholm), 1979, 360:56-70.

Spalteholz, W. *Hand Atlas of Human Anatomy*. Vol. 3 (5th ed.), Philadelphia: J. B. Lippincott Co.

Speckmann, E. J. (Ed.). *Origin of cerebral field potentials*. International Symposium, Muenster, Germany. Stuttgart: Thieme; Littleton, Mass.: P. S. G. Publishing Company, 1979.

Spelman, F. A., Pfingst, B. E., and Miller, J. M., et al. Biophysical measurements in the implanted cochlea. *Octolaryngology and Head and Neck Surgery*, 1980, 88(2):183-187.

Spoor, A. Apparatus for electrocochleography. *Acta Oto-Laryngologica* (Suppl) (Stockholm), 1974, 316:25-36.

Spoor, A., and Eggermont, J. J. Electrocochleography as a method for objective audiogram determination. In S. K. Hirsch, D. H. Eldredge, and I. J. Hirsh, et al. (Eds.), *Hearing and Davis: Essasys honoring Hallowell Davis*. St. Louis: Washington University Press, 1976.

Spoor, A., Timmer, F., and Odenthal, D. W. The evoked auditory response to intensity modulated and frequency modulated tones and tonebursts. *International Audiology*, 1969, 8:410-415.

Spreng, M., and Keidel, W. D. Separierung von Cerebroaudiogram (CAG), Neuroaudiogram (NAG) und Otoaudiogram (OAG) in der objectieven Audiometrie. *Archives für Klinische und Experimentelles Ohres Nases und Kehlkopf Heilkunde* (Munich), 1967, 189:225-246.

Squires, K. D., Chippendale, T. J., and Wrege, K. S., et al. Electrophysiological assessment of mental function in aging and dementia. In L. W. Poon (Ed.), *Aging in the 1980's: Selected contemporary issues in the psychology of aging*. Washington, D.C.: American Psychological Association, 1980.

Squires, K. C., Donchin, E., and Herning, R. I., et al. On the influence of task relevance and stimulus probability on event-related potential components. *Electroencephalography and Clinical Neurophysiology*, 1977, 41:2-14.

Squires, K. C., Wickens, C., and Squires, N. K., et al. The effect of stimulus sequence on the waveform of the cortical event-related potential. *Science*, 1976, 193:1142-1146.

Squires, N., Aine, C., and Buchwald, J., et al. Auditory brain-stem response abnormalities in severely and profoundly retarded adults. *Electroencephalography and Clinical Neurophysiology*, 1980, 50:172-185.

Squires, N., and Buchwald, J. S. Unpublished observations, 1980.

Squires, N. K., Donchin, E., and Squires, K. C., et al. Bisensory stimulation: Inferring decision-related processes from the P300 component. *Journal of Experimental Psychology: Human Perception and Performance*, 1977, *3*:299-315.

Squires, K. C., Petuchowski, S., and Wickens, C., et al. The effects of stimulus sequence on event-related potentials: A comparison of visual and auditory sequences. *Perception and Psychophysics*, 1977, *22*:31-40.

Squires, N. K., Squires, K. C., and Hillyard, S. A. Two varieties of long-latency positive waves evoked by unpredictable auditory stimuli in man. *Electroencephalography and Clinical Neurophysiology*, 1975, *38*:387-401.

Stapells, D. R., and Picton, T. W. Technical aspects of brainstem evoked audiometry using tones. *Ear and Hearing*, 1981, *2*:20-29.

Starr, A. Auditory brainstem responses in brain death. *Brain*, 1976, *99*:543-554.

Starr, A. Clinical relevance of brain stem auditory evoked potentials in brain stem disorders in man. In J. E. Desmedt (Ed.), *Progress in clinical neurophysiology. Vol. 2. Auditory evoked potentials in man: Psychopharmacology correlates of EPs.* Basel: Karger, 1977.

Starr, A. Sensory evoked potentials in clinical disorders of the nervous system. *Annual Review of Neuroscience*, 1978, *1*:103-127.

Starr, A., and Achor, L. J. Auditory brainstem responses in neurological disease. *Archives of Neurology*, 1975, *32*:761-768.

Starr, A., and Achor, L. J. The generators of the auditory brainstem potentials as revealed by brainstem lesions in both man and cat. In R. F. Naunton, and C. Fernandez (Eds.), *Evoked electrical activity in the auditory nervous system.* New York: Academic Press, 1978.

Starr, A., Amlie, R. N., and Martin, W. H., et al. Development of auditory function in newborn infants revealed by auditory brainstem potentials. *Pediatrics*, 1977, *60*:831-839.

Starr, A., and Hamilton, A. E. Brain regions generating auditory brainstem responses: Correlating between site of pathology and response abnormalities. *Neurology*, 1975, *25*:385.

Starr, A., and Hamilton, A. E. Correlation between confirmed sites of neurological lesions and abnormalities of far-field auditory brainstem responses. *Electroencephalography and Clinical Neurophysiology*, 1976, *41*:595-608.

Starr, A., Sohmer, H., and Celesia, G. G. Some applications of evoked potentials to patients with neurological and sensory impairment. In E. Callaway, P. Tueting, and S. H. Koslow (Eds.), *Event-related brain potentials in man.* New York: Academic Press, 1978.

Stephens, S. D. G., and Thornton, A. R. D. Subjective and electrophysiologic tests in brain-stem lesions. *Archives of Otolaryngology*, 1976, *102*:608-613.

Stevens, S. S., Davis, H., and Lurie, M. H. The localization of pitch perception on the basilar membrane. *Journal of General Psychology*, 1935, *13*:297-315.

Stillman, R. D., Crow, G., and Moushegian, G. Components of the frequency-following potential in man. *Electroencephalography and Clinical Neurophysiology*, 1978, *44*:438-446.

Stillman, R. D., Moushegian, G., and Rupert, A. L. Early tone-evoked responses in normal and hearing impaired subjects. *Audiology*, 1976, *15*:10-22.

Stockard, J. E., Stockard, J. J., and Westmoreland, B. F., et al. Normal variation of brainstem auditory-evoked responses as a function of stimulus subject characteristics. *Archives of Neurology*, 1979, *36*:823-831.

Stockard, J. J., and Rossiter, V. S. Clinical and pathological correlates of brain stem auditory response abnormalities. *Neurology*, 1977, *27*:316-325.

Stockard, J. J., Rossiter, V. S., and Wiederholt, W. C., et al. Brain stem auditory evoked responses in suspected central pontine myelinolysis. *Archives of Neurology*, 1976, *33*:726-728.

Stockard, J. J., and Sharbrough, F. W. Unique contributions of short-latency auditory and somatosensory evoked potentials to neurologic diagnosis. In J. Desmedt (Ed.), *Clinical uses of cerebral, brainstem and spinal somatosensory evoked potentials. Vol. 7. Progress in Clinical Neurophysiology*. Basel: Karger, 1980.

Stockard, J. J., Sharbrough, F. W., and Tinker, J. A. Effects of hypothermia on the human brainstem auditory response. *Annals of Neurology*, 1978, *3*:368-370.

Stockard, J. J., Sharbrough, F. W., and Westmoreland, B. F., et al. Screening for subclinical lesions with brainstem auditory responses—earlier diagnosis of multiple sclerosis (MS) and posterior fossa tumors. *Neurology*, 1978, *28*:409.

Stockard, J. J., Stockard, J. E., and Sharbrough, F. W. Detection and localization of occult lesions with brainstem auditory responses. *Mayo Clinic Proceedings*, 1977, *52*:761-769.

Stockard, J. J., Stockard, J. E., and Sharbrough, F. W. Nonpathologic factors influencing brainstem auditory evoked potentials. *American Journal of Electroencephalography and Technology*, 1978, *18*:177-209.

Stotler, W. A. An experimental study of the cells and connections of the superior olivary complex of the cat. *Journal of Comparative Neurology*, 1953, *98*:401-432.

Strominger, N. L., and Hurwitz, J. L. Anatomical aspects of the superior olivary complex. *Journal of Comparative Neurology*, 1976, *170*:485-498.

Streletz, L. J., Katz, L., and Hohenberger, M., et al. Scalp recorded auditory evoked potentials and sonomotor responses: An evaluation of components and recording techniques. *Electroencephalography and Clinical Neurophysiology*, 1977, *43*:192-206.

Sutton, S. P300—Thirteen years later. In H. Begleiter (Ed.), *Evoked brain potentials and behavior*. New York: Plenum Press, 1979.

Sutton, S., Braren, M., and Zubin, J. Evoked potential correlates of stimuli uncertainty. *Science*, 1965, *150*:1187-1188.

Sutton, S., Tueting, P., and Zubin, J., et al. Information delivery and the sensory evoked potential. *Science*, 1967, *155*:1436-1439.

Suzuki, T., Hirai, Y., and Horiuchi, K. Auditory brain stem responses to pure tone stimuli. *Scandinavian Audiology*, 1977, *6*:51-56.

Suzuki, T., and Origuchi, K. Averaged evoked response audiometry in young children during sleep. *Acta Oto-Laryngologica* (Suppl) (Stockholm), 1969, *252*:19-28.

Suzuki, T., and Taguchi, K. Cerebral evoked response to auditory stimuli in young children during sleep. *Annals of Otology, Rhinology and Laryngology*, 1968, *77*:102-110.

Suzuki, T., Yoshie, N., and Ohashi, T. Auditory nerve action potentials in man recorded by external auditory meatal electrodes. *Audiology*, 1966, *9*:172-174. (Japanese text.)

Tabb, H. G., Komet, H., and McLaurin, J. W. Cancer of the external auditory canal:

Treatment with redical mastoidectomy and irradiation. *Laryngoscope*, 1964, *94*:634-643.

Taguchi, K., Goodman, W. S., and Brummitt, W. M. Evoked response audiometry in mentally retarded children. *Acta Oto-Laryngologica* (Stockholm), 1970, *70*:190-196.

Taguchi, K., Picton, T. W., and Orpin, J., et al. Evoked response audiometry in newborn infants. *Acta Oto-Laryngologica* (Suppl) (Stockholm), 1969, *252*:5-17.

Tanguay, P. E., and Ornitz, E. M. Two measures of auditory evoked response amplitude and their relationship to background EEG. *Psychophysiology*, 1972, *9*:477-483.

Tanguay, P. E., Ornitz, E. M., and Forsythe, A. B., et al. Basic rest-activity cycle rhythms in the human auditory evoked response. *Electroencephalography and Clinical Neurophysiology*, 1973, *34*:593-603.

Tanguay, P. E., Taub, J. M., and Doubleday, C., et al. An interhemispheric comparison of auditory evoked response to consonant-vowel stimuli. *Neuropsychologia*, 1977, *15*:123-131.

Taub, J. M., Tanguay, P. E., and Doubleday, C., et al. Hemispheric and ear asymmetry in the auditory evoked response to musical chord stimuli. *Physiology Psychology*, 1976, *4*:11-17.

Teas, D. C., Eldridge, D. H., and Davis, H. Cochlear responses to acoustic transients and interpretation of the whole nerve action potentials. *Journal of the Acoustical Society of America*, 1962, *34*:1438-1459.

Tecce, J. J. Contingent negative variation (CNV) and psychological processes in man. *Psychological Bulletin*, 1972, *77*:73-108.

Terkildsen, K. Personal communication, 1974.

Terkildsen, K. Brain stem audiometry. Experiences and applications. *Scandinavian Audiology* (Suppl), 1978, *8*:29-31.

Terkildsen, K., Osterhammel, P., and Huis in't Veld, F. Electrocochleography with a far-field technique. *Scandinavian Audiology*, 1973, *2*:141-148.

Terkildsen, K., Osterhammel, P., and Huis in't Veld, F. Far-field electrocochleography, electrode positions. *Scandinavian Audiology*, 1974a, *3*:123-129.

Terkildsen, K., Osterhammel, P., and Huis in't Veld, F. Recording procedures for brainstem potentials. *Scandinavian Audiology*, 1974b, *3*:415-428.

Terkildsen, K., Osterhammel, P., and Huis in't Veld, F. Far-field electrocochleography. Adaptation. *Scandinavian Audiology*, 1975a, *4*:215-220.

Terkildsen, K., Osterhammel, P., and Huis in't Veld, F. Far-field electrocochleography. Frequency specificity of the response. *Scandinavian Audiology*, 1975b, *4*:167-172.

Terkildsen, K., Osterhammel, P., and Huis in't Veld, F. Recording procedures for brainstem potentials. In R. F. Naunton and C. Fernandez (Eds.), *Evoked electrical activity in the auditory nervous sytem*. New York: Academic Press, 1978.

Tew, J. M., Saul, T. G., and Mayfield, F. H. Neurosurgery. In M. M. Paparella and D. A. Shumrick (Eds.), *Otolaryngology. Vol. I*. Philadelphia: W. B. Saunders, 1980.

Thompson, R. F., and Patterson, N. M. (Eds.), *Bioelectric Recording Techniques: Part A. Cellular Processes and Brain Potentials*. New York: Academic Press, 1973.

Thomsen, J., Terkildsen, K., and Osterhammel, P. Auditory brainstem responses in patients with acoustic neuromas. *Scandinavian Audiology*, 1978, 7:179-183.

Thornton, A. R. D. Interpretation of cochlear nerve and brain stem evoked responses. *Scandinavian Audiology*, 1974, 3:429-442.

Thornton, A. R. D. The diagnostic potential of surface recorded electrocochleography. *British Journal of Audiology*, 1975a, 9:7-13.

Thornton, A. R. D. The measurement of surface-recorded electrocochleographic responses. *Scandinavian Audiology*, 1975b, 4:51-58.

Thornton, A. R. D. Statistical properties of surface-recorded electrocochleographic responses. *Scandinavian Audiology*, 1975c, 4:91-102.

Thornton, A. R. D. Electrophysiological studies of the auditory system. *Audiology*, 1976, 15:23-38.

Thornton, A. R. D., and Coleman, M. J. The adaptation of cochlear and brainstem auditory evoked potentials in humans. *Electroencephalography and Clinical Neurophysiology*, 1975, 39:399-406.

Thornton, A., Mendel, M. I., and Anderson, C. Effects of stimulus frequency and intensity on the middle components of the averaged auditory electroencephalic response. *Journal of Speech and Hearing Research*, 1977, 20:81-94.

Tietze, G. The acoustically evoked potential with inverse tone burst stimulation compared to a model experiment. *Audiology*, 1979, 18(5):403-413.

Tolbert, L. P., and Morest, D. K. Combined Golgi, horseradish peroxidase (HRP), and electron microscopic study of bushy cells in the cochlear nucleus. *Neuroscience (Abstract)*, 1977, 3:12.

Tolbert, L. P., Morest, D. K., and Yurgelun-Todd, D. A. The neuronal architecture of the anteroventral cochlear nucleus of the cat in the region of the cochlear nerve root: Horseradish peroxidase labelling of identified cell types. In press.

Tonndorf, J., and Khanna, S. M. Submicroscopic displacement amplitudes of the tympanic membrane (cats) measured by a laser interferometer. *Journal of the Acoustical Society of America*, 1968, 44:1546-1554.

Townsend, G. L., and Cody, D. T. R. The averaged inion evoked response by acoustic stimulation: Its relation to the saccule. *Annals of Otology, Rhinology and Laryngology*, 1971, 80:121-131.

Townsend, R. E., House, J. F., and Johnson, L. C. Auditory evoked potential in stage 2 and REM sleep during a 30-day exposure to tone pulses. *Psychophysiology*, 1976, 13:54-57.

Travis, L. E., and Dorsey, J. M. Mass responsiveness in the central nervous system. *Archives of Neurology and Psychiatry*, 1931, 26:141-145.

Travis, L. E., and Herren, R. Y. Action currents in the cerebral cortex of the dog and and rat during reflex activity. *American Journal of Physiology*, 1930, 93:693.

Trinder, E. Auditory fusion: A critical interval test with implications in differential diagnosis. *British Journal of Audiology*, 1979, 13(4):143-147.

Tsuchitani, C. Functional organization of lateral cell groups of the cat superior olivary complex. *Journal of Neurophysiology*, 1977, 40:296-318.

Tsuchitani, C., and Boudreau, J. C. Wave activity in the superior olivary complex of the cat. *Journal of Neurophysiology*, 1964, 27:814-827.

Tsumato, T., Hirose, N., and Nonaka, S. Analysis of somatosensory evoked potentials to lateral popliteal nerve stimulation in man. *Electroencephalography and Clinical Neurophysiology*, 1972, 33:379-388.

Tueting, P., Sutton, S., and Zubin, J. Quantitative evoked potential correlates of the probability of events. *Psychophysiology*, 1971, 7:385-394.

Tyberghein, J., and Forrez, G. Objective (ERA) and subjective (CVR) audiometry in the infant. *Acta Oto-Laryngologica* (Stockholm), 1971, 71:249-252.

Uziel, A., and Benezech, J. Auditory brainstem responses in comatose patients—Relationship with brainstem reflexes and levels of coma. *Electroencephalography and Clinical Neurophysiology*, 1978, 45:515-524.

Vaughan, H. G., and Ritter, W. The sources of auditory evoked response recorded from the human scalp. *Electroencephalography and Clinical Neurophysiology*, 1970, 28:360-367.

Vivion, M. C. Clinical status of evoked response audiometry. *Laryngoscope*, 1980, 90(3):437-447.

Vivion, M. C., Goldstein, R., and Wolf, K. E., et al. Middle components of human auditory averaged electroencephalic response: Waveform variations during averaging. *Audiology*, 1977, 16:21-37.

Vivion, M. C., Hirsch, J. E., and Frye-Osier, J. L., et al. Effects of stimulus rise-fall time and equivalent duration on middle components of AER. *Scandinavian Audiology*, 1980, 9(4):223-232.

Vivion, M. C., Wolf, K. E., and Goldstein, R., et al. Toward objective analysis for electroencephalic audiometry. *Journal of Speech and Hearing Research*, 1979, 22:88-102.

Vurkek, L. S., White, M., and Fong, M., et al. Opto-isolated stimulators used for electrically evoked BSER: Some observations on electrical artifact. *Annals of Otology, Rhinology and Laryngology*, 1981, 90 (Suppl 82):21-24.

Walter, W. G. The convergence and interaction of visual, auditory and tactile response in human nonspecific cortex. *Annals of the New York Academy of Sciences*, 1964, 112:320-361.

Walter, W. G., Cooper, R., and Aldridge, V. J., et al., Contingent negative variation: An electric sign of sensori-motor association and expectancy in the human brain. *Nature*, 1964, 203:380-384.

Warr, W. B. Fiber degeneration following lesions in the anterior ventral cochlear nucleus of the cat. *Experimental Neurology*, 1966, 14:453-474.

Warr, W. B. Fiber degeneration following lesions in the posteroventral cochlear nuclus of the cat. *Experimental Neurology*, 1969, 23:140-155.

Warr, W. B. Fiber degeneration following lesions in the multipolar and globular cell areas in the ventral cochlear nucleus of the cat. *Brain Research*, 1972, 40:247-270.

Warr, W. B. Olivocochlear and vestibular efferent neurons of the feline brain stem: Their location, morphology, and number determined by retrograde axonal transport and acetylcholinesterase histochemistry. *Journal of Comparative Neurology*, 1975, 161:159-182.

Watson, J. D. *The Double Helix: A Personal Account of the Discovery of the Structure of DNA*. New York: Atheneum, 1968.

Weber, B. A. Auditory brain-stem response audiometry in children. *Clinical Pediatrics* (Philadelphia), 1979, 18(12):746-749.

Weber, B. A., and Fletcher. G. L. A computerized scoring procedure for auditory brainstem response audiometry. *Ear and Hearing*, 1980, 1(5):233-236.

Weitzman, E., Fishbein, W., and Graziani, L. J. Auditory evoked responses obtained from the scalp electroencephalogram of the full-term neonate during sleep. *Pediatrics*, 1965, 35:458-562.

Weitzman, E., and Graziani, L. Maturation and topography of the auditory evoked response of the prematurely born infant. *Developmental Psychobiology*, 1968, *1*:79-89.

Weitzman, E., and Kremen, H. Auditory evoked responses during different stages of sleep in man. *Electroencephalography and Clinical Neurophysiology*, 1965, *18*:65-70.

Weinberg, H., Walter, W. G., and Cooper, R., et al. Emitted cerebral events. *Electroencephalography and Clinical Neurophysiology*, 1974, *36*:449-456.

Weiss, T. J. A model of the peripheral auditory system. *Kybernetik*, *3*:153-175.

Wepsic, J. G. Multimodal sensory activation of cells in the magnocellular medial geniculate nucleus. *Experimental Neurology*, 1966, *15*:299-318.

Wever, E. G., and Bray, C. W. Auditory nerve impulses. *Science*, 1930, *71*:215.

White, M. W., Merzenich, M. M., and Vivion, M. C. A noninvasive recording technique for evaluating electrode and nerve function in cochleas implanted with a multichannel electrode. In *Advances in prosthetic devices for the deaf*. Rochester, New York: National Technical Institute for the Deaf, 1980.

Wiederhold, M. L. Variations in the effects of electric stimulation of the crossed olivocochlear bundle on cat single auditory-nerve fiber responses to tone bursts. *Journal of the Acoustical Society of America*, 1970, *48*:966-977.

Wiederhold, M., and Kiang, N. Y.-S. Effects of electrical stimulation of the crossed olivocochlear bundle on single auditory-nerve fibers in the cat. *Journal of the Acoustical Society of America*, 1970, *48*:950-965.

Wiederhold, M. L., Martinez, S. A., and Paull, D. M., et al. Noninvasive chronic recording of auditory nerve potentials. *Annals of Otology, Rhinology and Laryngology*, 1978a, *87*:(Supp. 45)1-11.

Wiederhold, M. L., Martinez, S. A., and Paull, D. M., et al. Effects of eustachian tube ligation on auditory nerve responses to clicks. *Annls of Otology, Rhinology and Laryngology*, 1978b, *87*:(Supp 45)12-20.

Wiederhold, M. L., and Peake, W. T. Efferent inhibition of auditory-nerve responses: Dependence on acoustic-stimulus parameters. *Journal of the Acoustical Society of America*, 1966, *40*:1427-1430.

Wilkinson, R. T., and Morlock, H. C. Auditory evoked response and reaction time. *Electroencephalography and Clinical Neurophysiology*, 1967, *23*:50-56.

Williams, H. L., Tepas, D. I., and Morlock, H. C. Evoked response to clicks and electroencephographic stages of sleep in man. *Science*, 1962, *138*:685-686.

Williamson, P. D., Goff, W. R., and Allison, T. Somatosensory evoked responses in patients with unilateral cerebral lesions. *Electroencephalography and Clinical Neurophysiology*, 1970, *28*:566-576.

Williston, J. S., Jewett, D. L., and Martin, W. H. Planar curve analysis of three channel auditory brain-stem responses: A preliminary report. *Brain Research*, 1981, *223*:181-184.

Wilson, J. P., and Johnstone, J. Basilar membrane and middle ear vibration in guinea pig measured by capacitance probe. *Journal of the Acoustical Society of America*, 1975, *57*:705-723.

Wit, H. P., and Nijdam, H. F. On the combination of otometry with brainstem-evoked response audiometry. *Scandinavian Audiology*, 1980, *9*(1):59-61.

Witter, H. L., Deka, R. C., and Lipscomb, D. M., et al. Effects of prestimulatory carbogen inhalation on noise-induced temporary threshold shifts in humans and chinchilla. *American Journal of Otology*, 1980, *1*(4):227-232.

Wolf, K. E., and Goldstein, R. Middle component averaged electroencephalic response to tonal stimuli from normal neonates. *Archives of Otolaryngology*, 1978, *104*:508-513.

Wolf, K. E., and Goldstein, R. Middle component auditory evoked responses from neonates to low-level tonal stimuli. *Journal of Speech and Hearing Research*, 1980, *23*:185-201.

Wolpaw, J. R., and Penry, J. K. A temporal component of the auditory evoked response. *Electroencephalography and Clinical Neurophysiology*, 1975, *39*:609-620.

Wolpaw, J. R., and Penry, J. K. Hemispheric differences in the auditory evoked response. *Electroencephalography and Clinical Neurophysiology*, 1977, *43*: 99-102.

Wolpaw, J. R., and Penry, J. K. Effects of ethanol, caffeine, and placebo on the auditory evoked response. *Electroencephalography and Clinical Neurophysiology*, 1978, *44*:568-574.

Wong, W. C. The tangential organization of dendrites and axons in three auditory areas of the cat's cerebral cortex. *Journal of Anatomy*, 1967, *101*:419-433.

Wood, C. C., Allison, T., and Goff, W., et al. Intracranial distribution of the P300 component of human somatosensory and auditory evoked potentials. Paper presented at the American EEG Society, San Francisco, 1978.

Woody, C. D. Characterization of an adaptive filter for the analysis of variable latency neuroelectric signals. *Medical and Biological Engineering and Computing*, 1967, *5*:539-553.

Woolsey, C. Organization of cortical auditory system: A review and synthesis. In G. L. Rasmussen and W. Windle (Eds.), *Neural mechanisms of the auditory and vestibular systems*. Springfield, Illinois: Charles C. Thomas, 1960.

Worden, F. G., and Marsh, J. T. Frequency following (microphonic-like) neural response evoked by sound. *Electroencephalography and Clinical Neurophysiology*, 1968, *25*:42-52.

Worden, F. G., Marsh, J. T., and Bremner, F. J. Electrophysiological analog of the interaural time-intensity trade. *Journal of the Acoustical Society of America*, 1966, *39*:1086-1089.

Worthington, D. W., and Peters, J. F. Quantifiable hearing and no ABR: Paradox or error? *Ear and Hearing*, 1980, *1*(5): 281-285.

Yagi, T., and Kaga, K. The effect of click repetition rate on the latency of the auditory evoked brainstem response and its clinical use for a neurological diagnosis. *Archives of Oto-Rhino-Laryngology*, 1979, *222*:91-97.

Yamada, T., Kimura, J., and Young, S., et al. Somatosensory evoked potentials elicited by bilateral stimulation of the median nerve and its clinical application. *Neurology*, 1978, *28*:218-223.

Yamada, T., Kodera, K., and Hink, R. F., et al. Cochlear initiation site of the frequency following response: A study of patients with sensorineural hearing loss. *Audiology*, 1978, *17*:489-499.

Yamada, T., Kodera, K., and Hink, R. F., et al. Cochlear distribution of frequency-following response initiation. A high-pass masking noise study. *Audiology:*, 1979, *18*(5):381-387.

Yamada, T., Marsh, R. R., and Potsic, W. P. Generators of the frequency-following response in the guinea pig. *Otolaryngology and Head and Neck Surgery*, 1980, *88*(5):613-618.

Yamada, T., Yagi, T., and Yamane, H., et al. Clinical evaluation of the auditory evoked brainstem response. *Auris, Nasus, Larynx*, 1975, *2*:92-105.

Yamada, T., Yamane, H., and Kodera, K. Simultaneous recordings of the brain stem response and the frequency-following response to low-frequency tone. *Electroencephalography and Clinical Neurophysiology*, 1977, *43*:362-370.

Yanz, J. L. Frequency specificity of the auditory compound action potential. (Unpublished master's thesis, Univ. of Iowa, Iowa City, 1976.)

Yoshie, N. Auditory nerve action potential responses to clicks in man. *Laryngoscope*, 1968, *78*:198-215.

Yoshie, N. Clinical cochlear response audiometry by means of an average response computer; non-surgical technique and clinical use. *Revue de Laryngologie Otologie Rhinologie* (Bordeaux), 1971, *92*:646-672.

Yoshie, N. Diagnostic significance of the electrocochleogram in clinical audiometry. *Audiology*, 1973, *12*:504-539.

Yoshie, N., and Ohashi, T. Auditory nerve action potentials in man. *Japanese Journal of Otology*, 1967, *70*:920-931.

Yoshie, N., and Ohashi, T. Clinical use of cochlear nerve action potential responses in man for differential diagnosis of hearing loss. *Acta Oto-Laryngologica* (Suppl) (Stockholm), 1969, *252*:71-87.

Yoshie, N., and Ohashi, T. Abnormal adaptation of human cochlear nerve action potential responses—clinical observations by nonsurgical recording. *Revue de Laryngologie Otologie Rhinologie* (Bordeaux), 1971, *92*:673-690.

Yoshie, N., Ohashi, T., and Suzuki, T. Non surgical recording of auditory nerve action potentials in man. *Laryngoscope*, 1967, *77*:76-85.

Yoshie, N., and Okudaira, T. Myogenic evoked potential responses to clicks in man. *Acta Oto-Laryngologica* (Suppl) (Stockholm), 1969, *252*:89-103.

Yoshie, N., and Yamaura, K. Cochlear microphonic responses to pure tones in man recorded by a non-surgical method. *Acta Oto-Laryngologica* (Suppl) (Stockholm), 1969, *252*:37-69.

Zambelli, A. J., Stamm, J. S., and Maitinsky, S., et al. Auditory evoked potentials in formerly hyperactive adolescents. *American Journal of Psychiatry*, 1977, *134*:742-747.

Zerlin, S., and Naunton, R. F. Early and late averaged electroencephalic response at low sensation levels. *Audiology*, 1974, *13*:366-378.

Zerlin, S., and Naunton, R. F. Physical and auditory specifications of third-octave clicks. *Audiology*, 1975, *14*:135-143.

Zerlin, S., and Naunton, R. F. Whole-nerve response to third octave audiometric clicks at moderate sensation level. In R. J. Ruben, C. Elberling, and G. Salomon (Eds.), *Electrocochleography*. Baltimore: University Park Press, 1976.

Zerlin, S., Naunton, R. F., and Mowry, H. J. The early evoked cortical response to third octave clicks and tones. *Audiology*, 1973, *12*:242-249.

Zollner, C., Karnahl, T., and Stange, G. Input-output function and adaptation behavior of the five early potentials registered with the earlobe-vertex pick up. *Archives of Oto-Rhino-Laryngology*, 1976, *212*:23-33.

Zollner, C., and Pedersen, P. Problems of a frequency-specific threshold measurement with the brainstem potentials using the otometric sound pressure signal (damped wavetrain). *Archives of Oto-Rhino-Laryngology*, 1980, *226*(4):259-268.

Index

a
b
3 c
4 d
5 e
6 f
7 g
8 h
9 i
8 0 j